Medical Negligence in
Pediatrics

Medical Negligence in Pediatrics

Editor-in-Chief
Mahesh Baldwa
MBBS MD (Pediatrics) DCH LLB LLM PhD (Law) MBA FIAP MA (Psy)
Founder President
Medicolegal Group/Chapter of the Central Indian Academy of Pediatrics
Senior Medicolegal Author, Advisor and Senior Consultant Pediatrician
Baldwa Hospital, Mumbai
Former Assistant Professor of Pediatrics, TN Medical College and Nair Hospital, Mumbai
Former Assistant Professor, JJ Hospital, Grant Medical College, Mumbai
Former Visiting Professor, Paper Setter and Examiner
Department of Law, University of Mumbai
External Faculty for Maharashtra National Law university
Aurangabad, Maharashtra, India

Editors

Hemant R Gangolia
MBBS DCH DPH (Mum) LLB (Ist Class) Mum
Pediatrician and Medicolegal Consultant
(Niesbud Certified)
V R Day Care Center
Neral, Raigad, Maharashtra, India
Past President
Maharashtra Academy of Pediatrics (MAHAIAP)
State IAP Branch, 2022

Jyoti Kumar Gupta
MBBS DCH PMHS LLB (1st Class) LLM
National Chairman
Indian Academy of Pediatrics
Medicolegal Chapter
President, Neonatology Association Kanpur
Pediatrician and Medicolegal Consultant
Yashi Child Care Center
Kanpur, Uttar Pradesh, India

Dnyanesh DK MBBS MD LLB
Professor and Head
Department of Pediatrics
KAHER's JN Medical College, Belagavi
Consultant Pediatrician
KLE PK Hospital, Belagavi
Medicolegal Consultant
Belagavi, Karnataka, India

Foreword
GV Basavaraja

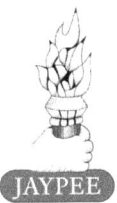

JAYPEE BROTHERS MEDICAL PUBLISHERS
The Health Sciences Publisher
New Delhi | London

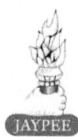

Jaypee Brothers Medical Publishers (P) Ltd

Headquarters
Jaypee Brothers Medical Publishers (P) Ltd
EMCA House, 23/23-B
Ansari Road, Daryaganj
New Delhi 110 002, India
Landline: +91-11-23272143, +91-11-23272703
+91-11-23282021, +91-11-23245672
Email: jaypee@jaypeebrothers.com

Corporate Office
Jaypee Brothers Medical Publishers (P) Ltd
4838/24, Ansari Road, Daryaganj
New Delhi 110 002, India
Phone: +91-11-43574357
Fax: +91-11-43574314
Email: jaypee@jaypeebrothers.com

Overseas Office
JP Medical Ltd
83, Victoria Street, London
SW1H 0HW (UK)
Phone: +44 20 3170 8910
Email: info@jpmedpub.com

EU GPSR Authorised Representative
Logos Europe, 9 rue Nicolas Poussin
17000, La Rochelle, France
Phone: +33 (0) 6 67 93 73 78
E-mail: Contact@logoseurope.eu

Website: www.jaypeebrothers.com
Website: www.jaypeedigital.com

© 2024, Jaypee Brothers Medical Publishers

The views and opinions expressed in this book are solely those of the original contributor(s)/author(s) and do not necessarily represent those of editor(s) or publisher of the book.

All rights reserved. No part of this publication may be reproduced, stored or transmitted in any form or by any means, electronic, mechanical, photocopying, recording or otherwise, without the prior permission in writing of the publishers.

All brand names and product names used in this book are trade names, service marks, trademarks or registered trademarks of their respective owners. The publisher is not associated with any product or vendor mentioned in this book.

Medical knowledge and practice change constantly. This book is designed to provide accurate, authoritative information about the subject matter in question. However, readers are advised to check the most current information available on procedures included and check information from the manufacturer of each product to be administered, to verify the recommended dose, formula, method and duration of administration, adverse effects and contraindications. It is the responsibility of the practitioner to take all appropriate safety precautions. Neither the publisher nor the author(s)/editor(s) assume any liability for any injury and/or damage to persons or property arising from or related to use of material in this book.

This book is sold on the understanding that the publisher is not engaged in providing professional medical services. If such advice or services are required, the services of a competent medical professional should be sought.

Every effort has been made where necessary to contact holders of copyright to obtain permission to reproduce copyright material. If any have been inadvertently overlooked, the publisher will be pleased to make the necessary arrangements at the first opportunity.

Inquiries for bulk sales may be solicited at: jaypee@jaypeebrothers.com

Medical Negligence in Pediatrics

First Edition: **2024**
ISBN: 978-93-5696-754-0

DEDICATION AND TRIBUTE TO OUR BELOVED PARENTS

Freedom fighter Shri Sohanlal Baldwa and Smt Sarladevi Baldwa –
Parents of Mahesh Baldwa

Shri Ramdas Gangolia and Smt Vidya Gangolia –
Parents of Hemant R Gangolia

Shri Laxmi Narain Gupta and Smt Suman Gupta –
Parents of Jyoti Kumar Gupta

Mr Duryodhan PK and Mrs Anusaya DK –
Parents of Dnyanesh DK

In the cherished memory of our beloved parents, whose unwavering love, support, and encouragement have illuminated our paths throughout our life's journey. With profound gratitude and deep appreciation, we dedicate this work to them.

Our parents instilled in us the timeless virtues of hard work, dedication, and resilience, which have led us to this significant moment.

To our fathers, whose wisdom, integrity, and unwavering strength have been our beacons of inspiration, we owe an immeasurable debt of gratitude.

To our mothers, whose boundless love, selfless sacrifices, and nurturing care have shaped our characters and fortified our spirits, we offer this work with the utmost appreciation.

Throughout every endeavor, you believed in us, offered unwavering support, and stood by our side. Your sacrifices and unwavering faith in our abilities have propelled us to this juncture in our journey.

As we dedicate this book to you, we do so with the knowledge that your love and enduring teachings continue to guide us in all that we do. Your legacy lives on through our work, and with each page we write, we endeavor to honor your memory and make you proud.

With all our love and heartfelt gratitude

Mahesh Baldwa
Hemant R Gangolia
Jyoti Kumar Gupta
Dnyanesh DK

DEDICATION AND TRIBUTE TO OUR BELOVED PARENTS

...

Contributors

AB Jaiswal LLB LLM PhD (BHU)
Professor and Head
Faculty of Law VSSD College
Kanpur, Uttar Pradesh, India

Abraham Paul MD DCH FIAP FNNF
Senior Consultant Pediatrician
Indira Gandhi Cooperative Hospital
Kochi, Kerala, India

Aishwarya Mantri MBBS MD
Senior Resident
Department of Pathology
Government Medical College
Akola, Maharashtra, India

Ambrish Gupta MD DCH
Head
Department of Pharmacology and Therapeutics
Government Medical College
Kanpur, Uttar Pradesh, India

Amit Padvi
MBBS MD Fellowship in Pediatric Anesthesiology
Former Assistant Professor
Faculty Member
Department of Pediatric Anesthesia
Seth GS Medical College and KEM Hospital
Mumbai, Maharashtra, India

Amrita Verma LLB LLM MPhil
Assistant Professor of Law
Faculty of Law VSSD College
Kanpur, Uttar Pradesh, India

Anita Sharma
MBBS (Medalist) MD (Pediatrics) DM
(Child Neurology -AIIMS New Delhi)
Professor Pediatrics and In-charge Child
Neurology
Faculty of Medical Sciences
SGT University
Gurugram, Haryana, India
Former Senior Professor Pediatrics and In-charge
Child Neurology
PGIMS
Rohtak, Haryana, India

Ankit Gupta BTech (IT)
Software Engineer
Melbourne, Australia

Anurag Mehrotra
BSc MBBS DCH DIP in Family Medicine
Diploma in Marketing Management
PG Certificate in Clinical Cardiology
Certificate in Evidence-based Diabetes Mellitus
LLB CSJM University Kanpur
Mehrotra Medical Center
Kanpur, Uttar Pradesh, India

Anurag Pangrikar MBBS MD (Ped, Gold Medal) LLB
Consultant
Shri Samarth Bal Rugnalay
Beed, Maharashtra, India

Ashish Jain MBBS DCH PGCC LLB
Consultant Pediatrician and Medicolegal Advisor
Tulip Chest and Child Care Clinic
Gurugram, Haryana, India
National President, Indian Medicolegal and
Ethics Association (IMLEA)
Member Board of District Medical Negligence
Committee, Gurugram (Haryana)
National Consultative Member IYCF Guidelines
2023, 2016

Ashok Baldwa BCom LLB
Advocate, Bombay High Court, Mumbai
Formerly SO, OIC AFMSD, AFMS
Minister of Defence, Government of India
Ex ADM (HQ), (Ret), MSO, DGHS
Minister of Health and FW Government of India

Atanu Bhadra MBBS MD
Consultant Pediatrician
Medical Superintendent ESI Hospital
Asansol, West Bengal, India

Bela Amichandra Verma MD DCH
Professor and Head
Department of Pediatrics
Grant Government Medical College
and Sir JJ Hospital Group of Hospitals
Mumbai, Maharashtra, India

Contributors

Bhvya Baldwa MBBS MD DNB DM (AIIMS New Delhi)
Pulmonary, Critical Care and Sleep Medicine
Assistant Professor at TN Medical College and
BYL Charitable Hospital
Formerly at Seth GS Medical College and
KEM Hospital
Mumbai, Maharashtra, India

C Nirmala MBBS DCH DNB (Pediatrics)
Professor of Pediatrics
Department of Pediatrics
Osmania Medical College
Hyderabad, Telangana, India

Devaraj Virupakshayya Raichur
MD (Pediatrics) MBA (Hospital Administration) LLB
Professor and Head
Department of Pediatrics
KAHER's JGMM Medical College, Hubballi
Consultant Pediatrician
Sushruta Multispecialty Hospital
Hubballi, Karnataka, India

Dnyanesh DK MBBS MD LLB
Professor and Head
Department of Pediatrics
KAHER's JN Medical College, Belagavi
Consultant Pediatrician, KLE PK Hospital, Belagavi
Medicolegal Consultant
Belagavi, Karnataka, India

Hemant R Gangolia
MBBS DCH DPH (Mum) LLB (Ist Class) Mum
Pediatrician and Medicolegal Consultant
(Niesbud Certified)
V R Day Care Center
Neral, Raigad, Maharashtra, India
Past President
Maharashtra Academy of Pediatrics (MAHAIAP)
State IAP Branch, 2022

Ishita Banerji
MBBS MD (Pediatrics) FIAE (Fellow Indian Academy of
Echocardiography) LLB PGDMLE (NLSIU Bengaluru)
Heartline Cardiac Care Center
Prayagraj, Uttar Pradesh, India

Jitendra Pratap Singh Chauhan BA LLB
President Civil Bar Association
Secretary—The Kanpur Dehat Bar Association
Kanpur, Uttar Pradesh, India

Jyoti Kumar Gupta MBBS DCH PMHS LLB
(1st Class) LLM
National Chairman
Indian Academy of Pediatrics
Medicolegal Chapter
President, Neonatology Association Kanpur
Pediatrician and Medicolegal Consultant
Yashi Child Care Center
Kanpur, Uttar Pradesh, India

Mahesh Baldwa MBBS MD (Pediatrics) DCH LLB
LLM PhD (Law) MBA FIAP MA (Psy)
Founder President
Medicolegal Group/Chapter of the Central
Indian Academy of Pediatrics
Senior Medicolegal Author and Advisor
Senior Consultant Pediatrician
Baldwa Hospital, Mumbai
Former Assistant Professor of Pediatrics
TN Medical College and Nair Hospital, Mumbai
Former Assistant Professor
JJ Hospital, Grant Medical College, Mumbai
Former Visiting Professor,
Paper Setter and Examiner
Department of Law, University of Mumbai
External Faculty for Maharashtra National Law
University
Aurangabad, Maharashtra, India

Marrisha Gupta MHA (IHM PUSA, New Delhi, India)
Corporate Relations Officer
Nova Benefits
Bengaluru, Karnataka, India

Namita Padvi
MBBS MD DNB Fellowship in Pediatric Anesthesiology
Emirates Hospital, Dubai
Former Assistant Professor
Department of Anesthesia
Topiwala National Medical College and BYL Nair
Charitable Hospital
Mumbai, Maharashtra, India

Pranjal Agarwal BA LLB (Hons)
Practicing Advocate
Supreme Court, New Delhi, India
Bombay High Court
Mumbai, Maharashtra, India

Raj Tilak MBBS MD (Pediatrics)
Associate Professor RAMA University
Medical College
GSVM Medical College Campus
Kanpur, Uttar Pradesh, India

Rajakumar Marol MBBS MD FIAP
Professor and Head
Department of Pediatrics
Karwar Institute of Medical Sciences
Uttara Kannada, Karnataka, India
Shivajyoti Institute of Child Health
Haveri, Karnataka, India

Rajat Dubey BSc MSc MA LLB LLM UGC Net Qualified
Advocate and Legal Consultant
District and Session Court
Kanpur, Uttar Pradesh, India

Ramesh B Dampuri
MBBS DCH PG Dip AP FPPC (Fellowship in Pediatric Palliative Care)
RMO, Nodal Officer, YUVA—State Centre of Excellence for Adolescent Health, Niloufer Hospital
Senior Consultant, Pediatrician and Adolescent Physician Pediatric Palliative Care Specialist
State Inspection Committee Member, Women Development and Child Welfare Department
Government of Telangana (2019–2023)

Ritu Kumar BDS MBA
Senior Health Planner
Sydney, Australia

Sameer Sadawarte MBBS DCH DNB MNAMS
Consultant Pediatrician and Pediatric Intensivist
Fortis Hospital
Mumbai, Maharashtra, India

Samik Basu DCH DNB MNAMS
Consultant, Pediatrician
Fortis, Woodlands, Iris Hospitals
Kolkata, West Bengal, India

Samir Hasan Dalwai MD DNB DCH FCPS LLB FIAP
National Treasurer, Indian Academy of Pediatrics
Developmental and Behavioral Pediatrician
New Horizons Child Development Center
Goregaon East
Mumbai, Maharashtra, India

Sanjay Mishra
Joint Director
Apex Group of Companies
Mumbai, Maharashtra, India

Sanjay Niranjan MD (Pediatrics) DCH
Former Pool Officer KGMU
Director Founder Neochild Clinic
Lucknow, Uttar Pradesh, India

Sanjio Borade
MBBS DGO DCH MD (Pharmacology) MCPS
Consulting Pediatrician, Gynecologist, Obstetrician and Clinical Pharmacologist
Joint Treasurer MLG, IAP, Amravati

Satish Agrawal MBBS (Nag) MD (Mum) DCH DNB (Ped)
Consulting Pediatrician
Agrawal Children Hospital
Amravati, Maharashtra, India

Satish Sharma MBBS MD (Ped) FIAP FIAMS FIACM
National Senior Vice President-North Zone
Indian Academy of Pediatrics (2024)
National Secretary IAP National Medicolegal Chapter 2023–2024
Past President
Indian Academy of Pediatrics, Haryana State
Medical Director, Arcus Superspecialty Medicenter
New Delhi, India

Satish Tiwari MD (Pediatrics) LLB FIAP
Founder President
Indian Medicolegal Ethic Association
Amrawati, Maharashtra, India

Shashikant Tripathi PhD LLM BCom
Specialization in Criminal Law Constitutional Law and Human Rights
Associate Professor and Director
Atal Bihari Vajpayee School of Legal Studies
Chhatrapati Shahu Ji Maharaj University
Kanpur, Uttar Pradesh, India

Suma Dnyanesh MBBS MD
Associate Professor
Department of Anatomy
KAHER'S JN Medical College
Belagavi, Karnataka, India

Contributors

Sushila Baldwa MBBS MD DGO
Consulting Obstetrician and Gynecologist
Baldwa Hospital and Apollo Clinic Nakoda
Foundation, Mumbai
Formerly Served as Faculty at BJ Medical College
and Sassoon General Hospital
Pune, Maharashtra, India

Varsha Baldwa MBBS MD FRCP (Australia)
Consultant, Clayton
Melbourne, Australia
Formerly, Seth GS Medical College and
KEM Hospital, Mumbai
Government Medical College, Surat
Government Medical College
Kota, Rajasthan, India

Vijay Arora LLB MBA
CEO
Apex Group of Companies
New Delhi, India

Vijay Baldwa
BDS (BOM) LLB LLM DIM DHRM PGDIM
Senior Dental Surgeon and Medicolegal Consultant
Architect, Prime Mover, Founder President of
IDA Mumbai WSB
Vice President, IDA Maharashtra SB
Author, Contributor, Invited Speaker on Legal
and Practice Management Issues
University Department of Law
Mumbai, Maharashtra, India

Vivek Saxena MD (Pediatrics) FIAP
President
Academy of Pediatrics Uttar Pradesh
Director and Pediatric Consultant
Vatsalya Hospital
Kanpur, Uttar Pradesh, India

VK Goyal MD (Pediatrics)
Director and HOD
Pediatrics Panchsheel Hospitals Pvt Ltd
New Delhi, India

Foreword

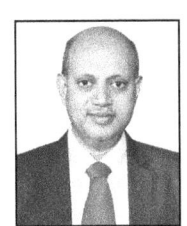

In the ever-evolving landscape of modern medicine, the dedicated individuals who shoulder the immense responsibility of healing and caring for our society find themselves navigating treacherous legal waters. The practice of medicine, once perceived as a noble art of compassion and healing, has transformed into a perilous legal battleground, where even the most well-intentioned physicians may find themselves ensnared in complex legal disputes. This shift not only poses a grave threat to the medical profession but also jeopardizes the quality of healthcare provided to patients.

The book you are about to delve into, "Medical Negligence in Pediatrics", underscores the urgent need to address the multifaceted challenges faced by physicians in today's healthcare environment. As physicians increasingly confront legal repercussions for errors or adverse outcomes, they are burdened with not only financial liabilities but also personal threats, acts of violence, professional sanctions, and even imprisonment. These consequences often arise from a lack of awareness and adherence to legal principles, casting a shadow over the noble mission of healthcare.

One of the remarkable strengths of this book lies in its dedication to keeping pace with the ever-changing legal landscape. It offers an in-depth exploration of recent legislative changes and landmark Supreme Court rulings, providing a thorough understanding of the legal framework governing medical practice in India. From new Consumer Protection Laws (2019) to the National Medical Commission Act (2019), Medical Termination of Pregnancy Regulations (2021), Passive Euthanasia Guidelines (2023), and State Laws and Regulations against Violence in Healthcare, this edition ensures that readers are equipped with the latest legal knowledge.

"Medical Negligence in Pediatrics" is a beacon of knowledge and guidance in a world where the medical and legal realms increasingly intersect. It provides a roadmap for physicians to uphold their commitment to patient care while safeguarding themselves from the perils of litigation. As we embark on this journey through the pages of this book, let us remember that the goal of modern medicine remains, at its core, the preservation of life, alleviation of suffering, and the restoration of health. May this book serve as a compass to help healthcare professionals navigate the challenging terrain of contemporary medicine, ensuring that the noble art of caring remains unwavering in its dedication to humanity.

GV Basavaraja
Professor
Pediatrics and Head PICU, IGICH
Bengaluru, Karnataka, India
National President IAP, 2024

**Endorsed by Medicolegal Chapter of
Indian Academy of Pediatrics**

Preface

"Wherever the art of medicine is loved, there is also a love of humanity."
—Hippocrates

In the words of the esteemed physician and medical educator, William Osler, "Medicine is a science of uncertainty and an art of probability". However, the contemporary landscape of medicine has strayed from this wisdom, driven by societal pressures and the pursuit of profit, demanding unwavering accuracy and guaranteed outcomes while disregarding the inherent complexities of the human body.

This modern approach to medicine comes at a significant cost. Physicians find themselves increasingly vulnerable to legal repercussions for any errors or adverse outcomes, facing financial burdens through substantial compensations, personal threats, and acts of violence, professional sanctions, and even imprisonment. These consequences often stem from a lack of awareness and adherence to legal principles, transforming the noble art of caring into a perilous legal battleground.

Even when driven by good intentions and acting in the best interests of their patients, physicians can become ensnared in legal disputes. This book emphasizes the paramount importance of practical and transparent communication strategies, including comprehensive risk disclosure during patient consent and meticulous documentation of medical records. By embracing these practices, physicians can proactively mitigate the risk of legal complications and adeptly navigate the intricacies of modern medical practice.

Acknowledging the ever-evolving legal landscape, this edition of "Medical Negligence in Pediatrics" provides comprehensive coverage of recent legislative changes and landmark Supreme Court rulings. These updates encompass a range of critical areas, including new Consumer Protection Laws (2019), the National Medical Commission Act (2019), Medical Termination of Pregnancy Regulations (2021), Passive Euthanasia Guidelines (2023), and State Laws and Regulations against Violence in Healthcare. Additionally, the book explores amendments in laws related to clinical establishments, the POCSO Act, child protection, and juvenile justice. Chimera of s. 106(1) of Bharatiya Nyaya Sanhita 2023 is apparently harsher than IPC 304A, a way away from complete decriminalization as promised on December 20th, 2023 by Union Home Minister. Only Judicial interpretation will make it more clear in time to come. The Indian Penal Code-IPC, criminal procedure code CrPC-1973, and Indian Evidence Act-IEA-1872 are to be replaced by brand new counterparts—the New Bharatiya Nyaya Sanhita 2023, Bharatiya Nagarik Suraksha Sanhita 2023, and Bharatiya Sakshya Adhiniyam 2023 respectively.

This comprehensive resource serves as a valuable tool for a diverse audience, including Indian doctors looking to understand their legal obligations and safeguard themselves from litigation, legal professionals engaged in healthcare litigation seeking a deeper understanding of medical contexts, hospital executives responsible for overseeing patient care and ensuring legal compliance, and the judicial system seeking clarification on the medical intricacies of litigation.

Through lucid explanations, meticulous references, and practical examples, "Medical Negligence in Pediatrics" provides a holistic understanding of the legal complexities entwined with medical practice. This book, when comprehensively explored, equips both medical professionals and legal practitioners with the knowledge and resources needed to navigate the intricate realm of healthcare litigation. By fostering a culture of legal awareness within the medical community, our aim is to reduce instances of negligence, ultimately creating a safer and more equitable environment for both patients and doctors.

With heartfelt gratitude to the dedicated team of Jaypee Brothers Medical Publishers, New Delhi, India, we proudly present "Medical Negligence in Pediatrics". We believe that by dispelling legal ignorance and promoting a culture of legal awareness within the medical community, we can collectively work towards a future where both patients and practitioners can reap the benefits of a more just and harmonious healthcare system.

Mahesh Baldwa
Hemant R Gangolia
Jyoti Kumar Gupta
Dnyanesh DK

Acknowledgments

The creation of "Medical Negligence in Pediatrics" represents the culmination of collective wisdom and the invaluable contributions of numerous individuals committed to advancing the fields of pediatrics and medical law.

We extend our heartfelt gratitude to all the contributors whose names grace the "List of Contributors" pages, for they have played pivotal roles in bringing this work to fruition.

Our deep appreciation goes out to the authors and editors who generously shared their knowledge, insights, and experiences in the realms of pediatrics and medical negligence law. Their combined expertise has enriched the content and depth of this book, establishing it as a comprehensive resource for professionals in the field of pediatrics.

We recognize the immeasurable support and understanding provided by our families and friends. To them, we owe a tremendous debt for dedicating a substantial part of their time to accommodate our writing commitments, maintaining normalcy at home, and offering unwavering encouragement. Their patience and belief in our endeavor have been our pillars of strength.

We also acknowledge the invaluable guidance and mentorship from our legal mentors and innumerable medical and legal teachers, which have profoundly shaped our professional journeys and contributed to the creation of this book. Additionally, we extend our gratitude to our colleagues and students in the fields of pediatrics and medical law, whose collaborative efforts have further enriched our collective knowledge.

We express our sincere thanks to Jaypee Publications, New Delhi, India, for recognizing the importance of this book and providing the platform to disseminate this critical information to the medical community and beyond. Your commitment to publishing excellence has been instrumental in transforming this project into reality.

Lastly, we acknowledge and appreciate our previous readers who engaged with our publications related to legal issues in medical practice, as well as prospective readers of "Medical Negligence in Pediatrics". It is the readers of medicolegal books who ignite our dedication to advancing legal and medical knowledge, as well as patient safety. Your motivation drives editors like us to continue our pursuit of excellence.

May this collaborative effort serve as a valuable resource and guide for medical professionals, legal experts, and anyone seeking a profound understanding of medical negligence in pediatrics.

With profound gratitude,

Mahesh Baldwa
Hemant R Gangolia
Jyoti Kumar Gupta
Dnyanesh DK

Contents

SECTION 1: Basis of Medical Negligence, Communication, Documentation, and Consent

1. Introduction to Medical Negligence 3
   Mahesh Baldwa, Namita Padvi, Amit Padvi, Ritu kumar
2. Effective Communication in Doctor-Patient and Medicolegal Contexts 11
   Devaraj Virupakshayya Raichur
3. Medical Documentation: The Only Defense for Doctors 26
   Dnyanesh DK, Suma Dnyanesh
4. Record Keeping, Making Easy 35
   Jyoti Kumar Gupta, VK Goyal, Anita Sharma, Marrisha Gupta
5. Medical Consent: The Best Friend of Doctor 54
   Mahesh Baldwa, Bhvya Baldwa, Namita Padvi, Varsha Baldwa
6. Logical Basis of Consent Formats 68
   Mahesh Baldwa, Namita Padvi, Varsha Baldwa, Ashok Baldwa
7. All About Medical Certificates 78
   Mahesh Baldwa, Namita Padvi, Vijay Baldwa, Ankit Gupta

SECTION 2: Consumer, Criminal Laws, Litigation Process, and Limiting Liability

8. Consumer Protection Act-2019 89
   Mahesh Baldwa, Varsha Baldwa, Aishwarya Mantri, Sanjay Mishra
9. Application of Criminal Law to Medical Practice 98
   Ishita Banerji
10. Dealing with Civil Pre-Litigation and Litigation Process 108
    Mahesh Baldwa, Varsha Baldwa, Namita Padvi, Vijay Arora
11. Limiting the Liability in Case of Alleged Medical Negligence 125
    Jyoti Kumar Gupta, Shashikant Tripathi, Amrita Verma, Rajat Dubey
12. Outdoor and Indoor Practice Giving Rise to Legal Liabilities in Medical Practice 140
    Ishita Banerji
13. Advance Deposit Before Admission and While Discharge Bill not Paid in Hospital 147
    Hemant R Gangolia, Ramesh B Dampuri, Sanjio Borade
14. Landmark Supreme Court Judgments and Their Importance in Medicolegal Litigations 152
    Jyoti Kumar Gupta, Ashish Jain, AB Jaiswal, Jitendra Pratap Singh Chauhan

SECTION 3: Various Scenarios in Medical Negligence

15. **Medicolegal Aspects of Difficult Situation of Unexpected Death** 181
    Mahesh Baldwa, Namita Padvi, Amit Padvi, Varsha Baldwa

16. **Prevention of Violence Against Doctors** 193
    Hemant R Gangolia, Bela Amichandra Verma, Samik Basu, Rajakumar Marol

17. **Medicolegal Issues in Pediatric Critical Care** 202
    Dnyanesh DK, Suma Dnyanesh

18. **Medicolegal Aspects of Vaccinations** 212
    Jyoti Kumar Gupta, Vivek Saxena, Raj Tilak, Sanjay Niranjan

19. **Medicolegal Aspects of Transferring the Acute Ill Patients, Transit Death, Inadvertent use of Expiry Drug** 225
    Jyoti Kumar Gupta, Anurag Mehrotra, Satish Sharma, Ambrish Gupta

20. **Legalities in Developmental Pediatrics** 248
    Samir Hasan Dalwai, Atanu Bhadra, Abraham Paul, Pranjal Agarwal

21. **Medicolegal Aspects for Pediatric Surgery** 255
    Mahesh Baldwa, Namita Padvi, Varsha Baldwa, Sushila Baldwa

22. **Legalities in Neonatology** 274
    Anurag Pangrikar, Hemant R Gangolia, Jyoti Kumar Gupta, Mahesh Baldwa

23. **Legal Hurdles of Police, RTI, Labor and Drug Inspectors, Fire NOC, Bio-Waste in Medical Practice etc.** 289
    Hemant R Gangolia, Satish Agrawal, Sameer Sadawarte, C Nirmala

SECTION 4: Miscellaneous

24. **Understanding National Medical Commission Act 2019 and Professional Conduct, Etiquette and Ethics and CEA 2010** 307
    Namita Padvi, Mahesh Baldwa, Varsha Baldwa, Sushila Baldwa

25. **Professional Indemnity and Out-of-Court Settlement** 325
    Satish Tiwari

Index *331*

SECTION 1

Basis of Medical Negligence, Communication, Documentation, and Consent

- **Introduction to Medical Negligence**
  Mahesh Baldwa, Namita Padvi, Amit Padvi, Ritu kumar

- **Effective Communication in Doctor-Patient and Medicolegal Contexts**
  Devaraj Virupakshayya Raichur

- **Medical Documentation: The Only Defense for Doctors**
  Dnyanesh DK, Suma Dnyanesh

- **Record Keeping, Making Easy**
  Jyoti Kumar Gupta, VK Goyal, Anita Sharma, Marrisha Gupta

- **Medical Consent: The Best Friend of Doctor**
  Mahesh Baldwa, Bhvya Baldwa, Namita Padvi, Varsha Baldwa

- **Logical Basis of Consent Formats**
  Mahesh Baldwa, Namita Padvi, Varsha Baldwa, Ashok Baldwa

- **All About Medical Certificates**
  Mahesh Baldwa, Namita Padvi, Vijay Baldwa, Ankit Gupta

CHAPTER 1

Introduction to Medical Negligence

Mahesh Baldwa, Namita Padvi, Amit Padvi, Ritu kumar

When trust is broken: Exploring the ethical and legal implications of medical negligence.

Keywords: Contact law, Criminal law, Duty breach causation damage, Jurisprudence, Medical negligence

Aim: This provides bird's eye view of liabilities which can arise under civil, criminal including consumer courts.

Objective: The rules governing civil, criminal including consumer courts forearms if doctor faces any case in court of law.

INTRODUCTION

The silent epidemic of medical negligence is a widespread yet often hidden danger, silently jeopardizing patient safety and healthcare quality. From missed diagnoses to botched surgeries, its tentacles reach far and wide. But we can fight back. By understanding its nuances, demanding accountability, and promoting best practices, we can combat this epidemic and usher in an era of safer, more reliable healthcare for all.

DEFINITION OF MEDICAL NEGLIGENCE

In India, medical negligence laws refer to a breach of duty of medical care by a physician/surgeon. This breach/failure of breach of duty of care can lead to harm or injury to the patient. This breach/failure of breach of duty of care can occur through an act of omission or commission by the physician/surgeon.

DIFFERENT PLATFORMS TO REDRESS GRIEVANCES

In India, patients can seek legal recourse for medical negligence by filing a complaint with the relevant State Medical Council (SMC), consumer court, or civil court. The complaint must provide details of the medical negligence, including the nature of the harm caused, the physician/surgeon's breach of duty, and the damages suffered by the patient.

SOURCES OF MEDICAL NEGLIGENCE LAW

Law of Tort and Civil Law

The Indian courts have developed the principle of "reasonable care" as the standard for physician/surgeon to adhere to when providing medical treatment to patients. This principle implies that a physician/surgeon must exercise a reasonable degree of skill and care while treating a patient. Failure to do so may result in legal action against the physician/surgeon may result in payment of unliquidated damages decided by consumer/civil courts using multiplier given in second schedule under Section 163-A MACT.[1]

CODE OF ETHICAL CONDUCT- LICENSE TO PRACTICE MEDICINE

National Medical Commission (NMC) in 2019[2] replaced the Indian Medical Council. NMC adopted Indian Medical Council (Professional Conduct, Etiquette and Ethics) Regulations in 2002;[3] outlines the duties and responsibilities of physician/surgeons, including the need to obtain informed consent from patients, maintain medical records, and adhere to medical ethics. A new code of conduct was rolled out on 02-08-2023[4] and rolled back on 24-08-2023.[5] SMC/NMC can warn, suspend, or cancel license. Cancellation of license to practice medicine leads to professional death.

> **CAUTION**
> Remember that IPC-1860 is set to be replaced by New Bharatiya Nyaya Sanhita 2023 (BNS), CrPC1973 by Bharatiya Nagarik Suraksha Sanhita act, 2023 (BNSS), IEA1872 by Bharatiya Sakshya adhiniyam 2023, so in future please refer to corresponding section before studying decided case laws.

CRIMINAL LAW ON MEDICAL NEGLIGENCE

Main four sections of Indian Penal Code (IPC)[6], 1860 (BNS 2023) relevant to physician/surgeon:

1. *Section 304 A IPC, 1860 (BNS 2023):* Death of any person by doing any rash or negligent act not amounting to culpable homicide, shall be punished with imprisonment of either description for a term which may extend to 2 years, or with fine, or with both.
2. *Section 336 IPC, 1860 (BNS 2023):* Any rash or negligent act that endangers human life or risks personal safety of people is punishable with imprisonment which may extend to 3 months and may even attract a fine up to INR 250.
3. *Section 337 IPC, 1860 (BNS 2023):* Whoever causes hurt to any person by doing any act so rashly or negligently as to endanger human life, or the personal safety of others, shall be punished with imprisonment of either description for term which may extend to 6 months, or with fine which may extend to INR 500, or with both.
4. *Section 338 of the IPC (BNS 2023):* This section deals with causing grievous hurt by an act endangering life or personal safety. If a medical professional causes grievous hurt to a patient due to negligence, they can be punished with imprisonment for up to 2 years or a fine, or both.

MEDICAL NEGLIGENCE UNDER CONTRACT

Even in the absence of an express stipulation to the effect that the physician/surgeon will exercise reasonable skill and care in treatment of a patient, it is taken as an implied duty arising out of the contract. Breach of this duty thus results in violation of the contract. Theoretically, the patient and doctor can pre-decide payment of liquidated damages in case of medical negligence not leaving it to courts to decide the total payment in such eventuality as per the Indian Contract Act 1872.[7]

JUDICIAL DECISIONS ON MEDICAL NEGLIGENCE

"Reasonable man" in Bolam case,[8] it was discussed that "In an ordinary case it is generally said you judge it by the action of the man in the street. He is the ordinary man". The courts used to "judge the conduct of any physician/surgeon by comparing it with that of the hypothetical ordinary man in that category".

The Supreme Court of India has delivered several landmark judgments related to medical negligence described Bolam test and its applicability of the consumer protection act.

CHAPTER 1: Introduction to Medical Negligence

WHAT IS THE JURISPRUDENTIAL CONCEPT OF NEGLIGENCE?

Negligence is the breach of a duty caused by the omission which a reasonable man guided by those considerations which ordinarily regulate the conduct of human affairs would do or doing something which is a prudent and reasonable man would not do.

WHAT ARE THE PRACTICAL ASPECTS OF CONCEPT OF NEGLIGENCE?

Negligence is the omission to do something which a reasonable man, guided upon those considerations which ordinarily regulate the conduct of human affairs, would do, or doing something which a reasonable man would not do.

PRINCIPLE OF "REASONABLE CARE" AS THE STANDARD

The physician/surgeon must bring to his task a reasonable degree of skill and knowledge and must exercise a reasonable degree of care. Neither the very highest nor a very low degree of care and competence judged in the light of the particular facts and circumstances of each case is what the law requires.

The law in India recognizes the right of patients to receive reasonable standard of medical care. When a physician/surgeon fail to render this legal duty of medical care, and a patient is harmed as a result, the patient may have a right to compensation for their injuries.

Onus of Proof

In order to establish medical negligence, it must be shown that the physician/surgeon breached their duty of care by failing to provide treatment that met the required standard.

ESSENTIALS OF MEDICAL NEGLIGENCE

To establish medical negligence, certain essential elements must be proven. These essentials include:
- *Duty of care:* The physician/surgeon must have had a duty of care to the patient. This means that physician/surgeon had a legal obligation to provide medical care that meets the expected standard of care.
- *Breach of duty:* The physician/surgeon must have breached their duty of care by failing to provide treatment that met the required standard. This breach of duty can occur through an act of omission or commission.
- *Causation:* The breach of duty must have caused harm or injury to the patient. It must be shown that the harm or injury was a direct result of the physician/surgeon's breach of duty.
- *Damage:* The patient must have suffered harm or injury as a result of the physician/surgeon's breach of duty. This harm or injury can be physical, emotional, or financial.

It is important to note that in order to establish medical negligence, all four of these elements must be proven. The burden of proof lies with the patient or their legal representative to demonstrate that the physician/surgeon breached duty of care and that this breach caused harm or injury to the patient.

TYPES OF INJURIES TO PATIENT DUE TO MEDICAL NEGLIGENCE

These can result in a wide range of injuries or harm to the patient, including physical, emotional, and financial damages.

COMPENSATION

The compensation awarded to patients in cases of medical negligence in India can vary depending on the severity of the harm caused as decided by judicial discretion as unliquidated lump sum damages or, as per multiplier system or principle of "restitutio ad integrum" which has no capping (limit) in India. The patient may be entitled to compensation for their damages, including medical expenses, lost income, pain and suffering, and other related expenses.

EXAMPLES OF MEDICAL NEGLIGENCE

These may include delayed diagnosis, misdiagnosis, incorrect treatment or medication, surgical errors, failure to obtain consent, inadequate follow-up care and advice for screening for retinopathy of prematurity (ROP), and birth injuries to mother and neonate such as brain damage and paralysis. Anesthesia errors can occur when a physician/surgeon administer too much or too little anesthesia, or fail to monitor the patient's vital signs during the procedure.

DEFENSES

- *Law of limitation:* Prescribes a time period of 2 years for consumer cases and for other cases 3 years. The patient party has right to sue with in that period originating from cause of action.
- *Error of judgment:* If a medical professional makes a reasonable and honest error in judgment while treating a patient, it may not be considered negligence.
- *Emergency situations:* If a medical professional acted in good faith to save a patient's life in an emergency situation, they may not be considered negligent.
- *Contributory negligence:* If the patient contributed to their injury or death through their own negligence, the medical professional may not be held entirely responsible.
- *Novus actus interveniens:* It is a Latin phrase which means there will be appearance of a new act or event in the causal chain between initial event, in a sequence and the result causing a break in the continuity of the same.

POTENTIAL LITIGANT

A prudent physician should view each patient as a possible legal adversary. This mindset serves as a reminder to the doctor to adhere to a set standard of care and avoid any risky endeavors. It is important for the doctor to take all accusations seriously, whether they are spoken or written, and respond to them with clarity and empathy.

What are antonyms of negligence?
It is due diligence with care and caution.

What are synonyms of negligence?
Synonyms are carelessness, lack of care, lack of proper care and attention, dereliction of duty, nonperformance of duty, nonfulfillment of duty, neglectfulness, neglect, laxity, laxness, irresponsibility, and delinquency.

Is negligence offence?
Negligence is an offense under tort, IPC (BNS 2023), Indian Contracts Act, Consumer Protection Act, and many more legal fields. Medical negligence basically is the negligence by a medical practitioner or doctor by not providing enough care resulting in breach of their duties and harming the patients. Bottom line is patient expects getting cured by treatment given by doctor at any cost. The expectation of law is never cure but its demonstration of medical care during treatment.

LAY CONCEPT OF MEDICAL NEGLIGENCE

To err is human. In legal parlance, diligence means medical carefulness. Opposite of diligence is negligence. Not every mistake is negligence nor all complications are negligence. Even poor, bad, or adverse result including death does not constitute negligence. Though patients see the doctors in high esteem as God and believe that disease will be cured and they will be healed by given treatment but there are exceptions due to peculiarity of medical paradigm.

STANDARD OF CARE, AMOUNT OF CARE, AND DEGREE OF CARE

"Being in such a profession where sick, ill, and sufferers look upon doctors as polymaths, almost in the place of almighty. Doctors also make last ditch efforts to save patients. In fact such an extreme care is not required legally. Law requires and expects average amount of care not heroisms".

REASONABLE MAN

In Bolam case, it was discussed that "In an ordinary case it is generally said you judge it by the action of the man in the street. He is the ordinary man". The courts used to judge the conduct of any defendant doctor by comparing it with that of the hypothetical ordinary doctor in the same field.

DEGREE OF NEGLIGENCE

The Delhi High Court laid down in 2005 that in civil law, there are three degrees of negligence in Smt. Madhubala versus Government of NCT of Delhi; Delhi High Court, DEL 209 = 2005 (118) DLT 515, W.P. No. 2011-03-03 Page No. 7:[9]
1. Lata culpa, gross neglect
2. Levis culpa, ordinary neglect, and
3. Levissima culpa, slight neglect.

CUSTOMARY PRACTICE

It can be pleaded in court of law.

In, Helling versus Carey 1974 183 wash 2d 514, 519 P. 2nd 981,[10] glaucoma—routine tonometry before 40 years not done—patient suffered due to nonmeasurement with tonometer—standard of practice reasonable or customary practice. Custom do not justify but court may be allowed customary practice.

LOCALITY OR GEOGRAPHIC PRACTICE

Locality rule of standard is justified because of rural urban divide.

LEVEL OF KNOWLEDGE THAT IS EXPECTED FROM A DOCTOR

Should it include the latest developments in the field, hence require constant updating or is it enough to follow what has been traditionally followed? It has been recognized by the courts that what amounts to reasonableness changes with time. The standard, as stated clearly herein before requires that the doctor possess reasonable knowledge. Hence, a doctor has to constantly update his knowledge to meet the standard expected of him. Since only reasonable knowledge is required, it may not be necessary for him to be aware of all the developments that have taken place in field on medicine.

No need to apply every latest modality of investigation/treatment of latest journals (Crawford's principle), use what is currently available locally.

In Crawford versus Board of Government of Charring hospital, 1953, The Times 8th

December (CA),[11] anesthetist causing malpositioning of arm causing paralysis. It is not necessary to follow every new modality of investigation or management, which is latest by reading journals at the same time outdated treatment should not be followed pig headedly, e.g., prescribing phynylbutazone for arthritis.

In Vinitha Ashok versus Laxmi Hospital, (Supreme Court of India) (SC) I (2002) CPJ, 4,[12] cervical pregnancy doctors did not do ultrasonography (USG). Supreme Court said not necessary to follow each and every latest investigation, held not negligent in spite of massive bleeding during MTP controlled by cesarean hysterectomy. Hysterectomy was done for saving life of patient.

LEGAL PRESUMPTION FOR SPECIAL PROFESSIONAL TASKS

Law presumes if any one holds out to public at large any task which is required to be performed with a special skill would generally be performed only if the person possesses the requisite qualifications, skills, and competence for performing that task by exercising reasonable degree of care and caution. If one does not possess requisite qualifications, skills, and competence then it is negligence per se.

COMPARISON OF CARE EQUIVALENT TO AVERAGE PRACTITIONER

Medical professional may be held liable for negligence even when possessed with requisite qualification and skill which he professed to have possessed but did not exercise, reasonable care equal to competence of an average person possessing similar skill. It is not necessary for every professional to possess the highest level of expertise in that branch which one practices. Where a profession embraces a range of views as to what is an acceptable standard of conduct, the competence of the professional is to be judged by the lowest standard that would be regarded as acceptable. The test is the standard of the ordinary skilled man exercising and professing to have that special skill.

STANDARD OF CARE CASE LAWS

Negligence Per Se

In Poonam Verma versus Ashwin Patel 1996 AIR 2111, 1996 SCC (4) 332[13] where doctor registered as homeopathic medical practitioner entitled to practice in homeopathy only not allopathy. Doctor prescribed an allopathic medicine to the patient. The patient died. The doctor was held to be negligent and liable to compensate the wife of the deceased for the death of her husband on the ground that the doctor who was entitled to practice in homoeopathy only, was under a statutory duty not to enter the field of any other system of medicine and since he trespassed into a prohibited field and prescribed the allopathic medicine to the patient causing the death, his conduct amounted to negligence per se actionable in civil law.

Standard of Care

Professionals are persons professing some special skill, who are trained to profess in that area especially and bear the responsibility of professing with due care. The SC in Jacob Mathew versus State of Punjab, AIR 2005 SC 3180,[14] explained that a professional entering into certain profession is deemed to have knowledge regarding that profession and it is assured impliedly by him that a reasonable amount of care shall be taken to profess his profession. The person can be held liable under negligence if he did not possess the required skills to profess or he failed to take essential amount of care to profess the said profession.

SUMMARY

Doctor will bring to his task a reasonable degree of skill and knowledge and must exercise a reasonable degree of care. Neither the very highest nor the very lowest degree of care and competence judged in the light of circumstances in each case is what the law requires. There is need to impose a higher degree of duty on a specialist. Higher the risk higher is degree of duty of care is imposed by law. Only reasonable knowledge is required, it may not be necessary for him to be aware of all the developments that have taken place in field on medicine. Court of law in India applies mainly *Bolam* principle when there two acceptable and reasonable standards procedures of care are available to doctor, one can follow one of the peer approved, accepted procedure in carrying out treatment. Even though, such procedure is followed by minority of doctors in profession. Whether Bolam principle is applicable to medical opinion, diagnosis, consent, and prognosis or not is left to judicial discretion. Now lot many judgments are questioning Bolam test.[15,16]

LEARNING KEY POINTS

- Medical practitioner will bring to his task a reasonable degree of skill and knowledge and must exercise a reasonable degree of care.
- Neither the very highest nor the very lowest degree of care and competence judged in the light of circumstances in each case is what the law requires.
- There is need to impose a higher degree of duty on a specialist. Higher the risk higher is degree of duty of care is imposed by law.
- Only reasonable knowledge is required, it may not be necessary for him to be aware of all the developments that have taken place in field on medicine.
- *Bolam* principle—when there two acceptable and reasonable standards procedures of care are available to doctor, one can follow one of the peer approved, accepted procedure in carrying out treatment. Even though, such procedure is followed by minority of doctors in profession. Whether Bolam principle is applicable to medical opinion, diagnosis, consent, and prognosis or not is left to judicial discretion.

MCQ

Choose one correct answer
1. What is Bolam test as applied by Indian courts?
   a. Doctor will bring to his task a reasonable degree of skill
   b. Reasonable knowledge
   c. Exercise a reasonable degree of care
   d. All of the above

Answer

1. d

TAKE-HOME MESSAGES

Medical negligence laws refer to a breach of duty of medical care by a physician *toward patient*.

MUST AVOID THINGS

Higher the risk higher is degree of duty of care is imposed by law, hence one should refer to appropriate specialist to avoid high risk patients.

DO NOT DO

Do not treat beyond one's knowledge and skill.

WARNINGS

It is not necessary to follow every new modality of investigation or management, which is latest but should never adhere to outdated modalities of treatment.

MESSAGES WHICH THE READER MUST BE AWARE

Negligence is unacceptable under tort, IPC (BNS 2023), Indian Contracts Act, Consumer Protection Act, and many more legal fields.

MUST DO THING

One can submit eye and expert witness without being asked by consumer court.

MEDICAL NEGLIGENCE PEARLS

If a medical professional acted in good faith to save a patient's life in an emergency situation, they may not be considered negligent by court of law.

ONLY ONE FACT TO REMEMBER

Negligence is the omission to do something which a reasonable man, guided upon those considerations which ordinarily regulate the conduct of human affairs, would do, or doing something which a reasonable man would not do.

REFERENCES

1. Motor Accident Claims Tribunal was established on 2nd December, 1959.
2. National Medical Commission Act, 2019.
3. Indian Medical Council (Professional Conduct, Etiquette, and Ethics) Regulations, 2002.
4. NMC's Professional Conduct for Registered Medical Practitioners, 2023 notified on 2nd August, 2023.
5. NMC's Professional Conduct for Registered Medical Practitioners, 2023 rolled back on 23-08-2023.
6. Indian Penal Code, 1860.
7. Indian Contract Act, 1872.
8. Bolam versus Friern Hospital Management Committee (1957) 1 WLR 583.
9. Smt. Madhubala versus Government of NCT of Delhi; Delhi High Court, DEL 209 = 2005 (118) DLT 515, W.P. No. 2011-03-03, Page No. 7.
10. Helling versus Carey 1974 183 wash 2d 514, 519 P. 2nd 981.
11. Crawford versus Board of Government of Charring Hospital, 1953, The Times 8th December (CA).
12. Vinitha Ashok versus Laxmi Hospital (Supreme Court of India) (SC) I (2002) CPJ, 4.
13. Poonam Verma versus Ashwin Patel 1996 AIR 2111, 1996 SCC (4) 332.
14. Jacob Mathew versus State of Punjab, AIR 2005 SC 3180.
15. Baldwa M, Baldwa V, Padvi N, Baldwa S. Legal Issues in Medical Practice, 2nd edition. New Delhi: CBS Publishers and Distributors Pvt. Ltd.; 2023.
16. Baldwa M, Baldwa V, Padvi N, Baldwa S. Legal Issues in Critical Care, 1st edition. New Delhi: CBS Publishers and Distributors Pvt. Ltd.; 2022.

CHAPTER 2

Effective Communication in Doctor-Patient and Medicolegal Contexts

Devaraj Virupakshayya Raichur

Effective communication is the cornerstone of patient-centered care, and is crucial to prevent and manage medicolegal litigations.

Keywords: Communication, Confidentiality, Language barriers, Nonverbal communication

Aim: Communication is the process of sending and receiving messages.

Objective: To ensure that communication between doctor and patient is 100% successful for better outcomes in medical treatment and patient satisfaction.

INTRODUCTION

Communication is the process of sending and receiving messages through verbal or nonverbal means.[1] Effective communication is vital in medical practice. It ensures accurate history-taking, fosters patient understanding, and supports healing. Interprofessional communication is crucial for teamwork, reducing care-gaps, building relationships, and promoting learning. In the medicolegal realm, poor communication underlies many cases, more than clinical quality, often leading to negligence claims.[2] For safe, effective, and patient-centered care, we must enhance our communication with patients in meaningful ways.[3-7]

ELEMENTS OF COMMUNICATION AND THEIR RELEVANCE IN MEDICOLEGAL CONTEXT

Communication Cycle and Basic Process Models of Communication

In 1949, mathematician Claude Shannon and engineer Warren Weaver developed a foundational model of communication that is still used today. David Berlo modified the Shannon and Weaver model in 1960 to better reflect the communication process. His model has four components, i.e., source, message, channel, and receiver. Each component has subcategories that describe it in more detail. The transactional model of communication, developed by Dean Barnlund (2008), is a simplified model that views communication as a circular process between participants, rather than a linear one.[8]

Elements of Communication Process

From the earlier mentioned models, we can summarize the elements of communication, which form components of the communication cycle (**Fig. 1**) as:

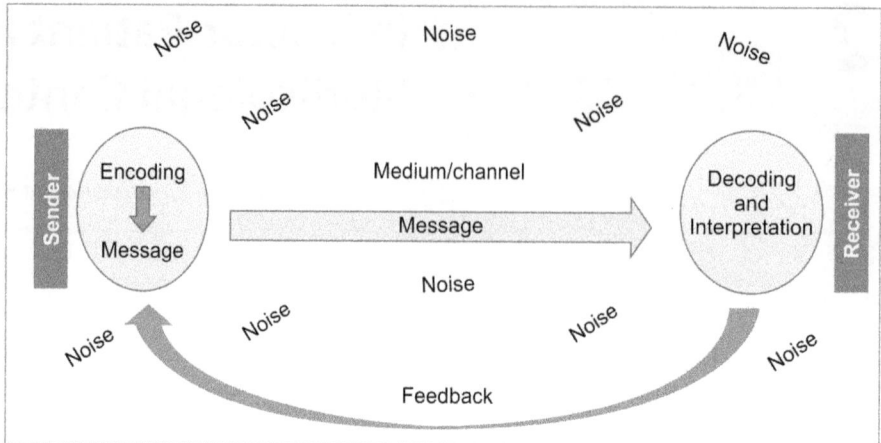

Fig. 1: Communication cycle.

- *Sender or source:* Represents the person intending to send a communication.
- *Encoding:* It is a process of creating a suitable form for the statement/idea to be transmitted.
- *Message:* It is the encoded statement/idea to be transmitted to the receiver.
- *Medium or channel:* It is the medium used for transmitting the message.
- *Receiver:* The person for whom the message was meant.
- *Decoding and interpretation:* The receiver decodes the message and interprets it.
- *Feedback:* The final part of a communication cycle, it is the response the receiver shows the received message. It enables the sender to assess if his message has reached and interpreted by the receiver, as intended. The feedback can be viewed as initiation of another communication cycle when a series of messages are being exchanged, forming a series of interwoven communication cycles where each feedback could form initiation of a next communication cycle by the receiver.
- *Noise:* It is a collective term representing various types of barriers for effective communication (physical noise, worries, distractions, unfamiliar language, attitudes, preconceptions, illness, etc.). Noise can exist at various stages of the communication cycle.

Core Elements of Communication in Medical Practice

With the understanding of the communication cycle and the elements of communication, they could be applied to the context of medical consultation, recognizing the following core elements—initiating the session, gathering information, explanation and planning, and closing the session. In addition, all through these steps, building the relationship and structuring the consultation also act as core elements for effective medical communication. The main part of the interview will be focused on gathering information and can be in the following steps: Asking questions, active-empathic listening, facilitation of patient's/parent's expression (with encouraging expressions, gestures, words, etc.), signposting (guiding the path of discussion), and summarizing (including the further plans and next visits, as appropriate).[9]

Challenges in Medicolegal Communication

Challenges in medicolegal communication, forming a part of "noise" in the communication process, can be complex and have significant consequences for patient care, legal proceedings, and professional relationships. Understanding these challenges is essential for healthcare professionals, legal professionals, and other stakeholders involved in the medicolegal context. Here are some common challenges in medicolegal communication.

Language Barriers

Patients with limited proficiency in the language spoken by healthcare providers may struggle to understand medical information and instructions. This can hinder effective communication and lead to misunderstandings or misdiagnoses. Healthcare professionals often use medical terminology that may be unfamiliar to patients (medical jargon).[4-7] Failure to explain medical terms in plain language can impede comprehension.[10]

Cultural Sensitivity

Patients from diverse cultural backgrounds may have unique beliefs and practices related to health and healthcare. Healthcare providers must be sensitive to these differences to avoid misunderstandings and potential conflicts. Some cultural or religious beliefs may affect a patient's willingness to accept certain treatments or procedures, leading to challenges in obtaining consent.[11,12]

Emotional Distress

Patients facing serious medical issues or legal proceedings may experience high levels of fear and anxiety. These emotions can make it difficult for them to absorb information effectively. In cases of medical negligence or adverse outcomes, patients and their families may experience grief and anger, which can complicate communication and trust.[13]

Information Overload

Healthcare providers may need to convey complex medical information to patients. Providing too much information at once can overwhelm patients and hinder their ability to make informed decisions. There is a legal expectation of detailed medical records and documentation. Balancing the need for thorough documentation with the risk of overwhelming patients or creating legal confusion can be challenging.[14]

Miscommunication and Misunderstanding

Miscommunication between patients and healthcare providers can result from rushed appointments, unclear explanations, or patients' reluctance to ask questions. In a medicolegal situation, the legal professionals may use legal terms and concepts that are unfamiliar to healthcare providers, potentially leading to misunderstandings.[12,15]

Confidentiality and Privacy Concerns

Confidentiality and privacy concerns act as barriers for effective communication. In this era of telemedicine, there is a plausible concern of confidentiality getting breached.[16-18] Further, patients may be concerned that sharing their medical information with legal professionals could compromise their privacy or be used against them in legal proceedings, leading to reluctance in providing necessary information. Similarly, for a medical practitioner, while sharing patient information with legal professionals, striking the right balance between patient privacy and legal requirements can be challenging.

Interprofessional Communication

During emergency department managements, patient transfers or shift changes, miscommunication between healthcare providers can lead to gaps in patient care, missed information, and potential medicolegal issues. Similarly, collaborating effectively between medical and legal professionals can be challenging, especially when their perspectives and objectives differ.[19,20]

Understanding and addressing these challenges in medicolegal communication is vital for improving patient care, preventing legal disputes, and maintaining the trust and confidence of patients and their families. Healthcare and legal professionals should receive training and guidance on how to navigate these challenges to ensure that communication remains clear, respectful, and patient-centered within the medicolegal context.

Effective Communication Strategies

Effective communication strategies in the medicolegal context are crucial for ensuring that information is conveyed accurately, clearly, and in a timely manner among healthcare professionals, patients, legal professionals, and other stakeholders. These strategies help prevent misunderstandings, errors, and can positively impact patient care and legal proceedings.

The following are some key effective communication strategies.

Clear and Compassionate Communication

Focus on the patient, using simple language and, when appropriate, use of visual aids during communication are important for effective communication. Patient-centered communication involves active listening, empathy, and addressing the patient's concerns and questions. It is essential for building trust and rapport. When communicating with patients, plain language avoiding medical jargon and complex terminology, helps them better understand their condition, treatment options, and risks. Effective use of visual aids, such as diagrams, charts, and images, can be valuable tools for explaining medical concepts to patients, especially when language barriers exist, to facilitate effective communication.[21]

Documentation and Record-keeping

As emphasized in documentation of communication section, accurate and timely documentation of communication and storing the documents are important aspects medicolegally. This includes documenting patient histories, diagnoses, treatment plans, medications, and any discussions with patients and their families. Timeliness in recording information is crucial for preserving the integrity of the medical record. To protect patient privacy and maintain data security, healthcare facilities should have robust record-keeping systems with restricted access to sensitive information.[22]

Interprofessional Collaboration

Almost always, medical practitioners manage their patients in collaboration with other healthcare workers. Further, there might be a need of coordination with other medical practitioners in the same setting, specialists,

CHAPTER 2: Effective Communication in Doctor-Patient and Medicolegal Contexts

referring medical practitioners and referral hospitals. This necessitates skills of a team player and an efficient manager; of these skills, communication is an important aspect. Effective communication among healthcare team members, including physicians, nurses, pharmacists, and specialists, is essential for coordinated patient care.[23]

Regular team meetings, updates, and clear delegation of responsibilities are crucial. During patient transfers or shift changes, clear handoff communication ensures that essential information about the patient's condition, treatment plan, and any critical concerns is passed on to the next responsible team.

Informed Consent/Real and Valid Consent

While informed consent, as practiced in the USA, is ideal for all invasive/surgical procedures, the Supreme Court of India in *Samira Kohli* case has decided that as of now, the real and valid consent, as practiced in the United Kingdom, is appropriate for the Indian conditions.[24]

However, it must be noted that on 2 August, 2023 the Regulation 19 of the National Medical Commission Registered Medical Practitioner (Professional Conduct) Regulations, 2023, had enforced informed consent in India but with a notification of the National Medical Commission dated 23 August 2023, these regulations have been kept in abeyance.

Informed consent places the focus on patient's right to information and autonomy, necessitating the medical practitioner to provide the patients with comprehensive information about the procedure, potential risks, alternatives, and expected outcomes before any medical procedure or treatment. Patients would have the opportunity to ask questions and provide informed consent voluntarily. Real and valid consent places the responsibility on the medical practitioner of deciding what all is necessary to inform to the patient based on the prevalent practice in the situation, and being sensitive to right to life of the patients and to various conditions impacting decision making by them.[24]

Consent discussions and agreements should be documented in the patient's medical record, confirming that the patient understood the information provided and agreed to the proposed treatment, duly signed by the medical practitioner, the patient, and two witnesses.

Confidentiality and Privacy

Confidentiality and privacy are components of the right to life, enshrined in the Article 21 of the constitution of India. Thus it is crucial that these are observed rigorously. Healthcare providers must adhere to all the relevant laws, including those related to insurance, to safeguard patient information. This includes maintaining patient confidentiality and ensuring secure communication methods. Healthcare providers should refrain from discussing patient cases or sharing sensitive patient information in public spaces or with unauthorized individuals. This is discussed in more detail in confidentiality issues section.

Cultural Sensitivity and Diversity Awareness

As noted in cultural sensitivity section, cultural variations could act as a barrier to the effective communication. Efficiently dealing with this goes a long way in optimal healthcare. Healthcare professionals should be culturally competent and aware of the diverse backgrounds and beliefs of their patients. Understanding cultural differences can help avoid misunderstandings and improve patient-provider relationships. In cases where patients have limited local language proficiency, healthcare facilities should provide language interpretation services to ensure effective communication.

These effective communication strategies are essential for promoting patient safety, preventing legal disputes, and maintaining the trust and confidence of patients and their families. By incorporating these strategies into their practice, healthcare professionals can enhance the quality of care they provide and reduce the risk of medicolegal issues stemming from communication breakdowns.

NONVERBAL, VERBAL, AND WRITTEN COMMUNICATIONS

In most medicolegal contexts, communication could be in the form of a nonverbal, or a verbal, or a written message. These form various channels used for communication.

Nonverbal Communication

Here no formal language is used but the message is conveyed by the sender to the receiver through a sign, or a gesture, or an action. For example, a parent bringing his/her child to the pediatrician, is a nonverbal communication of the consent for history taking and examination by the pediatrician. However, in case of examination of genitals or breasts, it is medicolegally appropriate for the pediatrician to explain what examination is contemplated and its relevance, and get a verbal consent from the parent. In addition, if the child is >12 years old an assent from the child is desirable.

Verbal Communication

It is in the form of a spoken conversation and has the advantage of simplicity and ease of message formation and transmission. It has its disadvantages too. It is more likely to be misinterpreted and unless a feedback is given by the receiver of the message and further corrected by the sender, it is likely to remain in the misinterpreted form. Further, unless there is some recording of the conversation it is difficult to prove exactly what was communicated. These disadvantages of verbal communication are lessened by written communication, though it is relatively tedious.

Verbal communication happens very commonly at various situations, including during the doctor-patient/parent interaction, between healthcare providers, and between medical and legal professionals in a medicolegal context.

Written Communication

It could be in the form of written information given from the sender of the message to the receiver, with or without any acknowledgement by the receiver. This mode of communication is resorted to communications which have important medical and medicolegal implications. Examples include the notes and prescriptions written by a medical practitioner, the notes and orders of a treating doctor and notes of nursing staff in the case paper of admitted patients, and consent documents from patients/parents for invasive/surgical procedures.

All official communications in case of medicolegal litigation between the patient/parent and the medical practitioner, as well as to and from the relevant legal authority also fall under this category.

DOCUMENTATION OF COMMUNICATION

Regulation 1.3 of the Indian Medical Council (Professional conduct, Etiquette and Ethics) Regulations, 2002 relates to maintenance of medical records and every medical practitioner in India must maintain medical documents as per the regulation and any further changes that could be brought in by the National Medical Commission.

Rising medical documentation requirements consume time but are crucial. Documentation facilitates accurate billing, protect against legal action, and serve as a vital patient history. Proper documentation can preempt adverse expert opinions, reducing legal risks.[25]

To be effective in the medicolegal context, all the issues related to patient care and communication need to be properly documented as courts tend to consider no documentation as no proof, poor documentation as a weak proof and good documentation as a strong proof of what happened, or was done. It is aptly said, "poor records mean poor defense, no records mean no defense".[26]

Types of Documentation of Communication

Mostly, medical documentation would be in the form of written documents, including the inpatient records, and the documents on consent. However, it could be in the form of video recordings with the consent of the patient, especially in the cases of patients in the intensive care unit when initial information and regular updates are given. In this case, consent of the patient/parent needs to be taken for the recording being done.

Dos of Medical Documentation

- *Record time and date of the notes:* This helps to know sequence of events. To rely on memory is not wise. "The palest ink is better than the best memory" is an old Chinese proverb that might be considered relevant even today.

  It includes presence and absence of important findings from the patient's history and physical examination.
- *Write legibly:* Courts have fined medical practitioners for not writing legibly considering it an obstruction in the court work.[27] Further, legible prescription is a requirement by the Regulation 1.5 of the Indian Medical Council (Professional conduct, Etiquette and Ethics) Regulations, 2002.
- Record you having reviewed all reports related to the patient management.
- Document details and reasons as for your plan of management.
- Mention any addition to the document as a "late entry" and sign with date and time. If the change is objective about what happened, courts are likely to accept it. If it is self-serving, it is less likely to be accepted.

Don'ts of Medical Documentation

- Refrain from commenting on other healthcare workers in the patient's record. It is proper that this is dealt with by hospital management.
- Do not destroy the evidence. It could be considered as an added offense.
- Do not change the record. Advancing technology could detect changes made in the records. This is detrimental for the medical practitioner in the court.
- Avoid personal opinions on the patient creeping into an objective professional

statement in the document. Legally, this could weaken the record.

JUSTIFIED COMMUNICATION

"Justified communication" in the medicolegal context denotes the legally sound and ethically valid exchange of information between healthcare professionals, patients, and relevant parties. This communication is considered appropriate, necessary, and defensible in the context of providing medical care and managing potential legal issues. It aims to minimize legal risks by ensuring that all communication and actions are well-documented, compliant with legal requirements, and in the best interest of patient care. Thus it typically involves ensuring patients have all necessary information to make informed decisions about their care, including risks and benefits, maintaining thorough and accurate medical records to support the care provided and justify decisions made, adhering to all laws and regulations related to patient privacy, confidentiality, and healthcare practices, sharing relevant patient information with other healthcare professionals involved in the patient's care; all through this respecting privacy and confidentiality and protecting patient information and only disclosing it when legally and ethically permissible.

DECISION MAKERS

The decision makers and their roles in relation to medical and medicolegal communication include:
- Medical professionals (e.g., physicians, nurses, and pharmacists) make care-related decisions and document patient information, influencing patient care and legal aspects.
- Patients are key decision makers in their care through informed consent and communication, impacting treatment outcomes and legal risk.
- Legal and compliance professionals (e.g., healthcare lawyers and compliance officers) advise on legal compliance and risk mitigation.
- Healthcare administrators shape communication protocols and resources to enhance staff-patient interaction.
- Government and regulatory bodies (e.g., Ministry of Health and Family Welfare and National Medical Commission) set communication standards and enforce them.
- Insurance companies influence documentation requirements for billing and can be involved in medicolegal cases.

These decision makers establish and enforce communication standards and legal compliance, facilitate informed consent and clear information exchange, document patient care for legal purposes, ensure patient privacy and compliance with regulations, and advise on reducing legal risks. Collaboration among these stakeholders ensures effective, lawful medical communication, enhancing patient care, and protecting legal interests.

CCTV RECORDING AND AUDIO RECORDING OF COMMUNICATION

Video (including CCTV) and audio recording of communication in the medical and medicolegal context involves ethical, legal, and practical considerations.

Ethical Concerns

Recording must respect patient privacy, and consent is vital except in emergencies or abuse cases. Potential distress to vulnerable patients should be balanced with recording benefits.

Legal Aspects

Adherence to local laws and regulations is crucial. In most cases, consent from all parties is needed, with exceptions for emergencies or suspected abuse. Recorded data must be securely stored and disposed of according to established protocols, which are likely to be evolving with time.

Practical Factors

The expense and logistics of implementing recording systems should be considered. Proper staff training ensures compliance with laws and regulations. Patients should be informed of potential recording through prominent notices, signage, education, or verbal consent.

Benefits of Recording

Recording can enhance patient safety by providing evidence for investigations, improvement areas, and legal disputes. At the same time, existence of a record of what happened could help a medical practitioner to prove not being negligent. Such recording aids in assessing care quality and communication skills and identifies areas for improvement. Recording is valuable for training healthcare providers in communication and patient safety.

Thus, the decision to record communication in the medical and medicolegal context should be made on a case-by-case basis, considering ethical, legal, and practical factors while balancing benefits with potential risks to patient privacy and well-being. Such recordings could help as defenses in medical negligence cases, and aid investigations of patient neglect, and abuse monitoring in healthcare setups.

COUNSELING

Counseling is the process of providing support and guidance to patients, and their families. In addition, in the realm of communication, it also involves providing support and guidance to healthcare professionals on how to communicate effectively in the medical and legal contexts.

Various Aspects of Counseling

Counseling could include the following topics:
- Understanding a disease, its impact on the future and its management.
- Counseling on informed consent helps patients to understand the risks and benefits of treatment options and to make informed decisions about their care.
- Counseling on medical communication skills can help patients to communicate their medical history and concerns effectively to their healthcare providers, and to ask questions and understand the information they receive.

Counseling on medicolegal communication can help patients to understand their legal rights and responsibilities, and to communicate effectively with healthcare providers and legal professionals in the event of a medicolegal dispute.

Professional Providing Counseling

Counseling can be provided by a variety of professionals. Healthcare professionals, such as physicians, nurses, and social workers, can provide counseling on medical condition to their patients. Mental health professionals, such as psychologists and counselors, can provide counseling to patients who are struggling to cope with the emotional challenges of illness or injury. Legal professionals, such as healthcare lawyers and patient advocates, can provide counseling on medicolegal situations to patients and their families.

For example, a counselor may counsel a patient on how to communicate their medical history and concerns to their healthcare provider in a clear and concise manner; a social worker may counsel a patient's family on how to support their loved one through a difficult medical diagnosis or treatment; a healthcare lawyer may counsel a patient on their legal rights and responsibilities in the event of a potential or actual medicolegal litigation.

In essence, counseling in medical and medicolegal communication can play an important role in improving patient outcomes and reducing medicolegal risks. By providing support and guidance on how to communicate effectively, counselors can help patients and their families to navigate the complex medical and legal system and to make informed decisions about their care.

PRACTICAL ASPECTS

Communication failures are associated with the medicolegal litigations. Disregarding or failing to recognize patient preferences puts medical practitioners at a higher risk of such litigation.[28]

Poor patient communication and lack of information are the leading causes of patient dissatisfaction and medicolegal claims.[29]

A few general observations about inadequate communication in medicolegal context in India are mentioned below.

- *Communication barriers:* There are a number of communication barriers that can exist between healthcare professionals and their patients in India, including language barriers, cultural differences, and educational disparities.
- *Lack of awareness:* Patients in India often lack awareness of their rights and responsibilities in the healthcare setting. This can make it difficult for them to communicate effectively with their healthcare providers and to make informed decisions about their treatment.
- *Fear of litigation:* Healthcare professionals in India are often hesitant to communicate openly with their patients about the risks and benefits of treatment, for fear of being sued. This can lead to patients being uninformed about their treatment options and, in some cases, to medical errors.

Healthcare professionals should strive to communicate effectively with their patients and their families at all stages of the treatment process. This will help to build trust, prevent misunderstandings, and reduce the risk of medical malpractice claims.

DOCTOR-PATIENT RELATIONSHIP

Effective communication holds a pivotal position within the doctor-patient relationship, as it enhances patient satisfaction, fosters compliance, and improves medical outcomes. Furthermore, proficient communication serves to lower healthcare expenses, thereby contributing to an overall elevation in the quality of healthcare.[30,31] All these have potential impact on reducing medicolegal litigations.

An "ideal" doctor is said to be the one who has capability for interpersonal relationships, excellence in knowledge, technical abilities, and benevolent intentions.[32] These qualities could be expressed with effective communication skills. While older patients are tolerant with medical "paternalism", younger patients tend to highlight doctors' skills in communication and in sharing decision-making.[33] Communication skill has been known to be an important characteristic of a "good" doctor.[34] Patients have specific expectations with regard to medical communication.[35]

Thus, having good communication skills is important in getting the patient's confidence and collaboration in disease management, which reflects in compliance to treatment and outcome, overall resulting in job satisfaction for the medical practitioner.[36-40]

Significance of effective communication skills is further emphasized due to the universal access to information through internet about health issues, which is disrupting the traditional doctor-patient relationship in fundamental ways.[41]

To facilitate better doctor-patient relationship, expanded training and assessment of physicians' communication skills has been suggested.[42]

For establishing medical negligence claims, the litigant needs to prove that a duty of care was there by the doctor to the patient. Such a duty is present when there is a doctor-patient relationship, which gets established when the patient seeks medical consultation by the medical practitioner, and the latter accepts it. However, when there is danger to the life of a person, even if there has been no doctor-patient relationship, the Supreme Court of India imposed a duty upon the doctor when it held, in *Parmanand Kataria versus Union of India*, "Every doctor, at the governmental hospital or elsewhere, has a professional obligation to extend his services with due expertise for protecting life".[43]

CONFIDENTIALITY ISSUES

Regulation 2.2 of the Indian Medical Council (Professional Conduct, Etiquette and Ethics) Regulations, 2002 compels the Registered Medical Practitioners (RMPs) to safeguard the patients' confidentiality.

As per Guideline 3.7.1.2 of Telemedicine Practice Guidelines, an RMP would be required to fully abide by Indian Medical Council (Professional conduct, Etiquette and Ethics) Regulations, 2002 and with the relevant provisions of the Information Technology Act, Data protection and privacy laws or any applicable rules notified from time to time for protecting patient privacy and confidentiality and regarding the handling and transfer of such personal information regarding the patient.

Further, it is the responsibility of the RMP to be cognizant of the current Data Protection and Privacy laws.

INFORMATION TECHNOLOGY ACT, 2000 AND MEDICAL COMMUNICATION

The following sections of the Information Technology Act, 2000 provide for privacy and punishment for privacy breach.

- *Section 43A:* This section prohibits the disclosure of personal information by any person who is in possession of such information, without the consent of the individual to whom the information relates.
- *Section 66C:* This section punishes any person who knowingly or intentionally intercepts, monitors or decrypts any electronic communication transmitted to or from a computer resource without the consent or knowledge of the sender or receiver of the communication.
- *Section 72A:* This section provides for punishment for the disclosure of information in breach of confidentiality.

The Information Technology Act is related to medical and medicolegal communication in the sense that it applies to all electronic communication, including communication that takes place in the medical setting. Thus, the provisions of the Act on privacy and punishment for privacy breach apply to healthcare providers, patients, and other stakeholders who are involved in medical communication.

For example, a healthcare provider in possession of a patient's electronic medical information who discloses the information without the patient's consent may be liable for violating Section 43A of the Act. A person who intercepts or monitors a patient's electronic communication without the patient's consent may be liable for violating Section 66C of the Act. And a person who discloses information in breach of confidentiality, such as a hospital employee who discloses patient information to the media, may be liable for violating Section 72A of the Act.

Patients can report healthcare providers who share their medical data without consent. Healthcare providers may be liable if they experience data breaches due to carelessness resulting in stolen patient records. However, according to the Guideline 3.7.1.3 of Telemedicine Practice Guidelines, a RMP will not be held responsible for breach of confidentiality if there is a reasonable evidence to believe that patient's privacy and confidentiality has been compromised by a technology breach or by a person other than RMP. The RMPs should ensure that reasonable degree of care is undertaken during hiring such services.

The Information Technology Act is vital in safeguarding medical data privacy and deterring breaches. Government enforcement of its provisions helps ensure that patient information remains confidential.

SUMMARY

Effective communication is important, as in any area of human interactions, for getting optimal outcomes in medical settings, too. Further, it has an impact on various aspects of patient-provider relationship including patient-satisfaction and reducing risk of medicolegal litigations. Knowing the basics of communication, and how various barriers for communication could affect the effectiveness of communication, enables formulate, and implement various strategies for effective communication.

LEARNING KEY POINTS

- Effective communication is crucial in reducing the risk of medicolegal litigations.
- For a medical practitioner, proper medical documentation, including the documentation of communication, would be a good defense against many medicolegal litigations.

TAKE-HOME MESSAGES/MUST AVOID THINGS/DO NOT DO/ WARNINGS/MESSAGES WHICH THE READER MUST BE AWARE

- Do not neglect in being trained in and committed to effective communication strategies.
- After any potential or actual medicolegal litigation situation arises, while a relevant and reasonable "late entry" (as described in dos of medical documentation section) might be legally acceptable, the medical practitioner should refrain from destroying or unduly modifying the documentary evidence.

MUST DO THING/MEDICAL NEGLIGENCE PEARLS/ONLY ONE FACT TO REMEMBER

- Empathetic and supportive communication and proper medical documentation are crucial in reducing risks of medicolegal litigations, and therefore a medical practitioners should practice them.

MCQs

Choose one correct answer
1. Feedback in a medical communication process involves:
   a. The patient expressing what he understood of what the doctor said
   b. The doctor expressing what he understood of what the patient said
   c. Both of the above
   d. None of the above
2. In today's age of telemedicine, the issue of privacy and confidentiality:
   a. Has been very well safeguarded with robust software
   b. Could act as a barrier for effective communication
   c. Is not really a problem, as otherwise also almost everyone's data is available with Google and other online service providers
   d. Both a and c are correct

Answers

1. c   2. b

REFERENCES

1. Barbosa Ide A, Silva KC, Silva VA, Silva MJ. The communication process in Telenursing: integrative review. Rev Bras Enferm. 2016; 69(4):765-72.
2. Hegan T. The importance of effective communication in preventing litigation. Med J Malaysia. 2003;58 Suppl A:78-82.
3. Singh M. Communication as a Bridge to Build a Sound Doctor-Patient/Parent Relationship. Indian J Pediatr. 2016;83(1):33-7.
4. Pitt MB, Hendrickson MA. Eradicating Jargon-Oblivion: a proposed classification system of medical jargon. J Gen Intern Med. 2020;35(6):1861-4.
5. Rosenberg K. Medical jargon may lead to confusion among patients. Am J Nurs. 2023; 123(3):61.
6. Rau NM, Basir MA, Flynn KE. Parental understanding of crucial medical jargon used in prenatal prematurity counseling. BMC Med Inform Decis Mak. 2020;20(1): 169.
7. Allen KA, Charpentier V, Hendrickson MA, Kessler M, Gotlieb R, Marmet J, et al. Jargon be gone—patient preference in doctor communication. J Patient Exp. 2023; 10:23743735231158942.
8. LibreTexts. Basic Process Models of Communication. [online] Available from: https://socialsci.libretexts.org/Bookshelves/Communication/Introduction_to_Communication/Communicating_to_Connect_-_Interpersonal_Communication_for_Today_(Usera)/01%3A_Fundamentals_of_Interpersonal_Communication/1.02%3A_Basic_Process_Models_of_Communication#:~:text=In%201949%20mathematician%20Claude%20Shannon,Shannon%20%26%20Weaver%2C%201949. [Last accessed December, 2023].
9. Perera HJM. Effective communication skills for medical practice. J Postgrad Inst Med. 2015;2(E20):1-7.
10. Dungu KHS, Kruse A, Svane SM, Dybdal DTH, Poulsen MW, Juul AW, et al. Language barriers and use of interpreters in two Danish paediatric emergency units. Dan Med J. 2019;66(8):A5558.
11. Betancourt JR, Green AR, Carrillo JE, Ananeh-Firempong O. Defining cultural competence: a practical framework for addressing racial/ethnic disparities in health and health care. Public Health Rep. 2003;118(4): 293-302.
12. Reiff M, Zakut H, Weingarten MA. Illness and treatment perceptions of Ethiopian immigrants and their doctors in Israel. Am J Public Health. 1999;89(12):1814-8.
13. Laronne A, Granek L, Wiener L, Feder-Bubis P, Golan H. "Some things are even worse than telling a child he is going to die": Pediatric oncology healthcare professionals perspectives on communicating with

children about cancer and end of life. Pediatr Blood Cancer. 2022;69(3):e29533.
14. Hwang SJ, Tan NC, Yoon S, Ramakrishnan C, Paulpandi M, Gun S, et al. Perceived barriers and facilitators to chronic kidney disease care among patients in Singapore: a qualitative study. BMJ Open. 2020;10(10):e041788.
15. Adelsjö I, Nilsson L, Hellström A, Ekstedt M, Lehnbom EC. Communication about medication management during patient-physician consultations in primary care: a participant observation study. BMJ Open. 2022;12(11):e062148.
16. Gibbs A, Gumede D, Luthuli M, Xulu Z, Washington L, Sikweyiya Y, et al. Opportunities for technologically driven dialogical health communication for participatory interventions: Perspectives from male peer navigators in rural South Africa. Soc Sci Med. 2022;292:114539.
17. Sekandi JN, Kasiita V, Onuoha NA, Zalwango S, Nakkonde D, Kaawa-Mafigiri D, et al. Stakeholders' perceptions of benefits of and barriers to using video-observed treatment for monitoring patients with tuberculosis in Uganda: exploratory qualitative study. JMIR Mhealth Uhealth. 2021;9(10):e27131.
18. Cochran GL, Lander L, Morien M, Lomelin DE, Brittin J, Reker C, Klepser DG. Consumer opinions of health information exchange, e-Prescribing, and personal health records. Perspect Health Inf Manag. 2015;12(Fall):1e. eCollection 2015.
19. Ong ZH, Tan LHE, Ghazali HZB, Ong YT, Koh JWH, Ang RZE, et al. A systematic scoping review on pedagogical strategies of interprofessional communication for physicians in emergency medicine. J Med Educ Curric Dev. 2021;8:23821205211041794.
20. Homeyer S, Hoffmann W, Hingst P, Oppermann RF, Dreier-Wolfgramm A. Effects of interprofessional education for medical and nursing students: enablers, barriers and expectations for optimizing future interprofessional collaboration—a qualitative study. BMC Nurs. 2018;17:13.
21. Hafner C, Schneider J, Schindler M, Braillard O. Visual aids in ambulatory clinical practice: experiences, perceptions and needs of patients and healthcare professionals. PLoS One. 2022;17(2):e0263041.
22. Glen P, Earl N, Gooding F, Lucas E, Sangha N, Ramcharitar S. Simple interventions can greatly improve clinical documentation: a quality improvement project of record keeping on the surgical wards at a district general hospital. BMJ Qual Improv Rep. 2015; 4(1):u208191.w3260.
23. World Health Organization. Framework for Action on Interprofessional Education and Collaborative Practice. Geneva: World Health Organization; 2010.
24. Samira Kohli versus Dr. Prabha Manchanda & ANR 1 (2008) CPJ 56 (SC).
25. Weaver JC. (2004). Appropriate Documentation: Your First (and Best) Defense. [online] Available from: https://www.reliasmedia.com/articles/7990-appropriate-documentation-your-first-and-best-defense. [Last accessed December, 2023].
26. Thomas J. Medical records and issues in negligence. Indian J Urol. 2009;25(3):384-8.
27. The Times of India. (2018). UP court fines doctors Rs 5,000 for poor handwriting. [online] Available from https://timesofindia.indiatimes.com/city/lucknow/court-fines-doctors-rs-5000-for-poor-handwriting/articleshow/66061795.cms. [Last Accessed December, 2023].
28. Joga Rao SV. Medical negligence liability under the consumer protection act: a review of judicial perspective. Indian J Urol. 2009;25:361-71.
29. Durand MA, Moulton B, Cockle E, Mann M, Elwyn G. Can shared decision-making reduce medical malpractice litigation. A systematic review? BMC Health Serv Res. 2015;15:167.
30. Stewart M. Effective physician-patient communication and health outcomes: a review. Can Med Assoc J. 1995;152:1423-33.
31. Kaplan RM. Shared medical decision making: a new tool for preventive medicine. Am J Prev Med. 2004;26:81-3.
32. Coulter A. Patients' views of the good doctor. BMJ. 2002;325:668-9.

33. Jung HP, Baerveldt C, Olesen F, Grol R, Wensing M. Patient characteristics as predictors of primary health care preferences: a systematic literature analysis. Health Expect. 2003;6:160-81.
34. Borracci RA, Álvarez Gallesio JM, Ciambrone G, Matayoshi C, Rossi F, Cabrera S. What patients consider to be a 'good' doctor, and what doctors consider to be a 'good' patient. Rev Med Chil. 2020;148(7):930-8.
35. Deledda G, Moretti F, Rimondini M, Zimmermann C. How patients want their doctor to communicate. A literature review on primary care patients' perspective. Patient Educ Couns. 2013;90:297-306.
36. Ong LM, de Haes JC, Hoos AM, Lammes FB. Doctor-patient communication: a review of the literature. Soc Sci Med. 1995; 40(7):903-918.
37. Stewart M, Brown JB, Donner A, McWhinney IR, Oates J, Weston WW, et al. The impact of patient-centered care on outcomes. J Fam Pract. 2000;49(9):796-804.
38. Jahng KH, Martin LR, Golin CE, DiMatteo MR. Preferences for medical collaboration: patient-physician congruence and patient outcomes. Patient Educ Couns. 2005;57(3): 308-14.
39. Härter M, van der Weijden T, Elwyn G. Policy and practice developments in the implementation of shared decision making: an international perspective. Z Evid Fortbild Qual Gesundhwes. 2011;105:229-33.
40. Härter M, Moumjid N, Cornuz J, Elwyn G, van der Weijden T. Shared decision making in 2017: International accomplishments in policy, research and implementation. Z Evid Fortbild Qual Gesundhwes. 2017;123-124:1-5.
41. Freckelton IR. Internet disruptions in the doctor-patient relationship. Med Law Rev. 2020;28(3):502-25.
42. Gallagher TH, Levinson W. A prescription for protecting the doctor-patient relationship. Am J Manag Care. 2004;10(2 Pt 1):61-8.
43. Parmanand Kataria versus Union of India. AIR 1989 SC 2039.

SUGGESTED READING

1. Baldwa M, Baldwa V, Padvi N, Baldwa S. Legal Issues in Critical Care, 1st edition. New Delhi: CBS Publishers and Distributors Pvt. Ltd.; 2022.
2. Baldwa M, Baldwa V, Padvi N, Baldwa S. Legal Issues in Medical Practice, 2nd edition. New Delhi: CBS Publishers and Distributors Pvt. Ltd.; 2023.

CHAPTER 3

Medical Documentation: The Only Defense for Doctors

Dnyanesh DK, Suma Dnyanesh

Court always says—"If it is not documented, then it did not happen"!

Keywords: Documentation, EHR systems, Expert testimony

Aim: Doctors must be ready to produce written documents which should be their ultimate defense for medical negligence is documentation in court of law.

Objective: Doctors are best givers of medical care but are lazy to document that care on paper. This is to wake up entire medical fraternity to shed lethargy and start documenting whatever good care they give to their patient's.

INTRODUCTION

Medical documentation is an essential component of modern healthcare practice. Beyond its role in patient care, medical documentation holds immense medicolegal significance. A medical document is a document containing the chronological account of patient's examination and treatment.[1] Medical documentation is the lifeblood of the healthcare industry, serving as both a record of patient care and a crucial defense for doctors. Medical evidence comprises a good proportion of civil and criminal law suits brought to trial in legal proceedings. Therefore the documents which are properly stored can become protective armors for doctors against the fiery darts of litigation in a court of law. This chapter explores the multifaceted world of medical documentation, delving into its importance in legal matters and healthcare systems.

THE ESSENCE OF MEDICAL DOCUMENTATION

Medical documentation is comprehensive repositories of patient information, encompassing a diverse range of data such as patient histories, diagnoses, treatment plans, test results, medication logs, surgical notes, and informed consent records.[2] They serve several pivotal functions:

- *Patient care continuity:* Medical documentation ensure the continuity of patient care. They provide a historical account of a patient's health, helping healthcare providers make informed decisions.
- *Adherence to standards:* Medical documentation reflect adherence to established medical standards and guidelines. They serve as a benchmark for evaluating the quality of healthcare provided.
- *Informed consent:* Proper documentation of informed consent is pivotal in

protecting both patient's rights and healthcare providers' interests.
- *Communication tool:* Medical documentation facilitate effective communication among healthcare professionals, reducing the risk of misunderstandings and errors.

MEDICOLEGAL IMPORTANCE OF MEDICAL DOCUMENTATION

Medical documentation plays a central role in medicolegal matters, encompassing areas such as:
- *Evidence in legal proceedings:* In legal disputes, medical documents serve as primary sources of evidence. They provide a detailed account of patient care and can significantly influence court decisions.
- *Standard of care:* Adherence to the standard of care is a crucial element in medical malpractice cases. Properly maintained documents can establish whether healthcare providers followed established protocols.
- *Informed consent documentation:* The absence of well-documented informed consent can expose healthcare providers to legal liabilities. Medical documents are instrumental in substantiating the consent process.
- *Chronology of events:* Medical documentation create a chronological timeline of a patient's medical journey. This timeline is essential for determining the sequence of events and assessing whether negligence occurred.

THE LEGAL IMPORTANCE OF MEDICAL DOCUMENTATION: A GLOBAL PERSPECTIVE

The medicolegal importance of medical documentation extends worldwide, with numerous legal systems recognizing its significance. Some prominent examples include:
- *United States:* In the United States, medical documents are governed by the Health Insurance Portability and Accountability Act (HIPAA). HIPAA not only regulates the confidentiality and security of medical documents but also emphasizes their legal importance in medical disputes. Courts often rely on medical documents to establish standards of care and evaluate the merits of medical negligence claims.
- *United Kingdom:* In the United Kingdom, the General Medical Council (GMC) issues guidance on documentation for healthcare professionals. Failure to maintain accurate and comprehensive documents can result in disciplinary action. In legal cases, medical documents are pivotal in establishing whether healthcare providers met their professional obligations.
- *Australia:* Australia's healthcare system emphasizes the importance of proper medical documentation. In legal proceedings, medical documents serve as primary evidence, shaping the outcomes of medical negligence claims. The Australian Medical Association (AMA) provides guidelines for maintaining quality medical documents.
- *Canada:* Canada recognizes the legal importance of medical documentation, and healthcare providers are expected to maintain accurate and complete documents. In medical malpractice cases, courts rely on these documents to assess the standard of care and determine liability.

CASE LAWS DEMONSTRATING THE MEDICOLEGAL IMPORTANCE OF MEDICAL DOCUMENTATION

White versus Brown (1981)—United States

In this landmark case, the court emphasized the crucial role of medical documents in medical malpractice claims. The plaintiff alleged negligence in the administration of anesthesia. The court relied heavily on medical documents to assess the standard of care and determine whether negligence had occurred.

Bolam versus Friern Hospital Management Committee[3] (1957)—United Kingdom

The Bolam test, established in this case, is widely used to assess whether a healthcare provider has met the standard of care. Properly maintained medical documents that reflect adherence to established medical practices can support a healthcare provider's defense in cases where the Bolam test is applied.

Rogers versus Whitaker (1992)—Australia[4]

This Australian case highlighted the importance of informed consent documentation. The court ruled in favor of the plaintiff, emphasizing that healthcare providers must provide comprehensive information to patient's and document the informed consent process adequately.

Snell versus Farrell[5] (1990)—Canada

In this Canadian case, medical documents played a pivotal role in assessing the standard of care. The court used the documents to determine whether the healthcare provider had followed established protocols, ultimately influencing the legal outcome.

Legal Importance of Medical Documentation—Indian Perspective

In the Indian healthcare landscape, comprehensive and accurate medical documentation serves as the primary line of defense for doctors facing allegations of malpractice and negligence.

CASE LAWS DEMONSTRATING THE ROLE OF DOCUMENTATION IN DEFENSE FOR DOCTORS IN INDIA

Jacob Mathew versus State of Punjab[6] (2005)

In this landmark case, the Supreme Court of India underscored the pivotal role of comprehensive medical documents. The court held that well-maintained documents provide essential insights into the treatment process and can protect healthcare providers from unfounded allegations of negligence. The case set a precedent for the importance of medical documentation in establishing the standard of care.

Samira Kohli versus Dr Prabha Manchanda[7] (2008)

This case reaffirmed the significance of informed consent documentation. The Supreme Court emphasized that consent must be properly documented. Failure to do so can expose healthcare providers to legal liabilities, even if the treatment was medically sound. This decision reinforced the importance of meticulous documentation of patient consent.

Martin F D'Souza versus Mohd. Ishfaq[8] (2009)

The court in this case stressed the importance of clear communication among healthcare professionals, which can be achieved through proper documentation. Effective communication can prevent misunderstandings and reduce the risk of medical malpractice claims. This case illustrates how proper documentation can foster a collaborative healthcare environment.

Malay Kumar Ganguly versus Sukumar Mukherjee[9] (2009)

This case underlines how medical documentation can serve as crucial evidence in court. The court heavily relied on medical records to determine whether negligence had occurred. The meticulously maintained records played a decisive role in shaping the legal outcome, showcasing the power of comprehensive documentation.

Maharaja Agrasen Hospital versus Rishabh Sharma[10] (2020)

Brief facts: Complainant, Pooja Sharma, mother of Master Rishabh Sharma, preterm child admitted in Maharaja Agrasen Hospital for preterm care nearly for 5 weeks. Doctors did not carry out retinopathy of prematurity (ROP) screening much later mother noticed baby's abnormal visual response. Eye checkup then showed total retinal detachment. Parents approached National Consumer Disputes Redressal Commission (NCDRC) for medical negligence. The hospital and its doctors denied allegation of negligence, claimed ROP screening was carried out and it had not revealed any problems. The NCDRC appointed expert medical board from AIIMS. Report said no negligence. The NCDRC in its order said that "we are not convinced whether the ROP screening was done by the ophthalmologist. The progress sheet is devoid of details about ROP examination, viz., who performed it, the method, instruments used, and drugs used during ROP testing. The discharge summary also has not mentioned ROP advice. Thus, "no record means, it was not done". Both the parties aggrieved by the NCDRC judgment, appealed to honorable Supreme Court. Honorable Supreme Court upheld the order of National Commission and awarded INR 76 lakh compensation.

CHALLENGES IN MEDICAL DOCUMENTATION

While medical documentation is undeniably crucial, several challenges persist:
- *Time constraints:* Healthcare providers often face time constraints, making it challenging to maintain meticulous records.
- *Electronic health records (EHRs):* While EHRs offer convenience, they come with their own set of challenges, including data security concerns and potential inaccuracies.
- *Interoperability:* Ensuring seamless sharing of electronic records across healthcare institutions remains a challenge, potentially hindering patient care continuity.
- *Legibility and completeness:* Illegible or incomplete entries in medical records can undermine their legal value.

ERRORS IN MEDICAL DOCUMENTATION

Errors in medical documentation can have consequences for patient care and safety.

Some common types of errors in medical documentation include:
- *Incomplete records:* Missing or incomplete information can lead to misdiagnosis or inappropriate treatment. This may include omitting essential patient history, medications, or test results.
- *Illegible handwriting:* Poor handwriting can result in misinterpretation of notes and medication errors. Many healthcare facilities have transitioned to EHRs to address this issue.
- *Incorrect information:* Entering incorrect information, such as patient demographics, can lead to confusion and potential harm. Verifying patient identity is crucial.
- *Abbreviation errors:* Using abbreviations without proper context can be confusing and lead to medication errors. There are standardized lists of medical abbreviations to reduce this risk.
- *Lack of date and time:* Failing to timestamp entries can make it challenging to track the timeline of a patient's condition and treatment.
- *Failure to document changes:* Failing to document changes in a patient's condition or treatment plan can result in miscommunication among healthcare providers.
- *Copy-paste errors:* Reusing text from previous notes without updating or verifying its accuracy can lead to misinformation.
- *Disorganization:* Poorly organized documentation can make it difficult for healthcare providers to find essential information quickly.
- *Privacy violations:* Unauthorized access to or disclosure of patient information violates privacy regulations and can lead to legal and ethical issues.

WHEN MEDICAL DOCUMENTATION IS VIABLE IN COURT OF LAW AND WHEN IT IS INVALID?

Medical documentation can be critical evidence in a court of law, especially in medical malpractice cases, personal injury claims, and other legal disputes involving healthcare. Whether medical documentation is considered viable or invalid in court depends on several factors:
- *Legibility and accuracy:* Viable medical documentation must be legible and accurate. Illegible or erroneous records can be challenged and may be considered invalid.
- *Timeliness:* Timely documentation is crucial. Courts may question the credibility of medical records if there are unexplained delays in recording information.
- *Authentication:* Medical records should be properly authenticated to ensure their validity. This often involves the signature of the healthcare provider or an authorized staff member.
- *Chain of custody:* In cases involving laboratory test results or medical imaging, maintaining a secure chain of custody is essential to ensure the integrity of the evidence.
- *Compliance with standards:* The documentation should adhere to established standards and protocols. Deviations from these standards may raise doubts about the validity of the records.
- *Documentation of informed consent:* In situations where medical procedures or treatments were performed, documentation of informed consent is vital. Patient's should be adequately informed about the risks and benefits before giving consent.

- *Hearsay:* Courts generally do not accept hearsay evidence, which includes second-hand accounts or statements. Medical documentation should primarily contain firsthand observations and assessments.
- *Patient privacy:* Healthcare providers must comply with patient privacy laws. Unauthorized disclosure of patient information can render documentation invalid.
- *Retrospective alterations:* Any alterations or additions to medical records should be properly documented, dated, and explained. Retrospective changes without clear justification can damage the credibility of the documentation.
- *Documentation by qualified personnel:* Medical records should be generated by qualified healthcare professionals or authorized personnel. Notes from unqualified individuals may not hold up in court.
- *Expert testimony:* In many cases, expert witnesses, such as medical professionals, are called upon to interpret and testify about the validity and significance of medical records.
- *Preservation of records:* Medical records should be preserved according to legal requirements and institutional policies to prevent loss or tampering.

In summary, viable medical documentation in a court of law is typically:
- Legible, accurate, and timely
- Properly authenticated and compliant with standards
- Generated by qualified personnel
- Free from unauthorized alterations or additions
- Protected patient privacy
- Supported by expert testimony when necessary.

Invalid medical documentation often involves issues with legibility, accuracy, authenticity, or compliance with legal and ethical standards. It is important for healthcare providers and institutions to maintain meticulous and legally compliant medical records to ensure their credibility and usefulness in legal proceedings.

DOCUMENTATION DURING MEDICAL EMERGENCY[11]

It should be done as comprehensively and accurately as possible, considering the urgency of the situation. Here is a general guideline on how and when to document a medical emergency:
- *Patient safety first:* In any medical emergency, the immediate priority is patient safety and providing necessary medical care. Ensure the patient receives appropriate and timely interventions without unnecessary delays.
- *Initial assessment:* Begin documenting as soon as possible after ensuring the patient's initial stabilization. This might involve assessing vital signs, starting treatment, or performing lifesaving interventions.
- *Continual updates:* Continuously document changes in the patient's condition, interventions performed, medications administered, and the response to treatments. Document with time stamps to create a chronological record.
- *Conciseness and clarity:* In emergency situations, brevity and clarity are essential. Use concise language to describe observations, interventions, and responses. Avoid unnecessary details that do not directly impact patient care.
- *Standardized forms or electronic records:* Use standardized forms or her,

if available. These systems often have predefined templates for emergencies, making documentation more structured and efficient.
- *Timestamps:* Always include timestamps for entries to establish a clear timeline of events. This is crucial for assessing the patient's progress.
- *Patient information:* Clearly document the patient's name, date of birth, and other identifying information. This ensures accurate identification.
- *Chief complaint:* Note the patient's chief complaint or reason for seeking emergency care.
- *Allergies and medications:* Document any known allergies and the patient's current medications. This information is vital to prevent allergic reactions and drug interactions.
- *Vital signs:* Record vital signs, such as heart rate, blood pressure, respiratory rate, temperature, and oxygen saturation, at regular intervals.
- *Interventions:* Document all interventions performed, including procedures, medications administered, and the rationale behind these actions.
- *Response to treatment:* Describe how the patient responds to interventions and any changes in their condition. This information guides ongoing care decisions.
- *Patient statements:* If the patient is conscious and able to communicate, document any statements or information provided by the patient. This may include allergies, medical history, or details about the onset of symptoms.
- *Witness information:* If there are witnesses or bystanders who provided assistance, document their names and contact information in case further information is needed.
- *Legal and ethical considerations:* Be mindful of legal and ethical considerations, such as patient confidentiality and informed consent. Ensure that your documentation complies with relevant laws and regulations.
- *Handoff communication:* When transferring care to another healthcare provider or facility, provide a clear and concise handoff report that summarizes the patient's condition and ongoing treatment plans.
- *Review and corrections:* After the emergency, review your documentation for accuracy and completeness. Correct any errors or omissions promptly.

In an emergency, the focus should always be on providing immediate care to the patient. However, maintaining good documentation practices throughout the process is essential for continuity of care, legal protection, and quality improvement efforts. Documenting critical information during or shortly after the emergency ensures that vital details are not lost.

Healthcare providers should prioritize documenting the most critical information while ensuring that the documentation process does not impede the delivery of lifesaving interventions.

MEDICAL DOCUMENTATION OF TELEPHONIC CONSULTATION AND TELE-CONSULTATION

Medical documentation of telephonic consultations and teleconsultations is essential for maintaining accurate and comprehensive patient records, ensuring continuity of care, and complying with legal and ethical requirements.

Remember that teleconsultations should be conducted with the same level of professionalism, confidentiality, and documentation diligence as in-person consultations. Thorough and accurate documentation is essential not only for patient care but also for legal and regulatory compliance when providing healthcare services through telemedicine.

BEST PRACTICES IN MEDICAL DOCUMENTATION FOR LEGAL DEFENSE

To overcome these challenges and maximize the role of medical documentation as a defense for doctors, healthcare institutions, and professionals can adopt best practices.
- *Training and education:* Providing training to healthcare professionals on proper documentation practices is essential.
- *Standardized templates:* Implementing standardized templates for documentation can ensure consistency and completeness.
- *EHR integration:* Ensuring that EHR systems are integrated seamlessly and securely can enhance the efficiency of documentation.
- *Quality assurance:* Conducting regular audits of medical records for legibility, completeness, and accuracy can help maintain high standards.
- *Legal review:* Involving legal experts to review and guide documentation practices can be beneficial.

SUMMARY

Medical record keeping is not a mere administrative task; it is a cornerstone of modern healthcare and a linchpin in medicolegal matters. As illustrated by case laws from various jurisdictions, comprehensive and accurate medical records provide critical evidence of patient care, adherence to standards, informed consent, and effective communication. In a healthcare landscape where legal claims are on the rise, healthcare institutions and professionals must recognize the paramount importance of meticulous documentation to safeguard their professional integrity and interests.

By embracing best practices and recognizing the legal significance of documentation, healthcare providers can ensure the highest standards of patient care while protecting themselves from unwarranted legal disputes. As technology continues to evolve, the digital transformation of medical documentation presents opportunities to enhance efficiency, security, and accessibility, further solidifying its role in both patient care and the legal arena.

LEARNING KEY POINTS

- *Legal safeguard:* Medical documentation serves as a crucial legal defense, providing a documented account of patient care that can protect doctors in case of legal disputes or malpractice claims.
- *Evidence of due diligence:* Comprehensive records demonstrate a doctor's commitment to thorough and diligent patient care, showcasing adherence to professional standards and guidelines.
- *Communication clarification:* Clear and accurate documentation enhances communication among healthcare professionals, reducing the risk of misunderstandings and ensuring a collaborative approach to patient treatment.
- *Risk mitigation:* Well-documented medical records serve as a proactive measure in risk management, minimizing the potential for errors, oversights, or misinterpretations in patient care.
- *Informed decision-making:* Thorough documentation provides a basis for informed

decision-making, offering a comprehensive overview of a patient's medical history, treatments, and responses, aiding both current and future healthcare providers.

TAKE-HOME MESSAGE

"Good documentation means a good defense, poor documentation means poor defense, and no documentation means no defense".

MUST AVOID THINGS

Reusing text from previous notes without updating or verifying its accuracy can lead to misinformation.

DO NOT DO

Do not fail to document any known allergies.

WARNINGS

Medical records should be preserved according to legal requirements and institutional policies to prevent loss or tampering.

MUST DO THINGS

Medical documentation is must even during emergency.

ONLY ONE FACT TO REMEMBER

Medical documentation is only defense available for doctors in case of medical negligence.

REFERENCES

1. Biswas G. Legal and ethical issues of medical records. In: Biswas G (Ed). Recent Advances in Forensic Medicine and Toxicology, 1st edition. New Delhi: Jaypee Brothers Medical Publishers (P) Ltd.;2015. pp. 140-59.
2. Indian Medical Council (Professional conduct, Etiquette and Ethics) Regulations, 2002.
3. Bolam versus Friern hospital management committee (1957) 1 WLR 582.
4. Rogers versus Whitaker (1992)175 CLR 479.
5. Snell versus Farrell (1990) 2 SCR 311.
6. Jacob Mathew versus State of Punjab (2005) 6 SCC 1.
7. Samira Kohli versus Dr Prabha Manchanda 2008 (1) CPR 237.
8. Martin F D'Souza versus Mohd. Ishfaq 2009 (1) CPJ 32.
9. Malay Kumar Ganguly versus Sukumar Mukherjee, AIR 2010 SC 1162.
10. Maharaja Agrasen Sharma Hospital versus Rishabh Sharma, (2020) 6 SCC 501.
11. Thomas J, Medical records and Issues in Negligence, Indian J urology, 2009;25:384-8.

SUGGESTED READING

1. Baldwa M, Baldwa V, Padvi N, Baldwa S. Legal Issues in Critical Care, 1st edition. New Delhi: CBS Publishers and Distributors Pvt. Ltd.; 2022.
2. Baldwa M, Baldwa V, Padvi N, Baldwa S. Legal Issues in Medical Practice, 2nd edition. New Delhi: CBS Publishers and Distributors Pvt. Ltd.; 2023.

CHAPTER 4

Record Keeping, Making Easy

Jyoti Kumar Gupta, VK Goyal, Anita Sharma, Marrisha Gupta

The current medical records system is this: Room after room after room in a hospital filled with paper files which are retrievable with difficulty.

Keywords: Confidentiality, Documentation, Evidentiary value, Medical record, Retention period

Aim: The primary purpose of the medical record is to facilitate patient care.

Objective: To allow yourself and or another practitioner to continue the management of the patient. Clinical observations, decision making, and treatment recommendations or plans should be recorded contemporaneously.

INTRODUCTION

Medical record is an important compilation of facts about a patient's life and health. It includes documented data on past and present illnesses, and treatment written by the healthcare professionals caring for the patient. As a written collection of information about a patient's health care, they are used in the management and planning of healthcare facilities and services, for medical research and the production of healthcare statistics. Moreover, it will also be of immense help in the scientific evaluation and review of patient management issues. This will be the only way for the doctor to prove that the treatment was carried out properly. In the era of increasing medicolegal litigations, record keeping has been one of the most important obligations on any medical professional. If one has no medical record, it simply means that he is barehanded in facing medicolegal litigation. Brad Cohn has rightly said "Nothing is more devastating to an innocent physician's defense against the allegations of medical malpractice than an inaccurate, illegible, or skimpy medical record". So it is imperative for all medical professionals not only make proper documentation but also learn the art of record keeping and its importance.

HISTORICAL ASPECT

Record keeping was never a consistent well-organized practice. It has received patchy support and inconsistent application. The records have been kept in a variety of ways. Medical records carved on wood, stone, and hieroglyphics have been discovered. The Atharvaveda gives the earliest documentation of medical records in India. An astrologer, horrendous quack doctor Forman recorded over 10,000 consultations between 1596 and 1603.[1] In the late 1590, Forman taught Napier his methods. Napier's record survives in full from 1598 to his death in 1634. These contain roughly 40,000 consultations. In 1880s, physicians at Mayo Clinic Minnesota kept the patient records in personal leather-bound ledger. This was replaced in 1907 with patient-based records, which is still used today. In 1928, the Associated for Record Librarians of North America was founded by the American College of Surgeons. They recognized the necessity of the comprehensive and long-term medical records on individual patients. In UK, the first major attempt to standardize medical record came in 1965 with publication of the Tunbridge report. Initially, the records were kept for physician's own epidemiological interest. Slowly as art and science of medical and surgical services getting complex and institutionalization approach developed, the records became mean of communication to other team members also. Public hospital and medical colleges started to have medical record department for research and statistical purpose. Today maintenance of records is mandatory from ethical and legal point of view.

RECORD KEEPING IN INDIAN CONTEXT

Despite knowing the importance of proper record keeping, it is still in a nascent stage in India. In India clinical establishments ranges from small clinics to big hospitals. Only larger hospitals have record keeping mechanism though in bad state. It is a well-established principle propounded by Indian Judiciary that "Poor records mean poor defense, no records mean no defense". This principle applies to every establishment and professional despite size of set up or nature of practice. Everybody must be sincere in record keeping. But neither doctors are well sensitized toward maintaining records nor hospitals take it seriously. Now time has come that apart from doctor paramedical and nursing staff also should be trained in proper maintenance of patient records.

The management and preservation of the hospital records in Indian context present a very gloomy picture. Despite the intensive effort at national and international level, the fundamental healthcare needs of the population of the developing countries are still unmet. The lack of basic health data renders difficulties in formulating and applying a rational for the allocation of limited resources that are available for patient care and disease prevention.

WHAT CONSTITUTES A MEDICAL RECORD?

The medical record is a legal document providing a chronicle of patient's medical history and care. The medical record is an important compilation of facts about a patient's life and health. It includes documented data on past and present illnesses and treatment written by the healthcare professionals and planned for future. The medical record "must contain sufficient data to identify the patient, support the diagnosis or reason for attendance at the healthcare facility, justify the treatment, and accurately document the results of that treatment".[2] The main purpose of the medical record is to record the facts about the patient's health history with emphasis on the events affecting the patient during the current admission or attendance at the healthcare facility, and for the continuing care of the patient when they require health care in the future. For good patient care, the patient should have one medical record with all admissions filed in the one record and kept in the one place. The physical medical record is the property of the hospital and the information in the medical record is the property of the patient, and cannot be released without the consent of the patient.

WHAT ARE THE CRITERIA FOR AN IDEAL MEDICAL RECORD

Always remember the five "C"s—Clean, Complete, Chronological, Comprehensive, and Correct. Records should be without manipulation and overwriting or tempering. If any changes have to be made, then it should be struck with single line and rewritten alongside with initials. Vital information needs to be highlighted like allergies and drug sensitivities, high-risk medical conditions, HIV status, history of violent tendencies, and known abuser of healthcare services.

Guidelines for Medical Record and Clinical Documentation by WHO-SEARO (World Health Organization South-East Asia Regional Office) coding workshop September 2007 has issued three guiding principles for medical record and clinical documentation:

1. *Guiding principle 1:* Comprehensive and complete record
2. *Guiding principle 2:* Patient centered and collaborative
3. *Guiding principle 3:* Ensure and maintain confidentiality.

WHAT IS THE PURPOSE OF A MEDICAL RECORD?

"Verba volant, scripta manent" (spoken words fly away, written words remain)—Caius Titus

Medical records serve many purposes. The main purpose of the medical record is to record the facts about the patient's health history with emphasis on the events affecting the patient during the current admission or attendance at the healthcare facility, and for the continuing care of the patient when they require health care in the future. Medical record documents the history of examination, diagnosis, and treatment of a patient. This information is vital for all providers involved in a patient's care and for any subsequent new provider who assumes responsibility for the patient.

IMPORTANCE OF RECORD KEEPING IN PRESENT SCENARIO

Medical records are important for two main reasons:

1. *Medical reason:* Medical record keeping is important to evaluate existing patient management strategies and to develop institute- and doctor-based disease statistics. For chronic disorders and old cases, records are of immense helping tools for treating clinicians. Multispecialty treatment concept cannot work out without proper medical record keeping.
2. *Legal reason:* Medical record keeping is not only an obligation on doctors and clinical establishments as per present Medical Council of India (MCI) Rulings and Clinical Establishment and other Acts but also a defense in modern era of litigations. "Poor Records means Poor Defense, No Record means No Defense". If any legal problem arises then properly maintained records are of utmost importance. They are the most important proof of what treatment was actually administered to the patient.

WHAT ARE THE TYPES OF MEDICAL RECORD?

Hospital records directly related to patient management (medical treatment records):
- Outpatient records
- In-patient record
- Record from diagnostic facility departments
- Copy of certificates issued, certificate register
- Medicolegal records.

Hospital records not directly related to patient management but necessary:
- Other administrative records and documents required under different laws
- Records under PNDT Act
- MTP Act
- Biomedical Waste, and Environment Protection Act, etc.

Other records not related to patient:
- Accounts and related records
- Service records of staff, leave, absence, qualifications, etc.
- Gratuity, Employee Provident Fund Act, under other labor laws
- Hospital housekeeping and maintenance record, lift and electric equipment maintenance, and ICU/NICU Sterilization roster
- Operation theater instruments and equipment list, autoclave schedule observed
- Asepsis maintenance protocol observed though out the hospital, etc.

ESSENTIAL COMPONENTS OF THE MEDICAL RECORD

- *Patient particulars:* Personal data of patient, detailed postal address, email, contact numbers, photo ID, and Aadhaar card
- *"Personal declaration proforma"* filled in writing of patient or attendant giving above details with essential past and personal history, socioeconomic status, and annual income.
- Admission assessment
- *History:* Chief complaint, history of (H/o) present illness, past medical history, family history, developmental history, dietetic history, and known allergy.
- *Examination finding:* Detailed complete physical examinations
- Progress notes/flow sheets
- Medicolegal case (MLC) notes/police information notes
- Surgical/procedure notes
- Anesthetic notes/preanesthetic check-up notes
- Vitals charting by doctors and nursing staff
- Nursing notes
- Resuscitation notes
- Diagnosis—provisional and final, differential diagnosis, patient care summary
- Investigation, charting, and reports
- Copy of past treatment and investigation record
- Serious consent, consent for procedure, daily prognosis explanation consent sheet
- Reference notes/transfer notes
- Treatment done and planned
- Telephonic consultation from senior doctors should also be noted down by junior doctors and nursing staff with date and time noting and endorsement afterward.
- Copy of discharge card/death summary/referral letter
- Document receiving by the patient at the time of leave
- High-risk screening notes/follow-up plan
- Certificate issued.

RISK AND WARNINGS

These need to be highlighted before start of treatment. H/o allergies or drug sensitivity and high-risk medical condition should be highlighted with red pen. H/o of violent tendency, HIV, hepatitis B and hepatitis C virus positive status, and known abuser of healthcare services should also be highlighted.

WHEN SHOULD THE DOCTOR START MEDICAL NOTES WRITING?

The medical note writing begins right from the time of admission of the patient. In fact even the outpatient department (OPD) case paper should have all the findings and treatment written in proper order. Whether the patient was admitted on outpatient basis or as an emergency also has to be mentioned very clearly. History in detail has to be recorded. Date and time is a very important record on case paper and name and signature of the treating doctor is mandatory.

DOCUMENTATION IN NEONATAL RESUSCITATION RECORD

The following things need to be documented for neonatal resuscitation:
- Time of arrival at the resuscitation
- Resuscitative procedures performed by others prior to your arrival
- Description of vital signs and APGAR (appearance, pulse, grimace, activity, and respiration) scores
- Procedure performed in resuscitation/ steps to be recorded
- Outcome of resuscitation, need of hospitalization, and referral to be documented with noting of time.
- Newborn status/disease with gestational age should be mentioned.
- If Do Not Resuscitation (DNR) situation arises, then proper informed consent with witness (video recording of DNR consent)
- Examination of congenital anomalies and injury sustained if any
- In case still born with congenital anomalies, samples must be sent for karyotyping and genetic evaluation
- Stopping of resuscitation in case of nonsurvival must be followed with standard norms with proper explanation to attendants.
- Last menstrual period (LMP), expected date of delivery (EDD), gestational age, mother blood group and thyroid status, antenatal history, and ultrasonography (USG) fetal well-being finding must be documented.

RECORD OF CERTIFICATE ISSUED

Many time medical professional has to issue various certificates, such as medical certificate, fitness certificate, certificate of child care leave, and experience certificate. Copy of all certificates issued should be preserved. Always remember that medical certificate should be issued on letterhead of doctor or hospital and a copy of the same must be preserved. It must contain date, time, identification mark, mobile number, and signature attested; it must be issued for legitimate purpose only on utmost need. As per clause 1.3.3 of Indian Medical Council Act Regulation 2002, register of medical certificates must be maintained by every physician. Medical professional should never issue a false certificate otherwise it will arise to medicolegal complication.

IMPORTANCE OF DISCHARGE CARD, REFERRAL, AND TRANSFER NOTES RECORD

Outpatient department papers, discharge card, referral letter, and death certificate are the most important record, because these are directly issued to patient party during the course of treatment, and there is no chance of making correction of mistakes. Receiving signed copies of these should be preserved with indoor records. Most of the times, these are the documents with which litigation is filed. Discharge card and transfer notes are the summary documents, which reflect the treatment received. The discharge card and transfer notes should mirror the case notes of the patient records with a brief summary. Discharge card must mention condition of the patient at the time of admission and at the time of discharge, treatment given in hospital and course of the stay of the patient, operation notes, complete diagnosis, treatment suggested at the time of discharge, investigation, follow-up schedule, prognosis, danger sign and care at home explained, and undertaking of patient/attendant on discharge card itself about understanding of the treatment prescribed, follow-up schedule, danger sign, prognosis, home care, and high-risk screening. Referral notes should mention prior information given to referred doctor or referral center and patient being referred under medical supervision by ambulance with resuscitation equipment including oxygen.

DISCHARGE CARD AND DISCHARGE/TRANSFER AGAINST MEDICAL ADVICE

Patients who get discharged against the advice of the doctor are also entitled to have a discharge card/transfer notes about the course of treatment. It is imperative to record the fact that the doctor has advised a course of action with all its implications if not followed. The fact that the patient has understood this and has refused it on his volition should be recorded. This should be signed by the doctor, patient, or relative and duly witnessed. This document has to be retained along with the patient records. It will help the doctor in situations where the patient alleges negligence later.

2013 case and 2016 case—leaving hospital—discharge against medical advice (DAMA)—no negligence

- "M. Sarala versus Sundaram Medical Foundation and another" 2016 (1) CLT 265
- "Union of India versus Sohan Lal Sharma" reported as 2013 (1) CPC 494

Leaving hospital against medical advice and the complainant having failed to follow the advice of doctor and having left the treatment midway, then the Hospital and the Doctor cannot be held negligent.

AVOID THOSE THINGS WHICH WOULD QUESTION CREDIBILITY OF MEDICAL RECORD

Improperly corrected medical records may give rise to issue of perjury and may put a question on credibility and evidentiary value of medical record. Always avoid overwriting, whitening, scratching, or scoring. In case corrections have to be made then strike the whole sentence and corrected notes should be written freshly with signature to avoid suspicion of tempering. Never leave OPD or indoor papers incomplete. All the columns of bed head ticket (BHT) should be properly filled, page should be numbered, and all the investigations, nursing notes, referral notes, copy of discharge card, death certificate, and bills should be properly annexed. Avoid leaving any paper loose. Always take informed consent on in-patient department (IPD) or OPD case paper rather than on any other paper and annexed it in BHT. Similarly, OPD case register should have no cutting, whitening, or erasing.

Altering Medical Record

- At the outset a mention may be made that altered records should never be presumed

to be manipulated. No one should draw any adverse inference from alteration, overwriting, or other changes made in medical records. Changes are made inadvertently rather than with any motive.
- While writing the medical notes, as far as possible do not overwrite. If the change is needed, strike the whole sentence. Do not leave ambiguity. Make a habit of signing if change is made. Preferably put the date and time below the signature.
- Do not alter the notes retrospectively. If something written was inaccurate, misleading, or incomplete then insert an additional note as a correction.
- Entries in a medical record should be made on every line. Skipping lines leave the room for tampering with the records.
- Amend on electric record by striking through rather than deleting and overwriting the original entry. After inserting the new note, add date, time, and doctor name.
- Correction of the personal identification data of the patient such as name, age, father/husband name, and address should only be made on the basis of affidavit attested by notary or first class magistrate.

CCTV RECORDING AND CALL/ VOICE RECORDING ON MOBILE AS RECORD

CCTV cameras are fitted in clinic and hospital by doctors mostly for safety purpose. But at times these may be needed as proof of treatment given or negligence committed. In privacy and criminal issues, such type of recording may be needed. Display sign board of under CCTV surveillance must be placed. In era of internet and smart phones, call recording may be done by either party and many times it is admissible in the court. So be cautious in telephonic interaction with attendants and anybody. Recording of consultation may be done where both parties agree. Audio-video consent has definitive added value in consent-taking procedure, and if done after consent of patient party and preserved properly, it may be good defensive tool in litigation. Many clinics and hospitals are now equipped with counseling room with in built audio-visual recording facility. DNR consent and organ transplantation consent must be audio-video recorded.

ISSUES IN OPD RECORD KEEPING

It has been a long tradition and still prevalent today that patient retains OPD records. All the OPD prescriptions, investigations, and imaging are handover to patient and attendants in original. Doctors are left with no documentation regarding OPD records. The patient is expected to preserve papers and bring it to clinic and hospital for follow-up consultation. Doctors are at mercy of patient party for OPD record. OPD records may actually be lost or may be hidden by patient at the time of litigation, which may prove disastrous to the defense of doctors. Preservation of OPD records is very cumbersome exercise for any doctor as it voluminous. Time restrain is also an issue which aid to reluctance in OPD record keeping.

ELECTRONIC RECORD KEEPING IN OPD

Although there is no obligation for private practitioner to preserve OPD records as of now, still preserving OPD records may prove to be useful at the time of litigations or any other medicolegal issues. OPD prescriptions may be prepared in two copies and one may be preserved by patient and another by doctor. But it is very difficult in practice. So, the best way would be to preserve record in electronic format, which is also admissible by courts under Section 65B of Indian Evidence Act. Now as per clause 1.3.4 of Indian Medical Council Regulation 2002 efforts shall be made to computerize medical records for quick retrieval. As per rule 13(d) National Medical Commission Ethics & Medical Registration Board (NMC EMRB) notifications published on 2nd August 2023, "Efforts shall be made to computerize patient's medical records for quick retrieval and security. Within 3 years from the date of publication of these Regulations, the Registered Medical Practitioner (RMP) shall ensure fully digitized records". So, time has come for every doctor and hospital to go for electronic record keeping.

■ TRAINING OF RECORD KEEPING

Record keeping is an important issue not only for hospitals and nursing homes but also diagnostic centers, clinics, and consultation chambers. There is enough scope in training regarding keeping. There should be orientation programs for all doctors and nursing staff for proper notes making and record keeping.

■ MEDICAL RECORD DEPARTMENT

Medical record department is needed for all hospitals and nursing homes. All large hospital and all public hospitals have medical record department for managing medical records. The Medical Record Department staff under the leadership of the medical record officer (MRO) or medical record clerk in-charge is responsible for the maintenance of medical records and medical record services. The hospital administration must provide security and sufficient storage space for medical records, and an adequate working area for medical record staff. The Medical Record Department staff must safeguard medical records from tampering, loss, and unauthorized use. They are responsible for seeing that the patient's right to privacy and the confidentiality of the information stored within the medical record are maintained at all times. The MRO or person in-charge of the Medical Record Department is responsible for the functions of that department and for seeing that the medical record is available when needed for the continuing care of the patient. They are also responsible for seeing that all forms relating to the care of a particular patient are in that patient's medical record; that the medical record has been completed by the doctor; diseases and operations are coded accurately; and all information produced for statistics is accurate and readily available when required by the administration, Ministry of Health or other government agency. To maintain an effective medical record service, MROs need the support of a medical record committee. They need to be able to bring important issues relating to medical record services to the committee for discussion.

■ PRESERVATION PERIOD FOR MEDICAL RECORDS

OPD Consultation Record by Registered Medical Practitioner: No Obligation to Preserve OPD Medical Record but INDOOR RECORD to be Reserved for 3 Years

As per clause 1.3.1 of Indian Medical Council Act Regulation 2002, "Every physician shall maintain the medical records pertaining to his/her indoor patients for a period of

3 years from the date of commencement of the treatment". NMC EMRB notification dated 2nd August 2023 also reiterate the same "Every self-employed RMP" shall maintain medical records of patient's (inpatients) for 3 years from the date of the last contact with the patient for treatment, in a standard proforma laid down by the NMC. So, it is apparent that there is no obligation on RMP to preserve OPD medical records as of now.

Teleconsultation by Registered Medical Practitioner

Telemedicine guideline has been regarded as annexure 5 of MCI regulation 2002 and is binding on every doctor. Section 3.7.2.1 of the guidelines mentions that it is incumbent on RMP to maintain Log or record of Telemedicine interaction (e.g. Phone logs, email records, chat/ text record, video interaction logs etc.) for the period as prescribed from time to time. Section 3.7.2.2 mentions that patient records, reports, documents, images, diagnostics, data, etc. (digital or nondigital) utilized in the telemedicine consultation should be retained by the RMP. Guideline 11 Telemedicine Guidelines of NMC ERB Notification 2023 in Duties and Responsibilities of RMPs reiterate the same "It is incumbent on RMPs to meticulously maintain the following records/documents for three years from the date of the last consult with the patient".

Retention Period for Government Hospitals

As per the Director General of Health Services (DGHS) vide letter No. 10-3/68-MH dated 31-8-68 (published in 'Hospital Manual' in 2002) medical records should be maintained as follows:
- Inpatient medical records—10 years
- Outpatient records—5 years
- Medicolegal registers—10 years.

As per office memorandum of DGHS, No. A-12034/3/2014-MH-II/MH-I dated 28th October 2014, hospital may store medical records in hard copy form:
- In-patient medical records for 3 years
- OPD records for 3 years
- Medicolegal register and case sheets for 10 years or till the disposal of ongoing case related to these records.

Director General of Health Services office memorandum also mentions that medical record of indoor patient's may be stored in digitized form for at least 10 years or as per availability. For future, all medical records of indoor patient should be digitized on regular and continuous basis and kept indefinitely for future reference since it contains valuable data, which may be required for research and policy planning purpose.

RECOMMENDATION OF RETENTION OF MEDICAL RECORDS AS PER NABH/NABL

- Outpatient case sheets—5 years
- Inpatient case sheets—7 years.

All other records, summaries, (admission, discharge, or death), laboratory reports, preanalytical reports, etc. are required to be retained for a minimum of 5 years.

RETENTION PERIOD OF MEDICAL RECORDS AS PER VARIOUS ACTS

Clinical Establishment Act

As per Uttar Pradesh Clinical Establishment Rule 30-1:
- Retention period is similar to MCI regulation 1.3.1 and 1.3.2

- No obligation to preserve OPD records
- Retention period for indoor medical record is 3 year.

PCPNDT Act 1994

Section 29 of PCPNDT Act 1994 requires proper maintenance of records for a period of 2 years or until disposal of proceeding.

MTP Act 1971 Regulation 2003

As per Rule 5 of MTP Act 1971 Regulation 2003, Form III or Admission register for termination of pregnancies should be kept for 5 year.

Retention of Record as per Income Tax Act 1961

As per Income Tax Act 1961, retention period is 6 year.

Section 44AA and Rule 6F mentions that professionals like doctors are obliged to maintain daily case register Form 3C, inventory, cash book, general ledger, carbon copies of bills issued, and original bills received for a period of 6 years from the end of relevant assessment year.

Section 271A mentions that "If professional failed to maintain said documents mentioned above, assessing officer may impose penalty up to rupees 25,000/-".

RECORD RETENTION PERIOD SHOULD NOT BE CONFUSED WITH LIMITATION PERIOD

Limitation period is often confused with record retention period while both are different entity with different legal meanings.

Record retention period is that period for which record has to be preserved as per duty defined in a statute.

Limitation period is that period during which person has right to file litigation.

There are two types of statute:
1. *Statutes in which specific limitation period is prescribed are governed by their own limitation provision*:

    Consumer Protection Act Section 69 of CPA 2019 clearly mentioned limitation period for filing complaint, which is 2 year and delay may be condoned by forum if forum is convinced by the complainant that there is sufficient cause for delay in filing litigation. Similar was provisioned in CPA 1986 section 24A.

    In Criminal Procedure Code (CrPC) 1973 also specific limitation period is prescribed under section 468 for filing criminal complaint.

    In such type of statutes, limitation act has no role to play.

2. *Statutes in which no specific limitation period is prescribed are governed by limitation Act 1961, e.g., Civil Procedure Code.*

    Section 29-2 of Limitation act 1961, specifically says that where any special or local law prescribes for any suit, appeal or application a period of limitation different from the period prescribed by the Schedule prescribed in Limitation Act, then specific limitation period provisioned in that statute will prevail.

    Supreme Court in Hukumde versus Narain Yadav versus Lalit Narain Mishra[3] has held that "where a Statute is a complete code in itself, meaning thereby that it is a substantive as well as procedural code, then the application of Limitation Act has to be seen from the scope of application of the Statute and not the Limitation Act".

RECORD MAINTENANCE FOR CONSUMER CASES

- In Consumer Protection Act, record maintenance period is not mentioned anywhere.
- Limitation Clause of Consumer Protection Act, i.e., Section 69 CPA 2019 or Section 24A Section 1986 say that a complaint may be filed within 2 year from the cause of action and delay may be condoned if forum is satisfied by the complainant that there was justified sufficient cause in filing litigation.
- Since Consumer Protection Act has its own limitation clause, preserving medical record till age of majority plus 2 year is not applicable in Consumer Cases.
- So maintaining medical record as per various abovementioned acts is recommended.
- Still it is wiser that medical record to be preserved for longer period in view of increasing number of consumer litigations.

RETENTION PERIOD OF INDOOR MEDICAL RECORD FOR CHILD PATIENT BY PEDIATRICIAN

It has been a great confusion that record preservation period for child is 21 years. Everybody should note that it is totally a myth. Section 6-1 of Limitation Act 1961 which is "disability section" says "Where a person entitled to institute a suit or make an application for the execution of a decree is, at the time from which the prescribed period is to be reckoned, a minor or insane, or an idiot, he may institute the suit or make the application within the same period after the disability has ceased, as would otherwise have been allowed from the time specified therefor in the third column of the Schedule". So, a minor may institute the suit after his disability period which is age of majority 18 years is over. This limitation clause is applicable only to those statutes in which specific limitation clause is not provisioned.

As per information received in RTI reply from MCI (MCI-211(2)(RTI)/2019-Ethics/17871 dated 02-01-2020 from MCI, retention period for indoor medical record of child patient for pediatrician is same 3 years as mentioned in MCI regulation 2002 clause 1.3.1.

ISSUING OF MEDICAL RECORD

As per clause 1.3.2 of MCI regulation 2002, if any request is made for medical records either by the patients/authorized attendant or legal authorities involved, the same should be duly acknowledged and documents shall be issued within the period of 72 hours by authorized person. As per Regulation 13-B of NMC ERB regulation 2023 medical record should be issued within 5 days of making request and as per regulation 13-C in case of medical emergencies, efforts should be made to make the medical records available at the earliest.

In *Raghunath Raheja versus The Maharashtra Medical Council and Ors., Bombay High Court*[4] held that doctors cannot hide behind confidentiality when the patient party demands medical records.

Precautions During Issuing Medical Record

- As soon as request of medical record is made, authority of record seeker must be checked and it must be issued to the patient or kin after verifying their relation and identity by ID proof otherwise it may give rise to confidentiality issues.

- Medical record may have to be issued to third-party administrator (TPA) company or police or may have to be submitted in court of law but whenever issued it must be issued to authorized person with proper receiving.
- Issued record must be complete, pages must be numbered, all columns must be filled, consultant notes and nursing notes must be complete, signatures must contain names of signee, and cutting over writing must be avoided as it will amount to tempering.
- As soon as request is made to issue medical record, consultants and concern nursing staff must be communicated immediately to fill up the vacant column and to complete the record by all means. So, it is advisable that every record must be completed at the time of stay of the patient as a healthy habit as one may not get time again to fill up shortcoming if any.
- Remember in criminal case, medical record would be forfeited by police official in no time. So, contemporaneous charting is must for all.

MEDICAL RECORD AND RTI ACT 2005

- RTI Act under Section 2(f) of the RTI Act, provided access to records held by private bodies through regulatory public authority as ordained by any law in force. Section 2(f) says: "information" means any material in any form, including records, documents, memos, e-mails, opinions, advices, press releases, circulars, orders, logbooks, contracts, reports, papers, samples, models, data material held in any electronic form and information relating to any private body which can be accessed by a public authority under any other law for the time being in force. With this definition, the right of the citizen is expanded beyond public bodies and extended to private bodies also provided there is any legal access.
- As per Clinical Establishment Act, clinics and hospitals are obliged to preserve medical records for 3 year and these needs to furnish district health authorities on demand. So, Clinical Establishment Act provides legal access to health record through district health authorities under RTI Act 2005.
- Chief Information Commission (CIC) held in NP Bhatia versus IHBAS[5] that the patient's right to obtain his medical record is not only protected under RTI Act, but also under the regulation of Indian Medical Council, which is based on world medical ethics, and also as a "consumer" under the Consumer Protection Act 1986.
- In Shri Prabhat Kumar versus Directorate of Health Services GNCTD, Delhi[6] case, the appellant claimed that the death summary of his father prepared by the team of doctors led by Dr Vivek Nangia of Fortis Hospital is insufficient, unsatisfactory, unsatisfactory, ambiguous, vague, and does not have complete facts and sought complete Death Summary Report and disclosure of the real facts and circumstances, leading to death of his father under the Right to Information Act. CIC directed Fortis Hospital to furnish certified copies of entire medical record including a note explaining the cause of death of the father of the appellant, certified copies of documents based on which the causes were ascertained. Rejecting the claim by Fortis hospital, CIC has held that malpractice by private hospitals amounting to medical terrorism.

The CIC called the government MCI and other regulatory authorities have to see that license to practice medicine will not become license to kill and extort and come to the rescue of the helpless patient.
- On tendency to ask information under RTI in Subjudice case, CIC in R K Moraraka versus Central Bank of India[7] has held that "This commission has consistently taken a view that if information sought relates to a pending proceeding before a competent court/tribunal, then the said information should be obtained only through court/tribunal and not under the provision of RTI Act".
- In case of nonavailability of record after prescribed retention period, CIC has held in T.V. Varghese versus BSNL[8] case that "When the records are not available due to the expiry of the period of preservation according to the departmental rules for destruction of old records, there is no question of providing such information even if the disclosure of such information is not prohibited under Section 8(1)(j) of the RTI Act".

PROTECTION OF RECORDS

Medical record should be protected from insects, fire, water, and theft. Insecticide spray must be used in record room and naphthalene balls may be used along with. Keep fire extinguisher available in record room. Records should be protected from dampness, water, and floods. To avoid theft windows and ventilators should be properly covered with frame. If record is lost in any manner then FIR must be lodged.

HOW TO DESTROY RECORDS?
- Give a public notice in English and Vernacular newspaper both with a time limit of usually 1 month from date of publication in which any one wants the relevant paper can come and take the copy of the medical record needed.
- After 1 month destroy record for everyone except where litigation is going on or prelitigation process of notice is going on.
- Always incarnate medical record. Never throw or sell as garbage.
- Maintain record of destroying process.

EVIDENTIARY VALUE OF MEDICAL RECORD

Whenever there is an issue of medical negligence or otherwise, Indian Legal system relies on documentary evidences, which has to be filed in the form of medical record. Medical records are medicolegal documents and treating doctor can be cross examined pertaining to such records. These are the most important evidence when compensation for damage or prosecution or acquittal has to be decided by court. Medical records are primary evidence under Section 62 of Indian Evidence Act. It is usually agreed that documentation of facts during treatment is genuine and unbiased. Erasing of entries is not permitted and questionable in court. Medical record can be summoned in court in original form in course of proceeding. Electronic records are also admissible under Section 65B of Indian Evidence Act. Under Section 91 of CrPC, it is required to handover medical record to the police. But one should keep a copy of receiving of handed over medical record.

MEDICOLEGAL CASES

Medicolegal cases is the case where attending doctor after taking history and clinical examination of the patient thinks that some investigation by law enforcing agencies are essential so as to fix the responsibility regarding the case in accordance with the law of land. Injuries due to accidents and assault, suspected or evident cases of suicides or homicides (even attempted cases), confirmed or suspected cases of poisoning, burns, cases of injuries with likelihood of death, sexual offences, suspected or evident criminal abortion, all patients brought to the hospital in suspicious circumstances/improper history (e.g., found dead on road), unconscious patients where cause of unconsciousness is not clear, child abuse, domestic violence, person under police custody or judicial custody, patients dying suddenly on operation table or after parenteral administration of a drug or medication, case of drunkenness, brought dead, natural disaster are some examples of MLC. The police should be informed under Section 39 of Criminal Procedure Code, the attending MO is legally bound to inform the police about the arrival of a MLC. Any failure to report the occurrence of a MLC may invite prosecution under Sections 176 and/or 202 of IPC (BNS 2023).

CONFIDENTIALITY OF MEDICAL RECORDS

Medical records can be used as a personal or impersonal document.
- *Personal document:* This information is confidential and should not be released without the consent of the patient except in some specific situations.
- *Impersonal document:* The record loses its identity as a personal document and patient permission is not required. These records could be used for research purposes.

Confidentiality is an important component of the rights of the patient. The hospital is legally bound to maintain the confidentiality of the personal medical records. The patient can claim negligence against the hospital or the doctor for a breach of confidentiality. The maintenance of confidentiality is an important issue in the era of electronic data storage. There should be checks in place so that only those who are authorized can access the patient data.

However, there are certain situations where it is legal for the authorities to give patient information. They are as follows:
- During referral
- When demanded by the court or by the police on a written requisition
- When demanded by insurance companies as provided by the Insurance Act when the patient has relinquished his rights on taking the insurance
- When required for specific provisions of workmen's compensation cases, consumer protection cases, or for income tax authorities.

ELECTRONIC HEALTH RECORD STANDARDS FOR INDIA 2016

In September 2013, the Ministry of Health & Family Welfare notified the Electronic Health Record (EHR) Standards for India. Ministry of Health and Family Welfare e-Health Section vide its Notification Q-11011/3/2015 e-Gov dated 30.12.2016 issued EHR Standard guidelines which says that preservation of medical records assume significant importance in view of the fact that an EHR of a person is an aggregation of all electronic medical records of the person from the very first entry to the most recent one. Hence, all records must compulsorily be preserved and not destroyed during the lifetime of the person, ever. Upon the demise of the patient where there are no court cases pending, the records can be removed from active status

CHAPTER 4: Record Keeping, Making Easy

and turned to inactive status. Healthcare service providers (HSPs) are free to decide when to make a record inactive; however, it is preferable to follow the "three (3) year rule" where all records of a deceased are made inactive 3 years after death. However these guidelines seem pertain to government hospitals only. More clarification from Ministry of Health and Family Welfare is needed.

Protected Health Information (PHI) would refer to any individually identifiable information whether oral or recorded in any form or medium that (1) is created, or received by a stakeholder; and (2) relates to past, present, or future physical or mental health conditions of an individual; the provision of health care to the individual; or past, present, or future payment for health care to an individual. Patients will have the sufficient privileges to inspect and view their medical records without any time limit. Patient's privileges to amend data shall be limited to correction of errors in the recorded patient/medical details within 30 days. Patients can demand from a healthcare provider a copy of their medical records, which should be provided within 30 days of receipt of communication of request. The existing Indian laws including IT Act 2000 and their amendments from time to time would prevail.

IMPORTANT CASE LAWS RELATED TO RECORD MAINTENANCE

Patient not admitted as indoor patient, hospital not required to maintain the medical record: In *Sh. Mahesh Prasad Aggarwal & Ors. versus M/S. Kamayani Patients Care India Original petition no. 39 OF 2003 NCDRC... on 3 January, 2013,* the important question was whether the deceased was indoor patient in the opposite party-hospital. Opposite party-hospital has proved that deceased was not admitted in the opposite party-hospital as indoor patient rather treated as outdoor patient. In these circumstances, Notification dated 11.3.2000 issued by the MCI is not applicable to the present case and opposite party-hospital was not required to maintain the medical record of deceased.

No negligence in failure to supply the medical records unless there is legal duty to issue it: In *Poona Medical Foundation versus Marutturao Tikare*[9] *case,* National Commission has held that there can be no question of negligence by the reason of failure to supply the medical records unless there is legal duty on the hospital to give the records.

Patient has right to claim medical records pertaining and hospitals are under obligation to maintain them and provide them. In *Kanaiyalal Ramanlal Trivedi versus Dr Satynarayan Vishwakarma,*[10] it was held by honorable court that without confusion patient has right to claim medical records pertaining to his treatment and the hospitals are under obligation to maintain them and provide them to the patient on request. The hospital and doctor were guilty of deficiency in service as case records were not produced before the court to refute the allegation of lack of standard care.

Duty to produce medical record in the court, adverse inference could be drawn for not producing the records. In *Dr Shyam Kumar versus Rameshbhai Harmanbhai Kachiya,*[11] it was held by honorable commission that it is the duty of the person in possession of the medical records to produce it in the court and adverse inference could be drawn for not producing the records. Not producing medical records to the patient prevents the complainant from seeking an expert opinion.

Destroying the case sheet is an attempt to suppress certain facts. In *SA Quereshi versus Padode Memorial Hospital and Research Centre*,[12] it was held by court that the plea of destroying the case sheet as per the general practice of the hospitals appeared to the court as an attempt to suppress certain facts that are likely to be revealed from the case sheet. The opposite party was found negligent as he should have retained the case records until the disposal of the complaint.

Issues of tampering of medical records needs to be examined in civil court: In *Harenbalal Das versus Dr Ajay*[13] it was held by court that issues of tampering of medical records need detailed examination in a civil court rather that in Consumer Court.

Not maintaining confidentiality of patient information can be an issue of medical negligence. In *Dr Tokugha Yeptomi versus Appollo Hospital Enterprises Ltd and Anr,*[14] it was held by Supreme Court that not maintaining confidentiality of patient information can be an issue of medical negligence. The HIV status of a patient was known to others without the consent of the patient.

Records show no pain, so not performing X-ray justified Dr S Ali versus Dr Lahari[15]*:* In an accidental injury doctor did not performed X-ray of shoulder as patient never complained pain. Patient alleged negligence and alleged no record was given. District forum dismissed the case as complainant did not specify that which fact was overlooked by doctor.

Bill suggested that treatment was given— PP Ismail versus KK Radha:[16] In this case patient with accidental fracture of leg operated in hospital. During operation left drill bits. Later on left out drill bits was removed by other surgeon. Hospital contended that surgeon was not attached to the hospital. But surgeon charges in bill suggested that surgeon was attached. So, hospital held vicariously liable.

Allegation of not informing negated by informed consent: In *C Anjani Kumar versus Madras Medical Mission case,*[17] it was alleged that possibility of vocal cord palsy was not informed but this allegation was negated as there was inform consent which showed that it was properly explained.

Incomplete record spell deficiency in service: In *Dr Paramjit Singh Grewal versus Charanjit Singh Chawla* NC 2006 case national commission observed that doctor recorded X-ray as OK even though separated chip of humerus was not rightly placed while performing the operation the doctor did or maintain proper written record of treatment given and rationale of treatment. Court held deficiency in service. The doctor in his admission stated that he had informed the complainant for the replacement of shoulder when he could not get relief even after open reduction. I orally informed but not mentioned in the discharge card. Court held not maintaining proper record amounts to deficiency in service.

Alleged Tempering/Manipulation of Record

In *Meenakshi Mission Hospital and Research Centre versus Samuraj and Anrs,*[18] National Commission held that hospital was guilty of negligence as name of anesthetic was not mentioned in operation notes though anesthesia was given by two anesthetics. There were two progress cards about the same patient on two separate papers.

Records Not Produced in Court

In *Kanhaiyalal Raman Lal Trivedi versus Dr Satya Narayan Vishwakarma,*[19] the hospital and doctor were guilty of deficiency of service as case records were not produced before the court to refute the allegations of lack of standard care.

Record destroyed: S. Qureshi versus Padode Memorial hospital and research center.[20] In this case arthroscopy was performed for knee ailment later on developed deformity. Doctor failed to explain cause as record destroyed. Court held that doctor is liable and observed that an educated person would not destroy record when case is pending.

SUMMARY

Best defense against medicolegal litigation has always been medical records. It is well established that poor record means poor defense, no record means no defense. So, when a medical record is incomplete or lost it may cost a much for defense. Somebody has rightly said that Dance like no one is watching, chart like it may be one day be read aloud in a deposition. So, it is vital for every medical personal not only chart with due diligence but also preserve the medical record. Always remember most of the time litigation is filed with medical records that are in hand with patients—OPD prescriptions, discharge card, referral letter, and investigations, so there will never be a chance to review it and some of vital documents may be hidden in oblique motives. So, it is prudent to prepare these documents with maximum care and always get a receipt while issuing them. To remove all the doubts, all doctors should preserve medical record for at least 3 years as per Medical Council Guidelines and Daily case register, etc. for 6 years as per Income Tax rules. Electronic record keeping is somewhat grey area and more clarity should be sought by medical professionals. Always better be safe than sorry in maintaining medical records. Records will always remember even if doctor and patient forget it.

LEARNING KEY POINTS

- Documentation of communication and communication of documentation is key to avoid medicolegal issues.
- Patient forgets, record remembers.
- Always take receiving of documents from attendant at the time of discharge/death/referral.
- Records pertaining to income tax like daily case register, inventory, cashbook, ledger, bill book etc. have to be retained for 6 years from end of financial year concerned.
- Medical practitioner are under domain of RTI act by the ways of clinical establishment Act.

TAKE-HOME MESSAGES

- Always remember the five "C"s: Clean, Complete, Chronological, Comprehencive, Correct, and without manipulation and overwriting hinting tapering of records.
- Records should not only show merely what is done but should explain and justify each and medical decision taken for every action or deviation from usual course.
- For destroying IPD records give a public notice in one English and other in vernacular newspaper, with a time limit of 1 month before actually destroying. Do not sell IPD papers to raddiwala for maintaining confidentiality.
- Issue discharge/transfer note/card even to patient who leave against medical advice (LAMA).
- One can do 24 × 7 CCTV audio-video recording as records.

MUST AVOID THINGS—DO NOT DO

- Do not handover medical records without written request or under RTI, 2005 or

third parties such as TPA and insurance companies.
- Do not leave records free for all IPD patients.
- Do not write undated prescription.
- Do not do overwriting, scratching, and scoring of notes.

MUST DO THINGS

- Always take receiving of documents from attendant at the time of discharge/death/referral.
- Always do FIR on stealing or loss of medical record.
- Always maintain the duplicate copy of every certificate.
- Documentation of allergy or hypersensitivity in medical record is must.

MESSAGES WHICH THE READER MUST BE AWARE

"Good records mean doctor has good defense, well explained records means winning the litigation".

WARNINGS

- Do not alter the notes retrospectively. If something written was inaccurate, misleading or incomplete then insert an additional note as a correction.
- Attempting to obliterate the erroneous entry by applying the whitener or scratching will raise the suspicion of perjury.

MEDICAL NEGLIGENCE PEARLS

- "Poor records mean poor defense, no records mean no defense".
- Patient forgets, record remembers.

ONLY ONE FACT TO REMEMBER

The legal system relies in the issue of alleged medical negligence mainly on documentary evidence in a situation where medical negligence is alleged by the patient or the relatives.

MCQs

Choose one correct answer

1. It is necessary to document allergy or hypersensitivity on:
   a. OPD paper
   b. IPD paper
   c. Discharge card
   d. In all of the above documents
2. Which document needs to be prepared in duplicate copies?
   a. Sick leave
   b. Death certificate
   c. MLC report
   d. All of the above
3. Record retention period for children is:
   a. 18 years
   b. 2 years
   c. 3 years
   d. 21 years
4. For RMP, retention period for OPD record is:
   a. 3 year
   b. 5 year
   c. 1 year
   d. RMP is not obliged to maintain OPD record
5. For destroying IPD record:
   a. Give a public notice in newspaper
   b. Sell IPD papers to raddiwala
   c. Destroying as you wish
   d. None of the above

Answers

1. d   2. d   3. c   4. d   5. a

REFERENCES

1. Wilkins A. How a pair of astrologers helped invent modern medical record-keeping. [online] Available from https://gizmodo.com/how-a-pair-of-astrologers-helped-invent-modern-medical-5850286 [Last accessed December, 2023].
2. Huffman EK. Medical Record Management, 9th edition. Physicians' Record Company, Berwyn: Illinois; 1990.
3. 1974 AIR 480 1974 SCR (3) 31 1973 SCC (2) 133.
4. AIR Bombay: 1996. P-198.
5. File No. CIC/AD/A/2013/001681-SA Date of decision 23.7.2014.
6. File No. CIC/SA/A/2014/000004 Date of decision 03.02.2015.
7. Appeal no 908/ICPB/2007/F.No.PBA/07/211 Date of decision 17th September 2007.
8. Appeal No. 251/ICPB/2006, Date of decision. 2.1.2007.
9. 1995 (1) CPR 991 (NC).
10. 1996 (3) CPR 24 (Guj); I (1997) CPJ 332 (Guj).
11. I (2006) CPJ 16 (NC).
12. II (2000) CPJ 463 (Bhopal).
13. Paul, 2001 (2) CPR 498.
14. III (1998) CPJ 132 (SC).
15. III (1997) CPJ 611.
16. 1997;2 CPR 171 (NC): (1998) CPJ 16 NC.
17. 1998; 2 CPR (Chennai); I (1998) CPJ 5333 (Chennai); 1998 CTJ 504 (CP) (SCDRC); 1999 CCJ 915 (TN).
18. I(2005) CPJ (NC).
19. 1996;3 CPR 24 (Guj); (1997) CPJ 332 (Guj).
20. II 2000 CPJ 463 Bhopal.

SUGGESTED READING

1. Baldwa M, Baldwa V, Padvi N, Baldwa S. Legal Issues in Critical Care. New Delhi, India: CBS Publishers & Distributors Pvt Ltd.; 2022.
2. Baldwa M, Baldwa V, Padvi N, Baldwa S. Legal Issues in Medical Practice, 2nd edition, 2 volume set. New Delhi, India: CBS Publishers & Distributors Pvt Ltd.; 2023.

CHAPTER 5

Medical Consent: The Best Friend of Doctor

Mahesh Baldwa, Bhvya Baldwa, Namita Padvi, Varsha Baldwa

"Consent is the key to patient autonomy—preserve it".

Keywords: Consent, Dissent, Implied consent, Informed consent, Real consent

Aim: Medical consent is aimed protect primarily to patient autonomy. Pediatrician may get protection when complications arise in any procedure or treatment modality. Medical consent includes assent, dissent, and video consent in procedures, consent for drug administration, and consent for injectables with off-label indications.

Objective: In a pediatric clinic, consulting room, nursing home, hospital, and institutions, there are invasive and noninvasive procedures requiring signed consent form. Consent form is by both parties. This consent form explains the goal of any procedure or treatment modality and vaccinations along with risks, dangers, and benefits.

INTRODUCTION TO INFORMED CONSENT, REAL CONSENT, ASSENT, RISK BOND, APPROVAL, AND PERMISSION

In India, informed consent, real consent, assent, risk bond, approval, and permission by patient party in medical practice is treated synonymously in legal parlance. Dissent or negative consent or refusal in medical practice is antonym of consent. But it is known as negative form of consent. Consent is usually required to protect doctor from alleged assault, battery, negligence, and breach of confidentiality. Usual scenario is what doctors name risks or complications of treatment or surgery; same is alleged to be caused by negligence of doctor by patient party.

CONSENT, ACCENT, APPROVAL, AND PERMISSION

It is sufficient to have a document that is tailored to the patient and the procedure, fully disclosing all information regarding the disease and treatment without any deception, manipulation, or pressure, and signed by an authorized individual with witnesses present.

WHY CONSENT?

Because every individual has a right to personal autonomy of choosing what is good means, method, modality for treating his illness. The law of consent originated from the intentional tort of battery. This law safeguards an individual from any uninvited physical contact with their body by someone who does not have their express or implied consent, nor a privilege to do so.

WHY IS IT AUTOMATIC GRANT OF PRIVACY TO PATIENT?

If individual communicates about illness with a doctor it is presumed to be fiduciary, confidential where such individual expects privacy in the matters related to health disclosed to medical professional.

WHAT IS CONSENT ABOUT?

Consent and confidentiality is all about patient party's autonomy of individual and privacy of individual in matters related to health disclosed to medical professional in confidence, which should not be breached without consent.

WHERE AND WHEN CONSENT IS NEEDED?

Implied or written consent may be needed for history writing, examination, noninvasive treatment like administering oral drugs, nondrug advise like advice about diet, exercise, work, rest, and general dos and don'ts. Written consent may be needed for invasive administering parenteral drugs, surgery, anesthesia, blood transfusion, and statutory consents. Patient's communication with doctor is privileged communication. Hence, patient confidentiality, privacy, or professional secrecy should not be breached without consent. Breach of secrecy may result in humiliation, suicide by patient, or patient may sue doctor for libel, slander, innuendo, or defamation.

HOW TO OBTAIN CONSENT AND AT WHAT TIME?

Consent should be obtained in consent form or format. Timing of consent is before undertaking patient for invasive administering parenteral drugs, procedure, surgery, anesthesia, blood transfusion, or like. A separate consent for each is preferable but even joint consent can be used for various procedures. After the procedure obtaining consent should be always avoided, as such it is illegal.

HOW INFORMED CONSENT PROTECTS?

The concept of informed consent is grounded in the idea that every person has the right to make choices that affect their own well-being. It is widely recognized that individuals should weigh the potential risks and benefits involved in their decisions. This requires having access to information about those risks and benefits. To safeguard the right to informed consent, the law mandates that the party requesting consent must disclose relevant information.

ELEMENTS OF THE CONSENT/PARTIES TO CONSENT

Usually there are two parties:
1. Patient party may be patient, spouse, relatives, attendants, school teacher, neighbor, court, police to name a few, or its combinations.
2. Medical team headed by consulting physician or surgeon, assistant doctors, nurses, compounders, supporting staff working under direction of medical team to name a few, or its combinations.

SUBJECT MATTER OF CONSENT

Patient counseling is crucial before obtaining informed consent for any treatment, procedure, surgery, or medication. It is important to disclose all risks and complications associated with the patient's condition and the proposed treatment. This chapter discusses the process of counseling patients about the risks involved before obtaining their consent.

WARNING TO DOCTORS FOR OVERSTEPPING AUTHORITY OF CONSENT EXCEPT IN EMERGENCY

Since consent itself falls in gray area of legal interpretation in case mishap or complication occurs. Hence, doctors are advised to act as per written consent. Do not use own discretion. Do not overstep consent given by legally authorized person. Doctors are warned for not using medical goodness and replacing it with legal authority given in consent. If doctors do so they will do that by undertaking undue legal risks. Exception to the rule is emergency lifesaving situations. Doctors is at liberty to go ahead with medical treatment to save life and limb of patient without consent.

VALIDITY OF CONSENT

Can Consent be Taken After the Surgery or Similar Invasive Procedure, etc.?

No. It will be invalid consent. Remember this is common allegation in law courts by patient party.

Can Consent be Taken Weeks or Months Before Procedure or Surgery?

No. It will be invalid consent. Remember this is one of the allegations in law courts by patient party that consent was not taken just prior to procedure. In one case patient came to outpatient department (OPD) for procedure which was not done on that particular day. When patient comes again for doing same procedure or surgery later on different day, is previous consent valid? Doctor cannot rely on previous consent taken on previous date. Though court may sometimes allow previous consent to be valid but it is advisable to take fresh consent.

CONSENT FOR DRUG ADMINISTRATION

Several drugs like oxidant drugs like sulfa drugs in G6PD may cause hemolysis, lowering of blood counts, Stevens–Johnson syndrome (SJS), or toxic epidermal necrolysis (TEN). Hence, special consent is required for same.

Some drugs can cause life-threatening sudden, rare, and unexpected anaphylaxis such as nonsteroidal anti-inflammatory drugs (NSAIDs) and beta-lactam antibiotics.

CONSENT FOR INJECTABLES IN PEDIATRIC

Vaccination injections can be injected after counseling forewarning and risk appraisal.

CONSENT IN PROCEDURES WITH LESS EVIDENCE AND OFF-LABEL INDICATIONS

"Off-label" or physician-directed use for prescription medications, biologics, and approved medical devices refers to any application that is not listed in the Food and Drug Administration (FDA)-approved labeling, e.g., repurposing of feeding tubes, red rubber catheters for chest and peritoneal, and even bladder drainage should be explained to patient party. Off-label uses of drugs are infrequent in pediatric such as use of tetracyclines in cholera, floxacins in typhoid, and aminoglycosides for serious infections in neonates. Consider using a medicine off-label only if all other options are unavailable, exhausted, not tolerated, or unsuitable.

TRANSFER CONSENT

Before transferring counseling, forewarning, risk appraisal, and need for transfer be told before obtaining transfer consent.

POLICE/ADMINISTRATIVE INFORMATION IN CASE OF REFUSAL OF TREATMENT AND INVESTIGATIONS

Before informing police/administrative if counseling, forewarning, risk appraisal, and need for information be told such as under communicable disease and epidemic act before obtaining police/administrative information consent but legally not needed. But police/administrative information in case of refusal of treatment and investigations becomes essential for protecting pediatrician

CONSENT IN TELECONSULTATION

The National Medical Commission (NMC) adopted 48 pages appendix 5 or guideline 11 on telemedicine prescribes the consent procedure.

Obtaining and duly recording the patient's consent is mandatory for any telemedicine consultation. Consent may be *implied* or *explicit*, depending on who has initiated the telemedicine consultation. *Explicit consent must be recorded* in any form. Electronic media can be used to provide information as in the written in-person informed consent process. Consent can be administered and documented using electronic formats such as text, graphics, audio, video, podcasts, or interactive websites. The Registered Medical Practitioner (RMP) should obtain the patient's signature or thumb impression and date of signing on the informed consent document either as a scanned document through email or as an image over the smart phone

Consent for Release of Medical Information to TPA and Mediclaim Insurance Companies

Medical records release to Third Party Administrator (TPA) and mediclaim insurance companies can be done with patient consent only.

CONSENT FOR MEDICAL RESEARCH

Consent for medical research is governed by the Indian Council of Medical Research (ICMR) and schedule Y guidelines under drugs and cosmetic act 1945.[1]

CONSENT FOR MEDICAL PUBLICATION

Medical publication with patient identity revealed can be done with patient consent only.

CONSENT TAKEN BY AUDIO AND VIDEOGRAPHY

Audio and videography for counseling before procedure, forewarning can be done with patient identity revealed but should be done with patient written permission and consent only. Section 65B of the Indian Evidence Act, 1872[2], to be replaced by Bhartiya Sakshya Adhiniyam 2023 (BSA-2023) is with respect of admissibility of electronic records, audio and videography, digital photography of diseases conditions for asking second opinion usually transmission of such recording is not permitted.

INFORMED CONSENT

Informed consent requires full disclosure of risks to patient before obtaining consent by way of preconsent counseling, forewarning about risks which can happen orally, in writing, audiography, videography, and digital photography.

IDEAL COMPONENTS OF VALID CONSENT

It is sufficient to have a document that is tailored to the individual patient and procedure, provides complete information about the disease and treatment, and is transparent, without concealing anything, misrepresenting, coercing, committing fraud, or exerting undue influence. The document should be in writing and signed by an authorized representative, with two witnesses present.

INDIAN DOCTORS GOING DIGITAL

In fact Indian doctors have fitted closed circuit television (CCTV) camera's in clinic displaying signs boards that the areas under CCTV surveillance for safety and security. In India, some doctors install CCTV cameras in their consulting rooms but not in examination rooms/area but recording requires consent of patient party.

AVOID OPD/IPD VISUAL AND AUDIO RECORDINGS OF PATIENTS ON PERSONAL SMART PHONES

Using personal mobile phones to take photos of patients or sending them electronically is not acceptable in any circumstance. Although there may be rare instances where a photo could assist in an emergency situation, such images should be sent through secure emails. In cases where images are needed for diagnosis or educational purposes, personal cameras and mobile phones should not be used. Taking patient images with a mobile phone, regardless of consent, is never justified except in emergencies and should be avoided.

GUIDELINES OPD/IPD—USE TECHNOLOGY WITH CONSENT TO MAINTAIN CONFIDENTIALITY

The utilization of video and picture messaging has made it simpler to capture, duplicate, and share recordings of patients. Medical professionals may want to use these technologies to assist in speedy diagnosis and consultation, ultimately benefiting the patient. It is important for doctors to remember that these recordings become part of the patient's medical record and therefore, the same confidentiality and consent standards apply.

SPECIFIC COMPLICATIONS REQUIRING DISCLOSURE

Any treatment modality leading to blindness, deafness, lameness, loss of limb or digit, gangrene, amputation, paralysis, and dysfunction of brain, heart, liver, kidney, or lungs needs to be disclosed as material risks. Very high and very low lab readings in any test needs rechecking of test. All fine-needle aspiration cytology (FNAC) need confirmation by biopsy. False-negative and false-positive reports do occur in any disease in any pathological and imaging procedure. If clinician is not able to corelate the reports, one should refer for redoing or refer to some other center to do same test or procedure to avoid mistakes emanating from false-negative and false-positive medical reports. This will avoid allegations of misdiagnosis, wrong diagnosis, and delay in diagnosis.

LOGIC AND REASONING FOR WRITTEN CONSENT

- The patient party is given complete freedom to decide as to what should be done to them when their child is inflicted medical/surgical problems.

- Legally invasive treatment without consent and most medical examinations, procedures, and surgery are liable for prosecution under assault, battery, or illegal touch.
- Consent absolves doctors by the principle of *"volenti non fit injuria"* meaning under law of tort says if patient is willing (consents), it shall be taken legally as if no injury is done to patient. This principle of risk applies to nature of complications arising out of treatment or surgery and in no way a defense for negligence.

PRECONSENT COUNSELING AND FOREWARNING

Preconsent are steps doctor should take before procedure, surgery by way of forewarning, counseling, describing dos and don'ts, cautions, precaution prior to surgery, and after surgery such as:
- Giving information brochure to patient party, regarding pediatrician physician or surgeon doctor, anesthetist if any, preanesthesia checkup, preoperative investigations, surgical or procedure details, cost, duration of surgery, extension of surgery if required, failure of surgery, recurrence of diseases, duration of hospital stay if required, most common complications which has incidence of >10%, signing of consent, and handover written consent format for patient party's study before signing
- Asking patient to surf Google or any other search engine and encourage participative debate.
- Explaining risks
- Disclosure of risk relating to surgery and procedure, disclosure of alternative methods, interaction with social, and monetary or time frame problems which are material to patient.
- Coming for follow-up, taking prescribed medicines, dos and don'ts about food, and exercise
- Capping of compensation in case of rare chance of litigation.
- Cashless mediclaim rejection is patient party responsibility.

TYPES OF CONSENT

Implied Consent (Tacit Consent)

The most frequently encountered form of consent in OPD practice is when a patient visits a doctor for a health issue, indicating their willingness to undergo a medical examination in a broad sense. However, this does not necessarily mean that the patient has given consent for any specific procedures or surgeries.

Express Consent

Consent is given in a way other than implying it, it is considered express consent. This can be given either verbally or in writing. Verbal consent is appropriate for minor procedures or examinations, and it is best to have a neutral party present. Written consent, on the other hand, is required for major procedures such as (1) biopsies, (2) general anesthesia, (3) surgery, and (4) intimate examinations.

Informed/Real Consent

Informed consent means giving relevant information to patient concerning a particular ailment/problem of patient. In the recent years, the idea of informed consent has gained prominence and many patients have filed lawsuits stating that they were not fully informed about the medical procedure they consented to. To prevent such situations, it is important to provide all information in clear and simple language, in the local language if possible. This should include the diagnosis, nature of treatment, potential risks, chances of success, possible outcomes if the procedure is not performed, and other available treatment options. The physician's duty to disclosure is subject to the exceptions: (1) if the patient prefers not be informed and (2) if the doctor believes in the exercise of coming to a sound medical judgment, that the patient is so disturbed or anxious that the information provided would not be processed rationally or that it would probably cause significant psychological harm. This is known as therapeutic privilege.

Proxy Consent (Substitute Consent or Surrogate Consent) for Minors by Parent or Decision Maker

Any person who has completed 18 years of age as per Indian Majority Act-1975[3] is considered an adult can sign proxy consent for minor or for person with legal disability. All the types of consent can take the shape of proxy consent are parent for child, close relative for mentally unsound/unconscious patient or decision maker, etc. To treat a minor without appropriate parental consent usually shall be construed "assault and battery" as per prevailing (1) legal philosophy and (2) customs and usage of common law and tradition. In general, in India parents pay for medical bills so again the wishes of parents prevail over adolescent. If adolescent is insured for medical treatment then emancipated or liberated adolescent's wish may have a say over parental say in medical treatment.

What is Blanket Consent?

In certain medical facilities, patients are asked to sign blanket consent forms, which indicate their willingness to receive any type of treatment or surgery without specifying a particular procedure. However, these forms hold no legal value since they do not address any specific procedures or their potential complications. This type of consent is referred to as mechanical consent, in which the patient does not actively consider the consequences of their decision.

Admission Consent

A general consent taken at the time of inpatient department (IPD) admission without specific purpose is admission consent. This consent has general value to protect the doctor for wrongful confinement but does not serve any purpose for doing surgery or procedure.

Printed Form Consent

All hospitals/nursing homes use pre-printed form consent. A controversy was created by national commission judgment in Vinod Khanna versus RG stone,[4] by raising objection to its use. The same is stayed by Supreme Court for now.

Real Consent or Real-time Specific Consent with Respect to Procedure and Complications Specific

This is outcome of Supreme Court's Samira Kohli judgment.[5] This is also known as real consent. The consent may be made procedure specific and complications specific where no extension or deviation from specific consent is permitted except in lifesaving emergencies. Any unforeseen risks which are not life-threatening will require patients consent. The doctors are advised to postpone operations or surgical extensions of such detected risks which are not life-threatening rather than taking authoritative positions invading patient's autonomy.

Consent for Complications

Consent for complication means commonly known, documented complications of surgery or procedure. Consent for complication does not mean unintended and accidental cutting of structure or organ or nerve, artery, and vein. Complications due to unmindful, unexplained, gross, and reckless procedures/surgeries done with whatever good intentions and which deviate grossly from the described procedures in textbooks unless situation is life-threatening are not permitted. Each and every deviation must be scientifically explained showing, emergency, or at least showing it benefitted the patient.

Consent with Disclaimers

- No 100% guarantee warrantee for cure
- No 100% assurance for success
- No assurance of "no cure no payment".

REFUSAL OF TREATMENT, DISSENT, AND NEGATIVE CONSENT

The patient has the right to control their own body and the legal concept of battery ensures that unwanted physical interference is prevented. If a competent adult decides to reject a particular treatment or all treatments, or choose an alternative option, they are entitled to do so even if the decision involves serious risks such as death.

A doctor must respect a patient's advance instructions, but in an emergency, they may act without consent under the doctrine of necessity. If a patient refuses treatment, the potential consequences should be explained to them with a witness present, and the refusal should be documented. The doctor may also refer the patient to another healthcare provider if they refuse treatment.

Patient Refusal or Negative Consent, Dissent or Part Refusal, or Best Option Refusal

Written refusal is required if patient does not want treatment in emergency as per *TT Thomas* (Dr) *versus Elisa,* Kerala HC, AIR 1987.[6]

SITUATIONS WHERE CONSENT MAY NOT BE OBTAINED

Hence let us enumerate situation where consent may not be obtained.

Emergency, Life-threatening, and Dying–dying Dead (Just on Verge of Death) Situation

The general rule with regard to informed consent in an emergency circumstance is that the standard informed consent rule still applies to cogent and conscious adults who require treatment. However, in most other situations in the emergency department (ED), informed consent is presumed for the patient.

Life-saving techniques give individuals the ability to survive and also save other people during life-threatening situations. First aid is as easy as ABC—airway, breathing, and cardiopulmonary resuscitation (CPR). Life support procedures include mechanical breathing (ventilation), CPR, tube feeding, dialysis, and more.

Legal Aspects Emergency, Life-threatening, and Dying–dying Dead Situation

- *No consent is required for lifesaving emergency treatment: A Practical legal aspect in court of law:* No consent is requires for emergency, life-threatening, dying–dying dead situations, and medical lifesaving emergencies like in medical emergencies. The well-being of the patient is of paramount importance; hence medical treatment precedes legal considerations. It is obligatory on part of doctor to treat emergency to save life as per Pt. *Parmanand Katara versus Union of India* SC, AIR 1989,[7] three judge bench of SC in *Paschim Banga Khet Mazdoor Samity* and *Ors. versus State of West Bengal* SC, AIR 1996.[8]

- *Written refusal* in emergency for not treating if patient does not want treatment in emergency as per *TT Thomas* (Dr) *versus Elisa,* Kerala HC, AIR 1987.
- Under the *therapeutic privilege,* the physician may withhold information if disclosure would be upsetting or otherwise would interfere with treatment or adversely affect the condition or recovery of the patient. Write reasons for withholding information to patient by taking relatives signatures.

NON-EMERGENCY STATE CONSENT

Non-emergency state or cold cases consent even when nonemergency deviation is found intraoperatively, one has to obtain consent till then postpone procedure or surgery. Three judge bench of SC in Samira Kohli versus Dr Prabha Manchanda 2008 2 SCC 1 says diagnostic procedure cannot be converted to therapeutic procedure without patient consent.

ASSENT VERSUS CONSENT

Neonatal intensive care unit (NICU) and intensive care consent when multiple interventions are needed during intensive care management.

Consent is not a single event during interaction with medical professional. Assent consent, dissent, forewarning, counseling, and refusal are continuous process. Consent or series of consent or multiple consents are required to be signed on the day/date when actually treatment, procedure, or surgery is done as a part of continuous process.

Consent is not a onetime spot ascent to doctor. Doctors daily take stock of medical situation/information on continuous basis from patient patients guiding doctors to do relevant physical examination and if needed relevant investigations. Since diagnosis is never written on the face of patient hence the progression of signs and symptoms doctors start with base line working diagnosis, for doctor advices single or multiple sittings of procedure/surgeries, single or multiple drugs, and or nondrug treatment in terms of diet, rest, exercise, abstinence from salt, and sugar as per situation for betterment of patient. Doctors should be always willing to revise diagnosis depending upon the therapeutic response or worsening of ailment. Diagnosis is not a goal post. It keeps changing if the nature of disease is such.

Each time the doctor has to wait for disease scenario to be clear and makes every day further evaluation of provisional diagnosis and or monitoring of disease. Ideally legally it may need separate fresh consent or continuity of same consent reaffirmed on each date patient is attended by doctor. Even though it is presumed by doctor that implied consent always existed by conduct of patient party hence doctor forgets to take written consent. This one time mistake may cost doctor dearly. If patient party does not get favorable results of treatment and asserts alleging that there was "no consent". Hence consent should form integral part of treatment process in tandem with each and every treatment, procedure, surgery, advices for investigations to evaluate recovery or worsening of disease vis-a-vis warn about side effects, adverse effects, complications of drug and/or nondrug, and/or surgical treatment. All refusals should be written on OPD/IPD paper and signed by patient party. All this algorithmic exercise of every treatment, surgery, and advices for investigations monitoring is done by medical professional to constantly done by doctor in an attempt to reduce health risks from disease, drugs, and surgery continuously hence doctors should not consider consent as one point activity in the beginning when patient submits and presents for treatment. Legally as we have seen it could be a continuous process requiring oral, written, and proxy consent depending upon facts and circumstances. In case of sin diseases, a number of times consent, reconsent, fresh consent, high-risk consent, etc., are required. Consent should not be considered a burden. Consent should not be mechanical. Consent should not be without application of mind.

Even informed consent is legally incomplete; it is time to switch to for contract for hiring of medical services to augment informed consent to restrict compensation granted by court.

PURPOSE OF REAL/INFORMED CONSENT

The main purpose of the informed consent process is to protect the patient to uphold autonomy of patient party. Primary purpose of consent is risk disclosures to patient. Consent form by itself is legally incomplete to protect doctor against allegations hurled by patient to seek compensation. Consent protects against patient voluntarily accepting risks of treatment/ surgery (*volenti non fit injuria*) cannot ask for compensation under law of tort.[9]

Purpose of Switching to "Contract for Hiring of Medical Services" is to Augment Informed Consent

"Contract for rendering/hiring of medical services" includes consent of patient party along with a number of terms and conditions which are usually not part of consent.

LEGAL CONTRACT

A contract is a legally binding agreement between two or more parties as per terms of contract, typically involving the medical services. Section 74 of Indian Contract Act (ICA)-1872,[10] governs liquidated damages. Parties at the time of contracting may stipulate an amount in the agreement itself, which shall become payable on the breach of contract, by doctor in favor of patient.

VALID CONTRACT FOR HIRING/PROVIDING OF MEDICAL SERVICES

Valid contracts to be legally enforceable if agreement contains all of the following legal criteria's:
- An offer (in form of proposed surgery/treatment)
- Acceptance by patient party by obtaining valid consent
- Clearly defined terms and conditions (about complications, disabilities, guarantee, warrantee, warnings, and disclaimers)
- Consideration (defined in terms of money and payment schedules)
- Intention to create legal relations (doctor-patient relationship)
- Capacity of the parties (competent to contract)
- Legality of purpose (standard surgery/treatment)
- Description of liquidated damages in case of breach of contract.

IS REAL/INFORMED CONSENT, A QUASI-CONTRACT AS PER SECTION 68–72 OF ICA-1872?

No. It is not a quasi-contract. Real/informed consent pave way for implied contract based on the conduct between doctor and patient.

WHAT IS CONSENT IN EYE OF LAW?

Section 13 of Indian Contract Act 1872 (ICA-1872) says "it is when two or more persons agree upon the same thing and in the same sense".

Consent means that patient party voluntarily and willfully agrees to doctors' proposition. The patient party who consents must possess sufficient mental capacity. Consent also requires the absence of coercion, pressure, force, fraud, misrepresentation, and trickery. Consent under Section 13 under ICA is an essential constituent of a contract (defined under Section 2 (h) of ICA) as an agreement enforceable by law. Consent is one of defenses available for doctor against allegations of tort (civil wrong) of negligence.

DOES CONSENT PROTECTS DOCTORS?

Yes, to some extent. Consent protects doctor by principle of *volenti non fit injuria* against allegation of tort of battery and assault. It is incomplete defense against allegation of negligence. Consent only allows describing risks about procedure, complications, and like.

IS CONSENT FORM LEGAL BINDING?

Consent form is not a legally binding contract. Consent is one of the legal the components of valid contract. A contract is an agreement which creates legally enforceable obligations between parties by obtaining valid consent. Hence, even informed consent is incomplete let aside real consent; therefore it is time to switch to "contract for hiring/rendering of medical services" to augment legal value of informed consent/real consent.

IS BREACH OF CONTRACT A TORT?

Even though contract law and tort law are similar, breach of contract is not a tort. In tort law, there is no contract between the parties involved. There is simply a duty of care that is imposed by the law upon the parties to take due diligence.

WHAT IS A TORT AND HOW DOES IT DIFFER FROM A BREACH OF CONTRACT?

Damages in torts are compensated by civil court as unliquidated. Damages in breach of contracts are decided by civil court as per terms and conditions of contract defined as liquidated damages.

CAN AN ACT BE BOTH A TORT AND A BREACH OF CONTRACT?

Yes, contract law and tort law can intersect in certain cases. If a breach of contract harms the other party, e.g., the wronged party (patient) could file a claim against defaulting party (doctor) in pursuit of financial compensation. Breach of contract intercepts with law of tort is obvious if unqualified doctor treats or when an instrument is left inside body, wrong gas for anesthesia used, and wrong side is operated upon leads damage to patient.

CAN YOU EXCLUDE NEGLIGENCE FROM A CONTRACT?

It is not possible to exclude or restrict liability for death or personal injury resulting from negligence. An exclusion clause, warning, or disclaimer should not be used to expressly exclude negligence.

COMPENSATION GRANTED CONSENT UNDER LAW OF TORT VERSUS CONTRACT AUGMENTING CONSENT UNDER INDIAN CONTRACT ACT—WHICH IS BITTER FROM DOCTORS POINT OF VIEW?

Consent versus contract for medical services from point of view of restricting compensation in consumer and civil jurisdiction.

Consumer and civil court usually decide one of the following aspects:
- Deficiency in medical service
- Was there unfair trade practice
- Was there medical negligence.

Hence, one should defend forcefully against alleged medical negligence and try and convert all allegations of negligence to deficiency of service for getting under liquidated damages under law of contract, since damages are defined and liquidated within the confines of contracted terms hence as per terms and conditions of contract civil court has to decide. Primary aim should be to convert all allegation of negligence to deficiency of service domain so as to align court granting liquidated compensation as per contract terms and conditions.

Medical negligence under law of torts paves way of civil court to grant compensation at court's own discretion as unliquidated with no holds barred on court to grant compensation. Choice is yours—which bitter pill to swallow—liquidated damages under contract law or unliquidated damages under law of tort.

SUMMARY

So in nutshell, obtaining consent in medicine is process that should include: (1) Describing the proposed intervention, (2) emphasizing the patient party's role in decision-making, (3) discussing alternatives to the proposed intervention, and (4) healthcare practitioner should be discussing the risks of the proposed intervention with reference to patient socioeconomic and cultural perspective.[11,12]

The main purpose of the informed consent process is to protect the patient to uphold autonomy of patient party. Primary purpose of consent is risk disclosures to patient. Consent form by itself is legally incomplete to protect doctor against allegations hurled by patient to seek compensation. Consent protects against patient voluntarily accepting risks of treatment/surgery (*volenti non fit injuria*) cannot ask for compensation. "Contract for rendering/hiring of medical services" includes consent of patient party along with a number of terms and conditions which are usually not part of consent. Does consent protect doctors—yes, to some extent. Consent protects doctor by principle of *volenti non fit injuria* against allegation of tort of battery and assault. It is incomplete defense against allegation of negligence. Consent only allows describing risks about procedure, complications, and like. Consent form is not a legally binding contract. Consent is one of the legal the components of valid contract. A contract is an agreement which creates legally enforceable obligations between parties by obtaining valid consent. Hence even informed consent is incomplete let aside real consent; therefore it is time to switch to "contract for hiring/rendering of medical services" to augment legal value of informed consent/real consent. Even though contract law and tort law are similar, breach of contract is not a tort. In tort law, there is no contract between the parties involved. There is simply a duty of care that is imposed by the law upon the parties to take due diligence. Damages in torts are compensated by civil court as unliquidated. Damages in breach of contracts are decided by civil court as per terms and conditions of contract defined as liquidated damages. It is not possible to exclude or restrict liability for death or personal injury resulting from negligence. An exclusion clause, warning or disclaimer should not be used to expressly exclude negligence. Medical negligence under law of torts paves way of civil court to grant compensation at court's own discretion as unliquidated with no holds barred on court to grant compensation. In future one has to switch to "contract for hiring of medical services" is to augment informed consent and restrict compensations from un-liquidated to liquidated damages as per contract.

LEARNING KEY POINTS

- Informed/real consent process is to protect the patient to uphold autonomy of patient party.
- Doctors take information from patients so it guides him in doing relevant physical examination and if needed relevant investigations. This process sometimes is short if disease is cured quickly. But it could be long if diagnosis and cure does not happen.
- Therefore, a short definition of consent is "doctor agreeing to give information or advice or warning to his patient or patient's natural parents/guardians/court who in turn agree with doctor.
- Assent is one sided, part consent of patient, means agreeing to few advices of doctor and dissent means one sided part disagreement with doctor's advice.
- Forewarning (better word is counseling) is needed where patient is likely to spread disease, or likely to commit suicide when human immunodeficiency virus (HIV) positivity is diagnosed.

KEY POINT AND PRACTICAL POINT TO REMEMBER

Informed/real consent process is primarily designed to protect the patient party to uphold autonomy of patient party and give information to decision maker who signs consent.

TAKE-HOME MESSAGES

Consent be obtained by competent patient party who is decision maker.

MUST AVOID THINGS

Avoid signature on blanket consent.

DO NOT DO

Do not force signing consent.

WARNINGS

Forewarning (better word is counseling) is needed where patient is likely to spread disease.

MESSAGES WHICH THE READER MUST BE AWARE

"Contract for hiring of medical services" be augmented by real/informed consent and restrict compensations from unliquidated to liquidated damages as per contract.

MUST DO THING

Consent for children is surrogate or proxy consent signed by competent decision maker on behalf of minor child.

MEDICAL NEGLIGENCE PEARLS

It is sufficient to have a document that is tailored to the individual patient and procedure, provides complete information about the disease and treatment, and is transparent, without concealing anything, misrepresenting, coercing, committing fraud, or exerting undue influence. The document should be in writing and signed by an authorized representative, with two witnesses present.

ONLY ONE FACT TO REMEMBER

One should not obtain signature on blank pre-printed consent form.

REFERENCES

1. Drugs and Cosmetic Act, 1945.
2. The Indian Evidence Act, 1872.
3. Indian Majority Act, 1975.
4. Vinod Khanna versus RG stone. Available from: https://indiankanoon.org/doc/179114819/
5. Samira Kohli versus Dr Prabha Manchanda 2008 2 SCC 1.
6. TT Thomas (Dr) versus Elisa, Kerala HC, AIR 1987.
7. Pt. Parmanand Katara versus Union of India SC, AIR 1989.
8. Paschim Banga Khet Mazdoor Samity and Ors versus State of West Bengal SC, AIR 1996.
9. Law of tort. Available from: https://en.wikipedia.org/wiki/Tort
10. ICA-1872. Available from: https://www.indiacode.nic.in/bitstream/123456789/2187/2/A187209.pdf
11. Baldwa M, Baldwa V, Padvi N, Baldwa S. Legal Issues in Medical Practice, 2nd edition. New Delhi: CBS Publishers and Distributors Pvt. Ltd.; 2023.
12. Baldwa M, Baldwa V, Padvi N, Baldwa S. Legal Issues in Critical Care, 1st edition. New Delhi: CBS Publishers and Distributors Pvt. Ltd.; 2022.

CHAPTER 6

Logical Basis of Consent Formats

Mahesh Baldwa, Namita Padvi, Varsha Baldwa, Ashok Baldwa

"The art of medicine consists of using consent forms while nature is made to obey the commands of medications and surgery to cures the disease".

Keywords: Benefits, Complications, Diagnosis, Risks

Aim: How to efficiently produce and translate knowledge about warning, disclosure, and counseling in consent formats for use in clinical practice. Even though attempt is made to dedicate formats to pediatricians but to get full insight in making formats is not possible without referring to doctors in general.

Objective: In a pediatric clinic, after proper communication, addressing answers to all questions, and doing medical counseling, forewarning about all complications and medical risk disclosure about invasive and noninvasive procedures, what to do? How to put it in writing? What should be the format of signed consent needs to be detailed. Here one will find logical basis of consent formats in pediatric.

INTRODUCTION

Informed consent is a cornerstone of medical ethics and practice, ensuring that patients have the autonomy to make informed decisions about their healthcare. The logical basis of consent formats in medicine is to provide a structured and standardized approach to obtaining and documenting informed consent.

Before preparing for the informed consent one should ask following questions in the process:[1,2]

- What is the diagnosis?
- How serious is this diagnosis?
- What method of treatment is recommended?
- Are other treatment alternatives available? What are they?
- What are the benefits and risks of the recommended and alternative treatments?
- What are the risks and complications of the recommended and alternative treatments?
  - How common are they?
  - What are the immediate, medium-term, and long-term side effects?
- Are there other discomforts associated with the treatments?
- Are these permanent or temporary?
- How long will treatment last?
- How long rest is required before relative of child/patient can resume normal activities?
- Any special precautions about diet, exercise, hygiene, bath, etc.
- How much does the treatment cost?
- What methods can be used to relieve the discomforts?

WHAT ARE THE COMPONENT CONTENTS OF CONSENT FORMATS?

Consent formats should contain typically four parts. Part I, II, III, and IV are more or less same for all pediatricians. Part II of consent documents describes what individual pediatricians may or may not need depending upon facts and circumstance of case as described earlier in questionnaire.

Part I

Part I is for personal information of relative of child/patient.

> Name (first-middle-surname):
>
> Age (date of birth dd/mm/yyyy format):
>
> Sex male/female, other:
>
> Address:
>
> (Flat/house no.-street name-village-tehsil-district-police station-post office–PIN code):
>
> Mobile number:
>
> Landline number:
>
> Email:
>
> Names of guardian or kith and kin with name and address and mobile numbers:
>
> Personal income:
>
> Family income:
>
> Documents submitted for identity, signature proof, birth date and address 1. .... 2. .... 3. ....

Part II

Details of Disease and Ailment under Treatment in Preferably in Brochure Format

Following logical legal points which should be kept in mind to avoid future allegations be included in consent forms in any suitable format of choice by carving out suitable sentences to cover:

- *Relative of child/patient's concerns which must be made known to pediatricians:*
  - Autonomy means relative of child/patient will decide what needs to be done to his/her body at his free will, relative of child/patient's will to do anything on his diseases is final.
  - Medically and scientifically documented safety of drugs, treatment, surgery/procedure, relative of child/patient party should be told about safest and riskiest procedure.
  - Security of life, security of limb, security of all faculties with which relative of child/patient is enjoying life, security of all life amenities of relative of child/patient, Security of all confidentiality by appropriate methods.
- *Pediatricians responsibility for not resorting to:*
  - Signature on blank page as consent—not a good practice
  - Taking signature on blank blanket printed consent—not at all good practice
  - Taking signature coercion—never be done in practice
  - Taking signature trickery—never be done in practice
  - Taking signature misrepresentation—never be done in practice
  - Taking signature fraud—never be done in practice
  - Taking signature by force or undue influence—never be done in practice
  - Taking signature by manipulation
- *Use legally/government guidelines/professionally recommended formats for mandatory consent forms:*
  - One can obtain permission and use readymade specific consents forms

are available. *A general model form is annexed at the end of this chapter.*
- Consent for hair transplant as per NMC guidelines (https://www.nmc.org.in/MCIRest/open/getDocument?path=/Documents/Public/Portal/LatestNews/20220927051220.pdf).
- Consent for research project—study ICMR guidelines (https://ethics.ncdirindia.org/asset/pdf/ICMR_National_Ethical_Guidelines.pdf).
- Informed consent as per the Indian Council of Medical Research (ICMR) guideline.
- ICMR guideline-4.1. 2-Informed consent is a continuous process involving three main components—providing relevant information, ensuring competence, ensuring comprehension, and voluntariness.

Legal Outlines/Ascent/Permission/Risk Bond for Invasive Procedures which should Find Place in Consent Form of Nonemergency Type

- Take written consent from mentally sound adult, preferably by asking for self-attested photocopy of photo ID, age, and address such as Aadhar card, PAN card, and passport.
- Written proxy consent taken from mentally sound adults assuming responsible (in writing) for minors, very old, mentally unfit, unconscious, drunk.
- Relative of child/patient is competent to written consent then do not take consent of spouse or relatives.
- Take written consent after medical disclosures of success, failure, and complications in percentages of surgery/procedure or treatment after proper explanation in a language which relative of child/patient party understands. Give idea of about expenditure. Write on outpatient department/inpatient department (OPD/IPD) paper and audio video recording, if possible.
- Surgery/procedure or treatment needs precounseling by explaining disease, surgery/procedure, and treatment. Write on OPD/IPD paper and audio video recording, if possible.
- Let relative of child/patient party decide after counseling regarding consent.
- If relative of child/patient party refuses, take refusal in writing.
- Disclose to the relative of child/patient and duly record in the consent:
  - Name of surgery/procedure and purpose in writing
  - Prognosis in writing
  - Risks involved in writing
  - Commonly occurring life-threatening and non-life-threatening complications in writing.
  - Even if complication is rare but likely to affect vision, hearing, motor and brain functions, lead to amputation, serious bleeding, and then document in writing.
  - Relative advantages and disadvantages of each of the available alternatives if any in writing.
  - Adverse consequences if any, in case of refusal by the relative of child/patient party in writing.
- Written consent for invasive investigations/diagnostic procedures in writing.
- In multistage treatment take specific and separate consent for each and every stage of treatment in writing.
- Take elaborate "high-risk" consent if:
  - The treatment/recovery are expected to take inordinately long time in a given situation in writing.

CHAPTER 6: Logical Basis of Consent Formats

- The surgery/procedure/procedure/procedure/treatment which has tendency for recurrence and has high failure rate. Explain if relapse of disease is common in writing.
- The technique/procedure/drug/protocol are not accepted mainstream surgery/procedure/procedure but relatively new.

- Two witnesses to written consent
- Name of consultant physician/surgeon doctor and anesthetist
- Consent of a literate relative of child/patient by affixing left hand thumb impression
- If it is commonly surgery/procedure/procedure in your hospital then provide relative of child/patient party with exhaustive brochure describing surgery/procedure/procedure, risks, prognosis, and advantages and mention in consent that patent party has read brochure. This can be done by printing on inside cover of file given to relative of child/patient.
- Mechanical formality of signing consent at the time of admission is "no consent"
- Do not change site of procedure, route of procedure/method for performing surgery/procedure/procedure, change surgery/procedure/procedure or extend or deviate from what is written in consent except in lifesaving situations like anaphylactic shock.
- No consent required for informing police and police can be requested to perform postmortem by pediatrician in case of rare event of death.

Relative of Child/Patient Giving Part Consent and Part Refusal

- Consent for one surgery/procedure/procedure should not come in way of surgery/procedure refused.
- Precounseling should be done for consequences of part consent.
- OPD/IPD paper and other medical records of relative of child/patient should mention precounseling and part refusal of surgery/procedure.
- Written signed refusal (dissent) with minimum two witnesses in writing.

Situations Requiring Extra Caution

Pediatricians should keep in mind certain high-risk situations, which are common causes for medical negligence actions; situations that require extra caution.

High-risk Consent

Specify what makes the consent to qualify to be high risk. Specify risk/s.

Part III

Part III are regarding declaration by relative of child/patient party and doctor.

Declaration about Social, Economic, and Other Comorbidities by Relative of Child/Patient

Claims by relative of child/patient:
- I have received, read, and understood the brochure about diseases (signed and annexed herewith) describing pros and cons of disease, treatment, surgery/procedure and procedure before signing the consent.
- I have revealed in writing about my personal details in the consent form and same are true.
- I have filled health status form after understanding it. (Signed and annexure herewith).

Disclaimers by pediatricians:
- Medical facility is registered with local authority and does not hold out any

assurance, guarantee, warrantee for cure.
- The treatment facility does not hold out 100% cure.
- The treatment facility does not hold out no to relative of child/patient as "no cure-refund of fees".
- Diagnostic opinion, reports, advice given or handed over to relative of child/patient may be false-positive or false-negative up to 1 in 100 (meaning having 1% error or incorrectness). Second opinion, repeat tests or follow-up is advised for such cases.
- Medical facility is registered with local authority and does not claim to conform to BIS, ISO, JHACHO, standards or otherwise.
- Medical facility is registered with local authority and does not claim to give latest, ultramodern, state of art facilities.
- The treatment facility does not hold out zero failures or zero complication rates. Complications and failure occur but can be suitably treated by referral.
- The treatment facility does not hold out zero recurrence of same disease, stones, swelling, pain, infection, inflammation, and abscess. Also nonunion of bone, malunion of bone, malocclusion, and disfigurement may occur after surgery/procedure or procedure.

Part IV

Part IV is signature and witness.
- Signature of relative of child/patient/guardian
- Signature of at least two witness with postal address, phone no, mobile no, emails
- Signature of doctor/s
- Date and time
- Place

MODEL CONSENT FORM ON LETTER HEAD OF INSTITUTION

Consent Form for Indoor Admissions-Model Consent Format-A

Part I—Model Consent Form

Relative of child/patient party's details	Guardian/relative's details
Full Name:	Full Name:
Sex: ☐ Male/☐ Female	Sex: ☐ Male/☐ Female
Age:	Age:
DOB: dd/mm/yyyy	DOB: dd/mm/yyyy
Address, email, mobile landline no.:	Address, email, mobile landline no.:
Provisional Diagnosis:	
Operation's Title:	Relationship with the relative of child/patient:

Doctor's details	Anesthetist's details
Name:	Name:
Degree:	Degree:
Risk Involved: ☐ Very High/☐ High/☐ Usual	Risk Involved: ☐ Very High/☐ High/☐ Usual
Provisional diagnosis:	Provisional anesthesia to be given:
Operation's title:	Fitness of the relative of child/patient for anesthesia:

Part II—Model Consent Form

I have read and understood the details here in above and here in below along with annexure 1 and 2 related to brochure on procedure and health status which forms integral part of this consent form.

I, _____
_____father/mother/uncle/aunt/grandfather/grandmother/guardian/other relationship _____ consent for _____ in my fully conscious state of my mind GIVE CONSENT after obtaining full discloser about surgery/procedure and anesthesia from above described pediatricians/doctors as below.

I _____
_____
_____ of my free will give consent for ☐ my own/☐ Aforementioned Relative of child/patient's abovementioned Operation and/or Medication/Investigation/Anesthesia/Operation/Therapy/Procedure etc.

- The necessity of this medication/investigation/anesthesia/operation/therapy/procedure, the ill effects if this is not performed; hazards and complications in the therapeutic modalities other than operation have been explained to me.
- I have been explained clearly that any medication/investigation/operation/therapy is not totally safe and that such procedure or Anesthesia can be a risk to life an otherwise healthy person also.
- Doctor have explained to me that excessive bleeding, infection, cardiac arrest, pulmonary embolism and complications like this can arise suddenly and unexpectedly while undergoing medication/investigation/operation/therapy/procedure.
- I give consent for any change in the anesthesia or operative procedure as well as removal of any digit or part of skin as organ as deemed necessary by the doctor at the medication/investigation/operation/therapy/procedure.
- I have been made aware that after the above operation/investigation/medication/therapy/procedure and Anesthesia, instead of desired benefit, some complications may arise, e.g., _____.
- About nature, type, and extent of sickness/diagnosis/disease pathology mentioned below and which is made after proper clinical, systemic examination and requisite investigations (Name of disease diagnosed _____ _____).
- About the nature and purpose of operation/surgical procedure/medical treatment.
- About proposed proper line of treatment which necessitate operation/surgical procedure in form of (Name of Surgical procedure _____ _____) with its need and necessity in the best interest of the relative of child/patient's health and life.
- About possible risks, consequences, unwanted and unexpected side effects or complications during and after said surgical procedure/medical treatment (some of which as following (i.e., _____ _____ _____).
- About alternative/other possible line of treatment with respective pros and cons benefits and hazards (i.e., _____ _____).
- About nature, extent and risks involved before, during and after anesthesia.
- About the fact that no drug whether used in form of oral, injection or infusion that will be given or injected to me/my

relative of child/patient before, during or after the said surgical treatment/procedure, are not free from its side effect and untoward results other then their benefits.
- About the prospects of success of the said procedure/operation and prognosis if the surgical procedure is performed or if not performed.
- That no guarantee has been given to me/us about result/prognosis of said surgical or medical treatment by the treating doctor.
- That my/our questions have been answered to my/our satisfaction prior to signing this form by the treating doctor/consultant concerned.
- That it has been specifically explained to me that the risk of the said procedure in my/my relative of child/patient case is high b/o following preexisting reasons/factor (i) _____
(ii) _____
(iii) _____
_____ (iv) _____ and I am ready to take this high risk involved at my own considered will.
- That I/we had been warned by the treating doctor/his associates concern specifically not to do following things i.e., _____ _____ during/after said procedure/operation and about other necessary precautions to be used in form of _____ etc.
- That any skin tissue/parts of skin removed surgically may be disposed of by consulting room, clinic, Nursing Home/Medical Centre in accordance with accustomed practice or according to direction of Doctor-In-Charge.
- That all infrastructures/instrumentations available in the consulting room, clinic, Nursing Home which are necessary to deal with any emergency health situation if occurred are also shown to me.
- That I know that hypersensitivity reaction (allergic response) to any drug is an unusual response of the live human body to the drug; it is not the fault of drug or doctor who prescribing the drugs.
- That I further authorize the treating doctor/phyician/surgeon doctor to —
- Employ or take help from Dr _____ _____ or any other doctor, to conduct aforesaid operation/surgical procedure/line of treatment, as his/her assistant/associate Doctor, on my/our behalf on extra payment payable as per applicable hospital's schedule.
- Employ or take help from anaesthesiologist Dr _____ as a anesthetist to gave anaesthesia in form of _____ which is necessary to conduct aforesaid operation/surgical procedure/line or treatment, and who has already declared me/my relative of child/patient fit for anesthesia and surgery/procedure at time of P.A.C. on my/our behalf on extra payment payable as per applicable hospital's schedule.
- That I/we have no reason to believe that's aforesaid doctor and his associates will acts negligently and without due care and without necessary precautions, before, during and after said treatment and further they will not act diligently and in good faith exclusively in the benefit of health and life of me/my relative of child/patient.
- That if any dispute arises between the parties to the contract/consent, the dispute forming matter shall refer to arbitration for final adjudication.
- So I/we hereby declare that I/we shall indemnify and not hold the doctor, his associates/assistants phyician/Surgeon doctor, anaesthetist, or other hospital

staff for any misfortune or accident or untoward incident or unwanted side effect or complications resulted out during and after said surgical treatment/procedure.
- I certify that I have read and fully understand which of the above consents, that the explanations therein referred to were made and that all blanks or statements requiring insert of completion were filled in before I signed.
- I/we further agreed to remit the charge of all hospitalisation treatment before leaving the hospital/nursing home which includes consultations fees, phyician/surgeon doctor's fees, boarding, lodging, nursing, investigations, medications and surgical procedure fee, etc. Applicable according to hospital norms, terms, conditions and schedule about which already informed and explained to me/us prior to hospitalization and further conduct, by the hospital authorities/personal and concerned doctor incharge; which is inconformity to the tariff as displayed at reception site.
- I have read the above writing and the same is explained to me in vernacular language in a manner understood by me.
- The above writing has been read out to me. I have understood the aforesaid and I am giving my consent willingly without any force, coercion and undue influence.

Jurisdiction: All disputes shall have local pecuniary or territorial jurisdiction.

Part III—Model Consent Form

Claims by relative of child/patient:
- I have received, read, and understood the brochure (signed and appended herewith) describing pros and cons of disease, treatment, surgery/procedure and procedure before signing the consent.
- I have revealed in writing about my personal details in part I of the consent form and same are true.
- I have filled health status form after understanding it. (Signed and appended herewith)
- Jurisdiction: All disputes shall have local pecuniary or territorial jurisdiction.

Disclaimers by pediatricians:
- Medical facility is registered with local authority and does not hold out any assurance, guarantee, and warrantee for cure.
- The treatment facility does not hold out 100% cure
- The treatment facility does not hold out to relative of child/patient as "no cure-refund of fees".
- Diagnostic opinion, reports, advice given or handed over to relative of child/patient may be false-positive or false-negative up to 1 in 100 (meaning having 1% error or incorrectness). Second opinion, repeat tests or follow-up is advised for such cases.
- Medical facility is registered with local authority and does not claim to conform to BIS, ISO, JHACHO, standards or otherwise
- Medical facility is registered with local authority and does not claim to give latest, ultramodern, state of art facilities.
- The treatment facility does not hold out zero failures or zero complication rates. Complications and failure occur but can be suitably treated by referral.
- The treatment facility does not hold out zero recurrence of same disease, stones, swelling, pain, infection, inflammation, and abscess. Also nonunion of bone,

- malunion of bone, malocclusion, and disfigurement may occur after surgery/procedure or procedure.
- Jurisdiction: All disputes shall have local pecuniary or territorial jurisdiction.

Part IV—Model Consent Form

Physician/surgeon doctor's acceptance	Anesthetist's acceptance
Sign of the Physician/Surgeon doctor :	Sign of the Anesthetist:
Registration No:	Registration No:
Relative of child/Patient's Acceptance/Signature	Guardian/Relative's Acceptance/Signature
Sign and/or L.H.T.I.	Sign and/or L.H.T.I.
Date: Time:	Date: Time:
Witness name in full Sign:	**Witness name in full** Sign:
Name:	Name:
Address, email, mobile landline no.:	Address, email, mobile landline no.:
Age:	Age:
DOB: dd/mm/yyyy	DOB: dd/mm/yyyy
Date:	Date:

SUMMARY

So in nutshell, obtaining consent in medicine is process that should include: (1) describing the proposed intervention, (2) emphasizing the patient party's role in decision-making, (3) discussing alternatives to the proposed intervention, and (4) healthcare practitioner should be discussing the risks of the proposed intervention with reference to patient socioeconomic, cultural perspective.[1,2]

LEARNING KEY POINTS

- Fill part I of format—the details of patient.
- Informed/real consent process is to protect the patient to uphold autonomy.
- Include risks in format.
- Include counseling in format.
- Include no 100% guarantee, warrantee clause as disclaimers.
- Fill Part IV of format—as signatures and witness.

KEY POINT AND PRACTICAL POINT TO REMEMBER

Informed/real consent process is primarily designed to protect the patient party to uphold autonomy.

TAKE-HOME MESSAGES

Consent be obtained by competent patient party who is decision maker.

MUST AVOID THINGS

Avoid signature on blank pages and fill details of consent behind the back of patient.

DO NOT DO

Do not force signing consent.

WARNINGS

Forewarning (better word is counseling) is needed where patient is likely to spread disease.

MESSAGES WHICH THE READER MUST BE AWARE

Consent may include a clause to restrict compensations in form of liquidated damages.

MUST DO THING

Consent for children is surrogate or proxy consent signed by competent decision maker on behalf of minor child.

MEDICAL NEGLIGENCE PEARLS

It is sufficient to have a consent document that is tailored to the individual patient and procedure.

ONLY ONE FACT TO REMEMBER

One should not obtain signature on blank preprinted consent form.

REFERENCES

1. Baldwa M, Baldwa V, Padvi N, Baldwa S. Legal Issues in Medical Practice, 2nd edition. New Delhi: CBS Publishers and Distributors Pvt. Ltd.; 2023.
2. Baldwa M, Baldwa V, Padvi N, Baldwa S. Legal Issues in Critical Care, 1st edition. New Delhi: CBS Publishers and Distributors Pvt. Ltd.; 2022.

CHAPTER 7

All About Medical Certificates

Mahesh Baldwa, Namita Padvi, Vijay Baldwa, Ankit Gupta

Fake medical certificate is a gun with bullets given to patient which many a times backfires on you.

Keywords: Duplicate certificates, Fake certificates, Psychiatric diseases certificates, Record keeping

Aim: Medical certificates should be stating truth.

Objective: Completing a medical certificate for a patient may be a common process, however it comes with particular responsibilities. This is not only the clinical responsibilities but ethical and legal requirements as well to be satisfied.

INTRODUCTION

It is nothing new for some dishonest patient parties to try and change the law to their advantage by taking medical certificates. Parents take sick certificates for submitting to school for unauthorized leave taken by their children. Typically, the legal system and the police are prepared to handle unearth such false certificates. Only in cases where a doctor issues a medical certification (for leave of absence or other nonmedical reasons), makes the doctor responsible for issuing false certificate. However, it would not be outrageous to suggest that the majority of doctors in India just have a cursory understanding of this subject and frequently rely on their own or their peers' opinions in issuing such "false" certificates. Since a sick leave certificate is a legal document with financial and administrative ramifications, there is a chance that it will be used as evidence in court, where the treating physician may be required to defend their position in accordance with both medical and legal norms. Therefore, physicians giving such certificates need to have a fundamental knowledge of the legislation.[1-3]

EXAMPLES OF "FAKE" MEDICAL LEAVE CERTIFICATES ISSUED BY REGISTERED MEDICAL PRACTITIONER

All of following were found to be unethical and illegal by the medical council:[4]

- In September 2017, five doctors in Delhi lost their registration for issuing "fake" medical leave certificates.
- One doctor had issued a 6-month medical certificate for a person. The diagnosis given was disk prolapse L4-L5. And no supporting diagnostic test was available.
- Medical leave certificate was issued for 62 days for a case of urinary tract infection (UTI).
- Medical certificate for a period of 11 months continuously. The patient who demands a

false medical certificate is also not without the chance of jeopardy. Production of false medical leave certificate can also be a ground for termination of service for the employee.[5]

ANATHEMA OF "FAKE" MEDICAL LEAVES CERTIFICATES

False medical certificates are abhorrent to both the patient and doctor. So the subject of how to draft an appropriate certificate by doctors for medical leave automatically arises.

DELHI MEDICAL COUNCIL GUIDELINES ON MEDICAL LEAVES CERTIFICATES

After the aforementioned incident in Delhi, the Delhi Medical Council (DMC) issued a guideline for this purpose. According to this, the following rules should be followed:[6]

- The medical certificate is a legal document. Any false certificates may expose a physician to punitive actions by the medical council and also the civil or criminal courts of law.
- Just writing that "this certificate is not for legal purposes" is not a valid statement and does not absolve a physician from the crime of a false certificate.
- The certificate should be legible.
- The certificates should be based only on facts seen by the doctor. If some of the facts of the illness are based on the patient's history only, that part should be clearly stated. It can be written as "reported by the patient and deemed to be true by the doctor".
- The certificate should have a clear date.
- The certificate should have registration number of the physician (even if written in a government hospital).
- The certificate should be prospective. That is, a doctor should state the probable period of absence from the date of issuance of the certificate. A certificate should not be retrospective normally. Sometimes, a short retrospective certificate may be issued, but in that case, the retrospective nature of the certificate must be stated clearly.
- The certificate should avoid abbreviations.
- The certificate should be addressed to the intended person (employer/school principal) (in other words, generic certificates with the heading "To whom it may concern" should probably be avoided).
- A doctor may write statements such as "suitable for light work" or "unfit for certain duties" if it is within the professional expertise of that doctor. For example, a gynecologist may not write whether a patient with leg fracture is suitable for work. Similarly, a physician cannot write whether bed rest is needed after radiotherapy. In the aforementioned Delhi case, the doctor writing the spinal disk prolapse certificate was a pediatrician!! (But he is not qualified to certify whether an adult with disk prolapse needs bed rest. For that an orthopedic specialist or neurosurgeon would be ideal).
- The DMC also states that normally, a certificate should be issued only for a maximum of 15 days. If further leave is needed, further certificates should be issued after that period of time. If a doctor thinks that a long period of absence is desirable, then it is better to refer the case to a medical board.
- The certificate should preferably contain an ID mark of the patient.

- And finally, the certificate must be accompanied by a *signature or thumb impression* of the patient. If it is a minor (in case of schoolchildren), the signature should be that of a guardian. It must be remembered that a doctor in India is not verifying authority. He/she has no way of knowing whether the name given by the patient for certificate purpose is correct. A doctor never asks for ID proof in India, especially in private chambers (in contrast, in the USA, when someone goes for a doctor consultation, social security number has to be provided). Thus, a person may register under a false name and get a certificate for sick leave. While it is true that a doctor–patient relationship depends on trust, still doctors need to take precautions against imposters. So, one insurance for doctors against such crime is the signature.
- The same rules will apply for government hospital certificates. A government doctor is also subject to harsh punishment if rules are violated.

RECORD KEEPING OF THE CERTIFICATES

The doctor should ideally retain a record of all sick and leave certificates. So that, in the event that the patient or a family member falsifies the certificate. It can be shown in to authority/court about such manipulation by patient. In clinic/hospitals, keeping records of the certificates is simple. However, it is particularly challenging to maintain records in private clinics managed by single doctor. At the very least, the doctor can store a photo image of the certificate on his smartphone. Use a pre-printed medical certificate though courts question pre-printed version. The storage period for duplicate copy for medical certificate retained by physician is usually for 3 years, same law is applicable like for any other medical records and documents.

DUPLICATE CERTIFICATES

- Certificates in duplicate should not be generally given. Before issuing a duplicate, if it is done in rare event, a written application from the patient should be obtained. On the top of the certificate, the word "duplicate" needs to be mentioned clearly.
- Use number of days in words well as figures.
- It is best to include both words and numbers when recommending the length of medical leave being prescribed. If the number of days is simply expressed as a number, it is simple to alter by appending a "0" or "1" before or after the figure. Thus, it is simple to convert 8 to 18. Even with a skilled graphologist, such minute alterations are quite challenging to spot later.

"FIT TO WORK" CERTIFICATE (MOSTLY FOR NONPEDIATRIC PATIENTS)

Finally, it should be kept in mind that a doctor's obligations are not terminated by a sickness certificate. The doctor must additionally give a "fit to work" certificate following the patient's recovery. "Fit to work" certificate is occasionally included on the sick note alone. Some people could choose to start working before the allotted time slot period has passed to take rest.[7]

CERTIFICATION OF HEALTH FOR A PHASED RETURN TO WORK (MOSTLY FOR NONPEDIATRIC PATIENTS)

- Modified hours
- Modified responsibilities

- Workplace modifications
- The doctor may note if the patient will need any special ongoing treatment, such as "patient needs physiotherapy three times a week".

MEDICAL CERTIFICATION THAT YOU CANNOT PERFORM HARD WORK (MOSTLY FOR NONPEDIATRIC PATIENTS)

Another request that Indian doctors frequently receive is this one. Particularly after having undergone a hysterectomy and been on lower segment cesarean section (LSCS) for a few months, housewives frequently make this request. After the fracture has healed, a male patient may request a certificate stating that he will be "unable to do heavy work" for, say, 3 months. The DMC standards, which state that certificates should not be issued for >15 days at a time, might put the doctor in a bind of not following guidelines.

MEDICAL DOCUMENTATION INDICATING INCAPACITY FOR NIGHTTIME DUTIES (MOSTLY FOR NONPEDIATRIC PATIENTS)

In India, a patient may ask their physician to "write a certificate" stating that their sickness prevents them from performing nighttime occupational tasks. While it is possible that a patient will face constraints in these situations, a doctor should not specify "night duties" or other clear prohibitions against performing nighttime occupational tasks. According to the aforementioned recommendation, the doctor may simply write "altered duty hours". Now, the employee and employer must discuss the subject of night shifts in specific occupational. Doctors do not have to use their judgment to determine exactly what work a patient is and is not permitted to perform.

MEDICAL CERTIFICATION FOR ALLEGED DUTY RESTRICTION (NONPEDIATRIC PATIENTS)

The alleged limitation on tasks may occasionally be hinted at. For instance, a doctor would note that a patient has back pain, which prevents them from bending forward. It is now up to the employer to analyze this report and make a decision.

DOCTOR'S CERTIFICATE INDICATING "BED REST" (MOSTLY FOR NONPEDIATRIC PATIENTS)

In the certificates, should "bed rest" be written? The use of that phrase is not required by law. Simply write "absent from work due to state details of illness in bracket (write diagnosis in this place)" on the certificate. Unless the patient gives written authorization, avoid writing the diagnosis and specifics of the prognosis with the diagnosis on certificates.

FITNESS-RELATED MEDICAL CERTIFICATION (MOSTLY FOR NONPEDIATRIC PATIENTS)

The issuance of a fitness certificate is not required prior to an individual returning to work following a medical leave, or when they enroll in school, college, a job, a gym, a swimming pool, etc. Typically, the doctor must sign the certificate. The fit certificate might be granted conditionally if a doctor feels that they should subsequently reevaluate a patient's fitness. After the next 15 days, Mr ABC must be reevaluated to determine whether he is still suitable for work.

DIAGNOSIS OF PSYCHIATRIC DISEASES

It is recommended to avoid including any specific psychiatric diagnoses in medical records.

The patient could experience prejudice after disclosing diagnosis of psychiatric diseases.

The employee has the choice of whether or not to disclose the psychiatric illness at work.

MEDICAL CERTIFICATE MENTIONING DURATION OF LEAVE

The doctor feels some rest is needed as per clinical judgment; one may issue medical certificate mentioning duration of leave. But since it is not written anywhere for what duration leave be prescribed for any particular patient. One has to be reasonable. Do not write excessive duration of leave, which may difficult to defend in court. If certificate is given longer than 15 days at a stretch, DMC guidelines will come in your way. If a patient is admitted to the hospital, a sick certificate may be written at the time of discharge. The case could be sent back to the general practitioner (GP) for further evaluation and a fit certification if the doctor is unsure. India has ambiguous laws. The majority of employers consider "medical leave" to mean presenting a medical certificate. However, there are numerous ailments for which a patient simply has to take a few days off from work to recover and does not even need to see a doctor.[8]

- A doctor should write the medical certificate only from the date he/she has seen the patient.
- The physician is responsible only from the time he/she has encountered the patient. However, the physician may include a note that he thinks the previous period of absence may be reasonable, based on the current condition of the patient.
- The patient may request the doctor not to write the actual diagnosis in the certificate. This wish for confidentiality must be respected. A doctor is not obliged to reveal the nature of the illness of the employee to the employer. In fact, if it is revealed against the patient's wishes, it may be ground for a legal dispute. Also, no employer has the right to demand medical diagnosis of his employee. (The US Equal Employment Opportunity Commission states that once a doctor certifies that a person is absent for medical reasons, the employer has no right to demand any more information. There is no reason why the same principle cannot be applied in India.)"

LEGAL CASES ON MEDICAL CERTIFICATES

Bombay High Court observed that "a medical certificate is not always sufficient proof of fitness. The court may decide to overturn it or call the medical expert in witness box for further clarification".[9,10]

Telgi allegedly obtained questionable medical certificates which enabled him to get bail on health grounds. Both the doctors who signed that medical certificate were sentenced to 7 years of rigorous imprisonment. Both were government doctors.

TYPES OF CERTIFICATES

Definition of Medical Certificate

A medical certificate is a document issued by a healthcare provider that verifies a person's medical condition, history, or status. It may be used for various purposes such as to confirm an individual's fitness to work, participate in sports, or travel among others. The content of the certificate typically includes information about the patient's diagnosis and treatment, any limitations or restrictions that need to be observed, and the healthcare provider's signature and contact details.

Treatment Certificate and Fitness Certificate

This gives format of certificate recommended for leave or extension or communication of leave and for fitness.[11]

Anesthesia Fitness Certificate

Preanestheia check is required before anesthesia fitness certificate. The American Society of Anesthesiology (ASA) score is a subjective assessment of a patient's overall health. ASA 1—normal healthy patient. ASA 2—patient with mild systemic disease. ASA 3—patient with severe systemic disease. ASA 4—patient with severe systemic disease that is a constant threat to life.[12]

Disability Certificate

Disability certificate is generally not issued by private pediatrician's hospital or clinic. Patient needs to be referred. Disability Certificate Issuing government Authorities (CMO Office/Medical Authority) will use this application to record the details of persons with disabilities (PwDs) and issue Disability Certificate/UDID Card electronically. Application from the PwD will be received by the CMO Office/Medical Authority.[13]

Estimated Treatment Cost Certificate

Estimated treatment cost certificate issued by private pediatrician's hospital or clinic if demanded by patient party in writing. One can give break up of all the estimated charges on pre-printed or hand written OPD/IPD paper.

Birth Certificate

Birth certificate is issued by local bodies like municipality or panchayat after receiving birth intimation form hospital or home delivery under birth and death registration act. Section 7(2) of the Registration of Births and Deaths Act, 1969[14] provides for the registration of every birth and death irrespective of nationality. The birth of the child of the foreign national may be registered by the local Registrar and a birth certificate to this effect may be issued under section 12 of the Act. Section 13 of the Act. Delayed registration of births and deaths—(1) any birth or death of which information is given to the Registrar after the expiry of the period specified therefor, but within thirty days of its occurrence, shall be registered on payment of such late fee as may be prescribed.

Death Certificate

Death certificate is issued by local bodies like municipality or panchayat after receiving Death intimation form hospital or from close relative in case of death at home. Documents needed in India for a death certificate is for providing a cause of death in Form No. 4 (institutional) and Form 4A (non-institutional) It is mandatory under the law (as per the Registration of Births and Deaths Act, 1969)[14] to register every death with the concerned State/UT Government within 21 days of its occurrence. If a death is not registered within 21 days of its occurrence, permission from the Registrar/Area Magistrate, along with the fee prescribed in case of late registration, is required.

Perinatal Death Certificate

When a baby is stillborn (born dead) after 24 weeks pregnancy, the stillbirth must be registered in the stillbirth register. The process for registering a stillbirth combines features of both birth and death registration in form 3.[14]

Death Declaration Certificate

Generally a physician must make the determination that a person is dead. The physician then makes a formal declaration of the death and a record of the time of death. In a hospital setting, the physician who declares the death may not be the one who signs the death certificate. The death certificate should document the immediate cause of death, which can be an event, clinical condition, or disease process, which is unsuitable for the continuation of life.[14]

Newborn Death Certificate

Birth and death dates may be very near to each other hence a goof up can take place. If death registration reaches before birth registration, problems may arise. See that birth is registered before death.[14]

Medical Certification of Death

Medical certification of cause of death is the medical doctor's responsibility for reporting of causes of death using a country's prescribed form that follows the World Health Organization standards. BDR Act Section 10(3) of the Act provides for issuing a certificate of the cause of death by the medical practitioner who has attended the deceased at the time of death. "Form of medical certificate of cause of death" is frequently incorporated into a form that includes other information required for administration purposes by national registration. It is sometimes referred to as "medical certificate", "cause of death certificate" or simply as "death certificate".[14]

■ SUMMARY

So in nutshell, obtaining consent in medicine is process that should include: (1) Describing the proposed intervention, (2) emphasizing the patient's role in decision-making, (3) discussing alternatives to the proposed intervention, and (4) healthcare practitioner should be discussing the risks of the proposed intervention with reference to patient socioeconomic and cultural perspective.

■ LEARNING KEY POINTS

- *False certificates:* Never issue fake certificates for absences, except for legitimate health reasons.
- *Unverified certificates:* Don't sign certificates without proper examination, especially for activities like sports, swimming, etc.
- *Epilepsy and water activities:* If a child has epilepsy, their swimming certificate should require lifeguard and coach supervision.
- *Certificates are legal:* They hold weight, treat them seriously.
- *Always record vitals:* Before signing health certificates, record weight, height, BP, pulse, and respiratory rate for children under routine medical care.
- *Vaccination records:* Ensure vaccination certificates for students traveling abroad match actual immunization records.

■ TAKE-HOME MESSAGES

- Medical certificate is legal document.
- Do not issue fake certificate. Do not issue >15 days period certificate at a time.
- It is not required to provide the diagnosis on a sick note if the patient does not wish so.
- A doctor should never issue a certificate that cannot be justified in court afterward.

- Clinical judgment must be used to determine the length of the absence.
- Repeat visits for issuing new certificates after 15 days necessary.

MUST AVOID THINGS

Never give false certificate to child to cover absence from school for other than health reasons.

DO NOT DO

Do not certify child without examining for permission sports or swimming or similar things.

WARNINGS

Certificate of waning epileptic child not swim without lifeguards and coach.

MESSAGES WHICH THE READER MUST BE AWARE

Certificates are not just a paper, they are legal documents.

MUST DO THING

Always record weigh, height, blood pressure (BP), pulse, respiratory rate, and head and chest circumferences before wring on school certificates needing them to be filled routinely.

MEDICAL NEGLIGENCE PEARLS

Vaccination certificates for adolescent traveling abroad for higher education should tally with actual records.

ONLY ONE FACT TO REMEMBER

Never ever oblige any parent with any kind of certificate unless in your opinion it should be given, otherwise do not give. Better refuse rather than be sorry later on.

REFERENCES

1. Baldwa M, Baldwa V, Padvi N, Baldwa S. Legal Issues in Medical Practice, 2nd edition. New Delhi: CBS Publishers and Distributors Pvt. Ltd.; 2023.
2. Baldwa M, Baldwa V, Padvi N, Baldwa S. Legal Issues in Critical Care, 1st edition. New Delhi: CBS Publishers and Distributors Pvt. Ltd.; 2022.
3. Scheil-Adlung X, Sandner L. Paid Sick Leave: Incidence, Patterns and Expenditure in Times of Crises. ESS paper: 27. Geneva: International Labour Office, Social Security Department; 2010.
4. Sharma P. (2017). Delhi Medical Council suspends doctors for issuing fake medical leave certs. [online] Available from: https://www.indiatoday.in/mail-today/story/delhi-medical-council-suspends-doctors-for-issuing-fake-medical-leave-certificates-1048361-2017-09-20. [Last accessed December, 2023].
5. The Economic Times. (2008). Employee can be sacked for unauthorized sick leave: SC. [online] Available from: https://economictimes.indiatimes.com/jobs/employee-can-be-sacked-for-unauthorised-sick-leave-sc/articleshow/2809286.cms?from=mdr. [Last accessed December, 2023].
6. Medical council of India. (2020) DMC guidelines for issuing a medical certificate. [online]. Available from: https://www.delhimedicalcouncil.org/images/New%20Doc%202019-11-29%2017.33.21.pdf. [Last accessed December, 2023].
7. NHS England. (2019). Fit Notes: A guide for hospital doctors. University Hospitals, Plymouth. [online]. Available from: https://www.england.nhs.uk/south/wp-content/uploads/sites/6/2019/03/fit-notes-briefing-a-guide-for-Hospital-Doctors.-V1.-FEB2019.pdf. [Last accessed December, 2023].

8. Medical Council of New South Wales. (2020). Medical certificates: what you should know. [online] Available from: https://www.mcnsw.org.au/medical-certificates-what-you-should-know. [Last accessed December, 2023].
9. Ganjapure V. (2012). Medical certificate not a complete proof of fitness: HC. [online] Available from: https://timesofindia.indiatimes.com/city/nagpur/Medical-certificate-not-a-complete-proof-of-fitness-HC/articleshow/17774953.cms. [Last accessed December, 2023].
10. Hindustan Times. (2007). Telgi, 2 doctors sentenced to 7 years in jail. [online] Available from: https://www.hindustantimes.com/india/telgi-2-doctors-sentenced-to-7-years-in-jail/story-QHbhmqlHxGpjBPiu1aRj0O.html. [Last accessed December, 2023].
11. Guideline 7 of National medical commission NMC's Professional Conduct for RMP-2023.
12. Daabiss M. American Society of Anaesthesiologists physical status classification. Indian J Anaesth. 2011;55(2):111-5.
13. Unique Disability ID. About Unique Disability ID. [online] Available from: https://www.swavlambancard.gov.in/. [Last accessed December, 2023].
14. The Registration of Births and Deaths Act, 1969.

SECTION 2

Consumer, Criminal Laws, Litigation Process, and Limiting Liability

- **Consumer Protection Act-2019**
  Mahesh Baldwa, Varsha Baldwa, Aishwarya Mantri, Sanjay Mishra

- **Application of Criminal Laws to Medical Practice**
  Ishita Banerji

- **Dealing with Civil Pre-Litigation and Litigation Process**
  Mahesh Baldwa, Varsha Baldwa, Namita Padvi, Vijay Arora

- **Limiting the Liability in Case of Alleged Medical Negligence**
  Jyoti Kumar Gupta, Shashikant Tripathi, Amrita Verma, Rajat Dubey

- **Outdoor and Indoor Practice Giving Rise to Legal Liabilities in Medical Practice**
  Ishita Banerji

- **Advance Deposit Before Admission and While Discharge Bill not Paid in Hospital**
  Hemant R Gangolia, Ramesh B Dampuri, Sanjio Borade

- **Landmark Supreme Court Judgments and Their Importance in Medicolegal Litigations**
  Jyoti Kumar Gupta, Ashish Jain, AB Jaiswal, Jitendra Pratap Singh Chauhan

2

Consumer, Criminal Law, Litigation and general personal liability

CHAPTER 8

Consumer Protection Act-2019

Mahesh Baldwa, Varsha Baldwa, Aishwarya Mantri, Sanjay Mishra

"As a doctor, you don't practice medicine; rather you become the medicine yourself".

Keywords: Consumer, Complaint, Dispute, Negligence, Services, Deficiency

Aim: To give bird's eye view of Consumer Protection Act.

Objective: A doctor who is aware of legal issues is forearmed in practice to prevent litigation in future with respect to Consumer Protection Act 2019.[1]

INTRODUCTION

The Consumer Protection Act, 2019 (CPA, 2019) is a landmark legislation in India that aims to protect the rights of consumers and establish a comprehensive framework for consumer protection. It repeals and replaces the CPA, 1986, and introduces several significant changes to strengthen consumer protection measures.

CONSUMER PROTECTION ACT

Mere repeal of the CPA 1986 Act by the CPA 2019 Act, without anything more, would not result in exclusion of "healthcare" services rendered by doctors to patients from the definition of the term "service" of "healthcare services" are not explicitly excluded unders. 2(42) of the CPA, 2019.[1] Hence "healthcare services" are within ambit of CPA, 2019.

No sooner CPA, 2019[1] is notified on 20th July 2020, its bad effects on doctors have become evident by seeing filing of cases against them for astronomical sum of money asked as compensation as can be seen by following example.

CPA 2019: COURT'S ATTITUDE IN VIEW OF ORIGINAL CPA 1986 AND AMENDED 2019

The CPA was implemented in 2019. Medical services were brought into its purview since 1995. Since then the doctor-patient relationship has deteriorated faster. Depending on the jurisdiction or scope of the claim, a consumer may go before the District Commission, State Commission, National Commission, and lastly the Supreme Court. The 2-year limitation period may be extended at the courts' discretion starting from cause of action. Recently in 2021 a PIL "Medicos Legal Action Group (MLAG) versus Union of India[2] (through Secretary, Department of Consumer Affairs, Ministry of Consumer Affairs, Food and Public Distribution) (High Court of Judicature at Bombay) Public Interest Litigation No. 58 OF 2021" was filed by a group "MLAG" seeking exemption of healthcare professionals from CPA 2019.

This PIL was rejected by Bombay High Court on 25-10-2021[2] and reaffirmed IMA versus V.P Shantha and Ors. III, (1996) CPJ I (SC).[3] The Bombay High Court even imposed the fine of ₹50,000/- against this group MLAG. This cleared the position of CPA 2019 that it still covers healthcare professional. The matter as SLP under article 136 was rejected by Honorable Supreme Court of India on 29-04-2022.[4]

Following sections are important from point of view doctors:

- *Section 2 (6) "complaint"* means any allegation in writing. An unfair contract or unfair trade practice or a restrictive trade practice has been adopted by any trader or service provider; the services hired or availed of or agreed to be hired or availed of by him suffer from any deficiency;
- *Section 2 (7) "consumer"* means any person who hires or avails of any service for a consideration which has been paid or promised or partly paid and partly promised.
- *Section 2 (8) "consumer dispute"* means a dispute where the person against whom a complaint has been made, denies, or disputes the allegations contained in the complaint;
- *Section 2 (11) "deficiency"* means any fault, imperfection, shortcoming, or inadequacy in the quality, nature, and manner of performance. Any act of negligence or omission or commission by such person which causes loss or injury to the consumer; like disclosing confidential information.

This means:
- New causes of deficiency of service
- Disclosing confidential information of patient
- Not giving indoor case paper, discharge card

- Consumer Protection (E-Commerce) Rules, 2020[5] shall guide advertisements and how it will affect doctors?
  - Penalties for misleading advertisements 2(28)
  - Penalties for endorsing services s. 2(18)
  - No cure-no fees–as such it is illegal
  - Beware—in vitro fertilization (IVF) and hair transplant
  - First offense—10 lakh fine with 2 years jail
  - Subsequent offense—50 lakh fine with 5 years prison.

IMPORTANCE OF SECTION 2(42) FROM DOCTOR'S POINT OF VIEW—SERVICE, NEGLIGENCE, DEFICIENCY OF SERVICE, AND UNFAIR TRADE PRACTICE

- *Section 2 (42) "service"* means service of any description which is made available to potential users and includes, but not limited to................... but does not include the rendering of any service free of charge or under a contract of personal service.
  - "Healthcare" not defined and omitted by legislative wing not binding on judicial wing.
  - Legislative wing omitted healthcare in new CPA 2019 is not binding on judiciary.
  - Definition of Service Under section 2(42) of CPA 2019.
  - In 1995, three judges bench the Supreme Court in the IMA versus VP Shantha case held that patients are consumers as long as they are making some form of payment for the medical service rendered. So this judgment

is not repealed by CPA 2019. Under article 141 of constitution all previous judgments shall remain in force till they are overruled by the Supreme Court. Hence, CPA 2019 is applicable to doctors. A PIL of 2021,[2] filed by a group that healthcare professionals are not under CPA 2019 which was rejected by Bombay High Court and imposed the fine of ₹50,000/- and same was upheld by Supreme Court of India in 2022.[4]

- *Constitutional validity of CPA*: Judicial wing SC decided constitutional validity of CPA 1986 in 2003, State of Karnataka versus Vishwabarathi CHSL, AIR 2003 SC 1043: (2003) 2 SCC 412,[6] DB bench of HC Karnataka upholding constitutional validity of the CPA 1986, which was challenged in SC-applies to CPA 2019.
- CPA 2019 also applies to "unfair trade practice" as per Section 2 (47) wherein "unfair trade practice" means a trade practice which, for the purpose of promoting the sales.
- Procedures for doctors with respect to jurisdiction, written statement, evidence, and written arguments in section 34, 47.
- *Revised pecuniary jurisdiction*:[7] Limit up to which money actually spent by complainant as in CPA 2019, it does not depend upon "compensation asked" as was in old CPA 1986 **(Table 1)**.

- The following change will occur because of new CPA:
  - Patient can file case in territorial jurisdiction of where one lives or works for gain as per section 34 for district, 47 for state.
  - Charges borne by Insurance Company/Employer/Mediclaim/Ayushman Bharat/RSBY are not service rendered free of charge.
  - So, expect increase in cases against doctors.
  - No capping on filing on amount of claim capping on filing on amount of claim—now it will be nearing to 1 crore.
- Every complaint shall be disposed of as expeditiously as possible and endeavor shall be made to decide the complaint within a period of 3 months.

WHAT DOCTORS CAN DO TO TAKE ADVANTAGE OF CPA 2019

- To avoid the awkward commission holding you responsible as "res ipsa loquitur" kindly submit degree, registration, outpatient department/inpatient department (OPD/IPD), discharge card, medical literature, eye witness, and expert witness.
- To avoid the awkward commission holding you responsible as "negligence", "Deficiency of service" and "unfair trade practice" for a known complication, kindly explain the complication and

TABLE 1: Revised pecuniary jurisdiction.

Revised from 30-12-2021-new limits[7]	Consumer commission	Section of CPA 2019	Old limits from 20-07-2020 to 29-12-2021
Up to ₹50 lakh	District Commission	Section 34	Up to ₹1 crore
50 lakhs to ₹2 crore	State Commission	Section 47	Up to ₹10 crore
More than ₹2 crore	National Commission	Section 58	More than ₹10 crore
(CPA: Consumer Protection Act)			

support it with the medical literature and expert witness.
- Is commission justified in levying interest on awarded amount beyond 3 months?
- Doctor cannot be held responsible for delay? *Answer is NO.*
- New India Assurance Co. Ltd. versus Hilli Multipurpose Cold Storage Pvt. Ltd.[8]—5 JJ, Constitution bench, of the Apex Court in March, 2020 said with respect to old CPA 1986 for s. 13 (iii) (3a) provides for deciding every complaint as expeditiously as possible and endeavor shall be made to decide the complaint within a period of three months from the receipt of notice by the opposite party. This is similar to Section 37(7) of CPA 2019, reaffirmed in Dr A. Suresh Kumar versus Amit Agarwal (SC), 2021(225) AIC 141: 2021(148) ALR 693: 2021(4) KLT 338.[9]

PROVISIONS FOR REVISION PETITION IS REMOVED AND REPLACED BY APPEALS BY SECTION 41, 47, 58

- *Expert witness:* Doctors point of view experts to assist-Section 66 for class action-experts to assist National Commission or State Commission.
- *Limitation Period-Section 69:* The District Commission, the State Commission or the National Commission shall not admit a complaint unless it is filed within 2 years from the date on which the cause of action has arisen.
  - Normally all cases—2 years mandatory
  - Optional—children limitation—reaching age of 18 years + 24 months depends on case
  - Appeals from District Commission to State Commission-45 days-mandatory
  - Appeals from State Commission to National Commission-30 days-mandatory
  - Appeals from National Commission to State Commission-30 days-mandatory
  - Kindly preserve the records for the period of 24 months from the point of CPA 2019-mandatory
- *Mediation:* The Consumer Protection (Mediation) Rules, 2020 shall guide about it along with following sections:
  - Mediation not available for medical negligence cases with death and grievous injury but is available for other cases-one has to apply within 5 days of launching of case or submission of written statement.
  - The decision reached if any by mediation shall be the order
  - If no decision is reached then continue hearing as usual
- *These sections have been removed from New CPA 2019 which is bad for doctor.*
  - No punishment for false and vexatious complaint.
  - Removal of Section 26 of old CPA 1986.[10]

CRIMINAL LAW AND CIVIL LAWS AND COMPLAINT TO OTHER AUTHORITIES CAN RUN SIDE BY SIDE

In many situations, criminal law and civil laws can both apply simultaneously without canceling each other out. These two legal options are not opposites, but rather complement each other and have distinct differences in their application and outcomes.

NEGLIGENCE AS A TORT

A tort is a type of civil wrong that does not fall under any specific category. The law dictates the duties that must be upheld and followed in tort, with the primary duty being to not cause harm to others. These duties are owed to the general public, known as rights in rem. If a tort has been committed, compensation can be sought through filing for unliquidated damages. It is also possible for a situation to involve both tort and contract liability, such as when a doctor has a contract with a patient and is also found to be negligent, resulting in liability under both contract and tort law.

NEGLIGENCE OF OMISSION AND COMMISSION UNDER TORT

Negligence in tort law can be defined in various ways. It refers to either failing to do what a reasonable medical professional would do in a similar situation or doing something that a prudent and reasonable medical professional would not do. The determination of negligence depends on the knowledge and circumstances of the parties involved. Conduct that does not meet the "standard of care" and poses an unreasonable risk of harm can be considered negligent.

NONINTENTIONAL NEGLIGENCE UNDER TORT CANNOT REDUCE COMPENSATION

Intention of doctor in not causing injury is unimportant. Intention or no intention of doing the wrong under law of tort makes no difference. If tort is proved then it needs to be equitably compensated.

CASE IN MEDICAL COUNCIL

If there is a complaint against a doctor, it can be filed with the relevant medical council. However, these councils do not have the authority to provide compensation or imprisonment. They can only issue warnings, suspend, or revoke the doctor's license.

WHAT IS VICARIOUS LIABILITY?

Literally vicar means a member of the clergy deputizing for another in church. Vicarious, literally means substitute. Vicarious liability is an important legal principle. It is the liability you may have for the acts and omissions of an employee or some other individual for whose conduct you are legally responsible. He who does an act through another is in law deemed to have done it himself. Liability for another's wrongful acts or omission can arise in following:

- When the liability is ratified
- When the liability accrues by abetment
- When the liability arises out of a special relationship.

Delegation of medical work to junior medical professionals, compounders, nurses (be those qualified or unqualified staff), employed or contracted or on profit sharing basis, the medical professional owes vicarious liability to patient on the basis of sound legal principle that one can delegate medical work not responsibility.

DOCTRINE OF RESPONDENT SUPERIOR

The legal concept of vicarious liability and the Doctrine of Respondent Superior occurs when the servant (employee) commits a tort or civil wrong within the scope of employment and the master (employer) is held liable although the master may have done nothing wrong. Physicians as employers need to be aware of this doctrine in the supervision of their staff and their day-to-day medical practice.

How to handle free service, not charged, government hospitals where free service given, semi-private hospitals, corporate with reserved free beds, charitable hospitals, and charitable OPDs?

1. Indian Medical Association versus VP Shantha, AIR 1996 SC 550[3] and Union of

India and Ors. versus N. K. Srivastava and Ors. 2020 SCC OnLine SC 636[11] makes it clear that free medical services across the board in all departments are not within ambit of *CPA, 2019*.
2. Some free medical services, some charged, or partially charged medical services in all departments are within ambit of *CPA, 2019*.
3. Just one patient is not charged does not make you to wriggle out of the ambit of *CPA, 2019*.
4. Corporate with reserved free beds are within ambit of *CPA, 2019*.
5. Government hospitals where free service given are not within ambit of *CPA, 2019*.
6. Charitable hospitals and charitable OPDs are not within ambit of *CPA, 2019*.

Differences between CPA, 1986 and CPA, 2019 are given in **Table 2**.

SUMMARY

The CPA of 2019 has no positive move for doctors. The act contains a number of new concepts that were urgently required. In the world of digitalization, steps like proceedings through video conferencing, and e-filing of cases will significantly improve, develop, and

TABLE 2: Differences between Consumer Protection Act, 1986 and Consumer Protection Act, 2019.[12,13]

S. No.	Basis	Consumer Protection Act, 1986	Consumer Protection Act, 2019
1	Ambit of law	All goods and services for consideration, while free and personal services are excluded	All goods and services, including telecom and housing construction, and all modes of transactions (online, teleshopping, etc.) for consideration. Free and personal services are excluded
2	Unfair trade practices (defined as deceptive practices to promote the sale, use or supply of a good or service)	Includes six types of such practices, like false representation, misleading advertisements	The new Act adds three types of practices to the list, namely: Failure to issue a bill or receipt; refusal to accept a good returned within 30 days; and disclosure of personal information given in confidence, unless required by law or in public interest. Contests/lotteries may be notified as not falling under the ambit of unfair trade practices
3	Product liability	No provision	Claim for product liability can be made against manufacturer, service provider, and seller. Compensation can be obtained by proving one of the several specified conditions in the Act
4	Unfair contracts	No provision	Defined as contracts that cause significant change in consumer rights. Lists six contract terms which may be held as unfair
5	Central Protection Councils (CPCs)	CPCs promote and protect the rights of consumers. They are established at the district, state, and national level	The new Act makes CPCs advisory bodies for promotion and protection of consumer rights. Establishes CPCs at the District, State, and National Level

Contd...

Contd…

S. No.	Basis	Consumer Protection Act, 1986	Consumer Protection Act, 2019
6	Regulator	No provision	Establishes the Central Consumer Protection Authority (CCPA) to promote, protect, and enforce the rights of consumers as a class. CCPA may issue safety notices; pass orders to recall goods, prevent unfair practices, and reimburse purchase price paid; and impose penalties for false and misleading advertisements
7	Pecuniary jurisdiction of commissions	District: Up to ₹20 lakh; State: Between ₹20 lakh and up to ₹1 crore; National: Above ₹1 crore	District: Up to ₹50 lakhs; State: Between ₹50 lakhs and ₹2 crore; National: Above ₹2 crore
8	Composition of commissions	District: Headed by current or former District Judge and two members. State: Headed by a current or former High Court Judge and at least two members. National: Headed by a current or former Supreme Court Judge and at least four members	District: Headed by a president and at least two members. State: Headed by a president and at least four members. National: Headed by a president and at least four members
9	Appointment	Selection committee (comprising a judicial member and other officials) will recommend members on the commissions	No provision for selection committee. Central Government will appoint through notification
10	Alternate dispute redressal mechanism	No provision	Mediation cells will be attached to the District, State, and National Commissions
11	Penalties	If a person does not comply with orders of the commissions, he may face imprisonment between 1 month and 3 years or fine between ₹2,000 and ₹10,000, or both	If a person does not comply with orders of the commissions, he may face imprisonment up to 3 years, or a fine not less than ₹25,000 extendable to ₹1 lakh, or both
12	E-commerce	No provision	Defines direct selling, e-commerce and electronic service provider. The central government may prescribe rules for preventing unfair trade practices in e-commerce and direct selling

upgrade consumer rights to great heights. In order to make any law successful, it is pertinent to see that it is implemented hassle-free and effectively for both doctors and patients.

Doctors should neither injure nor aggravate preexisting ailments or illnesses. And if they do, court wants them to explain what bad repercussions can occur. Simultaneously, good doctors should not be punished for doing nothing wrong. While these ideas appear simple, they are more challenging in practice. There are several defenses available to medical professionals accused of malpractice. The doctor may claim that his treatment was in conformity with medical standards or that the patient's injuries were not caused by a medical error.

Medical doctors cannot be blamed for injury due to negligence. If a medical professional can demonstrate that the damage would not have occurred if the patient had not been careless, he or she may have a legitimate defense against a malpractice claim.

Of course, the doctor must first inform the patient of the risks (failing to fully notify a patient about potential dangers can lead to a lack of informed consent charge). This is referred to as Bolam law. If a doctor helps someone in an emergency, he or she is immune from civil liability if something goes wrong during the rescue. In principle, a medical professional who voluntarily serves another person owes that person the same duty of care and treatment that a reasonably competent physician would under the same or similar circumstances.[4,5]

LEARNING KEY POINTS

- If doctors *conduct which falls short of "standard of care" leading to unreasonable risk of harm is negligence.*
- Intention of doctor in not causing injury is unimportant. Intention or no intention of doing the wrong under law of tort makes no difference. If tort is proved then it needs to be equitably compensated.
- To demonstrate causation in tort law, the patient party must establish that the loss they have suffered was caused by the defendant doctor.
- Novus actus interveniens (new intervening act), this may break the chain of causation removing liability from the defendant doctor. The legal test applicable will depend upon whether the new act was that of a third party or an act of the patient party.
- Medical negligence calls for a comparative high degree of care which is expected from a doctor of a reasonable degree.
- The standard of care is not of an ordinary prudent man but of an ordinary prudent doctor who belongs to that category to which the doctor belong who is to be judged by that standard.
- A balance is required to be made between the rights of the patients and the rights of the doctors.
- It is essential to open the doors for the new ways of treatment and for securing the rights of the patients.

MUST AVOID THINGS

Avoid low standard of care as to compare ordinary prudent doctor who belongs to that category.

DO NOT DO

Doctor's conduct should not falls short of "standard of care" lead to unreasonable risk of harm is negligence.

WARNINGS

Intention of doctor in not causing injury is unimportant. Intention or no intention of doing the wrong under law of tort makes no difference. If tort is proved then it needs to be equitably compensated.

MESSAGES WHICH THE READER MUST BE AWARE

Look for if the complaint is time-barred.

MUST DO THING

One can submit eye and expert witness without being asked by consumer court.

MEDICAL NEGLIGENCE PEARLS

Novus actus interveniens (new intervening act), this may break the chain of causation removing liability from the defendant doctor. The legal test applicable will depend upon whether the new act was that of a third party or an act of the patient party.

ONLY ONE FACT TO REMEMBER

No punishment for false and vexatious consumer complaint.

REFERENCES

1. Consumer Protection Act, 2019.
2. Medicos Legal Action Group (MLAG) versus Union of India.
3. IMA versus V.P Shantha and Ors. III, (1996) CPJ I (SC).
4. Medicos Legal Action Group (MLAG) versus Union of India in Supreme Court of India 29-04-2022.
5. Consumer Protection (E-Commerce) Rules, 2020.
6. State of Karnataka versus Vishwabarathi CHSL, AIR 2003 SC 1043: (2003) 2 SCC 412.
7. Revised pecuniary jurisdiction of Consumer Protection Act 2019 from 30-12-2021.
8. New India Assurance Co. Ltd. versus. Hilli Multipurpose Cold Storage Pvt. Ltd.
9. Dr A. Suresh Kumar versus Amit Agarwal (SC), 2021(225) AIC 141: 2021(148) ALR 693: 2021(4) KLT 338.
10. Removal of Section 26 of old Consumer protection act 1986.
11. Union of India and Ors. versus N. K. Srivastava and Ors. 2020 SCC OnLine SC 636.
12. Baldwa M, Baldwa V, Padvi N, Baldwa S. Legal Issues in Medical Practice, 2nd edition. New Delhi: CBS Publishers and Distributors Pvt. Ltd.; 2023.
13. Baldwa M, Baldwa V, Padvi N, Baldwa S. Legal Issues in Critical Care, 1st edition. New Delhi: CBS Publishers and Distributors Pvt. Ltd.; 2022.

CHAPTER 9

Application of Criminal Law to Medical Practice

Ishita Banerji

Law is like a Rubik's Cube—just when you think you have solved it, it twists again.

Keywords: Criminal, Fine, Gross and reckless, Imprisonment, Mens rea

Aim: This chapter aims to equip doctors with an understanding of criminal law in order to avoid criminal liability for medical negligence as per the law thus far, under Section 304 A Indian Penal Code (IPC), 1860, which is being replaced by section 106 subsection 1 of the Bharatiya Nyaya Sanhita, 2023.

Objective: In the duty of medical care doctors should always be diligent in their conduct and never be mindlessly reckless to cause any harm or injury to their patients.

INTRODUCTION

This chapter highlights the criminal laws applicable to medical practice that will help medical professionals stay abreast of the problem and be aware of the privileges and defenses available to them. While Criminal Law applies to all individuals and doctors are no exception to it, the circumstances under which a physician attracts criminal proceedings against himself are peculiar. A physician usually attracts criminal negligence when a patient dies in the course of his treatment if malafide intention or gross negligence can be proved. So far, criminal liability could be fastened pursuant to the provisions of the Indian Penal Code (IPC), 1860, which were general in nature and did not provide specifically for "medical negligence". The Code of Criminal Procedure (CrPC), 1973 provided for the procedure for arrest, prosecution, and bail for offenses under various sections of the IPC, 1860.

A NEW ACT

On August 11, 2023 the Central Government introduced three new Bills in the Lok Sabha, namely, Bharatiya Nyaya Sanhita (BNS), 2023 to replace the Indian Penal Code (IPC), 1860; Bharatiya Nagarik Suraksha Sanhita (BNSS), 2023 to replace the Code of Criminal Procedure (CrPC), 1973; and Bharatiya Sakshya Sanhita, 2023 to replace the Indian Evidence Act, 1872. The bills were subsequently referred to the Standing Committee of the Parliament for review. Pursuant to the recommendations of the Standing Committee the Bills were withdrawn from the Parliament and revised versions were introduced as the Bhartiya Nyaya Sanhita (Second) Bill, 2023 (BNS II) and the Bhartiya Nagarik Suraksha (Second) Sanhita Bill, 2023 (BNSS II), and the Bhartiya Sakshya Sanhita Bill, 2023.

On the 20th of December 2023, the Union Home Minister announced a proposed official amendment aimed at freeing doctors from criminal prosecution under Section 304A, which had been treated as a charge almost equivalent to murder. The proposed amendment sought to decriminalize cases of death resulting from medical negligence. It is worth noting that a significant number of criminal cases involve doctors in situations where patients have passed away due to medical negligence. The decriminalization of medical negligence was seen as a positive step that could enable doctors to make appropriate and confident treatment decisions, especially for critically ill patients.

The announcement of this legislative intent, particularly coming from the Union Home Minister, brought considerable relief and optimism within the medical community. Doctors wondered whether this intent would be reflected in judicial interpretations in a manner aligned with their own perception.

Similar excitement had been observed previously among the medical community when there was speculation about the legislative intent to exclude Healthcare Services from the scope of the Consumer Protection Act. However, this hope was dashed when subsequent judicial pronouncements clarified the situation, confirming that such exclusion was not in place.

Once again, the optimism and hope within the medical community were short-lived, as the final bill passed by both houses did little to alter the existing criminal law concerning medical negligence. Finally, the act received the assent of the President on the 25th of December, 2023 and it was published in the Gazette of India.

It is crucial to clarify that even if "causing death by medical negligence" had been removed from the legal framework, it would not have made the entire criminal justice system irrelevant, nor would it have eliminated all potential criminal actions against doctors within the system. Various other acts, such as PCPNDT, MTP, POCSO, surrogacy, adoption, and more, still remain in effect and continue to govern criminal law cases. These sections of criminal law regulations remain operational and play a significant role in addressing various aspects of medical and legal matters.

Meanwhile, the fate of doctors in relation to potential criminal proceedings for medical negligence remains unchanged by the Act and its applicability. The relevance of this chapter continues to persist in the light of these ongoing developments.

CAUTION

Bharatiya Nyaya Sanhita (BNS), 2023 is to replace the Indian Penal Code (IPC), 1860; Bharatiya Nagarik Suraksha Sanhita (BNSS), 2023 is to replace the Code of Criminal Procedure (CrPC), 1973; and Bharatiya Sakshya Sanhita, 2023 is to replace the Indian Evidence Act, 1872.

CRIMINAL LAWS

Neither the IPC, 1860 nor the BNS, 2023 provide any specific law for "medical negligence" per se. So far, the most common section applicable to medical negligence was Section 304A of IPC, which dealt with the death of a person by any rash or negligent act leading to imprisonment of up to 2 years or fine. It was primarily used to deal with cases of rash and negligent motor vehicle driving and eventually implied on medical negligence cases leading to the death of a patient as well.

Previously, the BNS, 2023 proposal under clause 104 imposed a harsher 7-year sentence for deaths caused by negligence. Thankfully, after considering Parliament Standing Committee recommendations, the penalty has been reduced to 5 years under clause 106(1) of the revised BNS II. Additionally, a tougher sentence of up to 10 years is specified in clause 106(2) for negligent acts involving failure to report the offense or fleeing the scene in cases of rash and negligent driving.

The inclusion of the phrase "rash and negligent driving of a vehicle" within the aggravated offense under clause 106(2) offers a clarity that this harsher penalty will not apply to medical negligence cases.

However, a crucial ambiguity remains in the lesser offense defined under clause 106(1). This subsection lacked the specific limitation to driving, which caused initial concern among the medical community about the possible loopholes for criminal prosecution in negligence-related deaths.

Fortunately, subsequent amendments to clause 106(1) addressed this uncertainty. Media reports confirmed the addition of a clause specifically stating that "registered medical practitioners performing medical *procedures*" will face a maximum 2-year imprisonment *and* fine upon causing death through negligence. Though the amendment provides the much needed reassurance, two things remain uncertain. One, if it is specified for "registered medical practitioners performing medical procedures" then what about other cases? Second, "... 2 year imprisonment and fine upon causing death through negligence". implies that the option of fine has been removed and now imprisonment and fine both shall be slapped.

Therefore, while the revised BNS II offers some positive developments regarding medical negligence and potential criminal charges, it is essential to remain aware of the nuances and potential interpretations of the law. Consulting legal professionals for further guidance is recommended for those seeking a deeper understanding of their rights and responsibilities within the new legal framework.

Several other general provisions of IPC, such as Section 337, causing hurt and Section 338, causing grievous hurt, both covered under section 125 of the BNS are also often deployed in medical negligence cases.[1] Thus, to assume that doctors will never be liable under criminal law for medical negligence shall remain a wishful thinking.

IPC SECTIONS 304 AND 304A

In the judgment of the Bombay High Court in *Dr Mrs Mrudula S Deshpande vs. State of Maharashtra*, Section 304 was converted to 304A. In the said case judgments passed by the Orissa High Court in *Dr Debendranath Tripathi versus State of Orissa*, by the Allahabad High Court in *Ram Niwas versus State of UP*, and by the Supreme Court in *Juggan Khan versus The State of Madhya Pradesh* were relied upon citing that the courts have consistently been of the view that if a patient dies on account of the negligence of doctors, during operation or medical treatment then the case would generally come under section 304A of IPC. The basic difference is in mens rea or criminal intent to cause death in Section 304 of IPC.[2]

FIRST INFORMATION REPORT

First information report (FIR) may be lodged at the police station for a cognizable offence on the face of it under Section 154 of CrPC (Section 173 BNSS II), by patients or relatives against medical professionals, which initiates criminal proceedings. Complaints for non-cognizable offences may be made in the court of the Judicial Magistrate. The police may detain the doctor without a warrant for a cognizable offence. Article 22 of the Constitution of India bestows the right to the detainee to be informed about the grounds of arrest and the right to consult and be defended by a lawyer of his choice. Section 38 of the BNSS states that any person arrested by the police shall be entitled to meet an advocate of his choice during interrogation. Further, Section 48 of BNSS has recommended an obligation on the person making an arrest to inform about the arrest to a relative or friend. Further under Section 162 of CrPC (Section 181 BNSS) statement made to police should not be signed nor can it be used in trial. Article 20(3) of the Constitution of India protects against self-incrimination, i.e., not be compelled to witness against himself.

PRIVILEGE TO MEDICAL PRACTITIONER IN ARREST AND LODGING FIR

In the landmark judgment of *Jacob Mathew versus State of Punjab, (2005) 6 SCC 1*, Hon'ble Supreme Court in order to protect the doctors from frivolous and unjust prosecutions held that the investigating officer before proceeding against a doctor should obtain an independent medical opinion preferably from a doctor in government service qualified in that branch of medical practice that a prima facie case exists, for an impartial and unbiased opinion applying Bolam's test to the facts. Medical professionals have the therapeutic privilege to adopt a particular course of treatment that finds acceptance amongst a reasonable body of medical men skilled in that art, even though there is another body of medical men who opine differently or hold adverse opinions. This in the legal world is called the Bolam's test. The Apex Court also held that the arrest may be withheld unless inevitable for furthering the investigation, collection of evidence, or when the doctor is not cooperating. In another landmark judgment of *Lalita Kumari versus Government of UP*, it was held that while registration of FIR was mandatory under Section 154 of CrPC (Section 173 BNSS) for cognizable offences, an exception was taken for cases of allegations of medical negligence wherein preliminary inquiry was permitted. Subsection 3 of clause 173 added in the BNSS includes a preliminary inquiry in certain cognizable offences. In a medical negligence case, the Tis Hazari Court opined that an FIR could not be lodged on the whims and fancies of the complainant guided by unfounded and unsubstantiated assumptions only to satisfy his discontentment with the treatment of his child.[3]

In the wake of the tragic incident of the suicide of Dr Archana Sharma following an FIR against her after a patient's death at her hospital in Dausa, the Rajasthan government has issued a new Standard Operating Procedure (SOP) for the state regarding the registration of FIR mandating approval of senior police officers and an opinion of medical board, suggesting gross medical negligence before arrest of medical professionals. The SOP further requires videography of postmortem examination.[4]

While the amended clause 106(1) of BNS 2023 is explicit on prescribing punishment for deaths due to medical negligence, no corresponding procedural change is noted in the BNSS 2023, for lodging of FIRs against doctors in such cases as advocated by the Supreme Court in the above landmark judgments.

LEGAL REMEDIES

Several IPC sections protect doctors from allegations of negligence yet none is specific enough to hold teeth. Currently, the legal remedies revolve around two landmark judgments of the Supreme Court, namely *Dr Suresh Gupta versus NCT of Delhi* and *Jacob Mathew versus State of Punjab*,[5] the guidelines of which were later reiterated in 2009 in the *Martin D'Souza versus Mohd Ishfaq* case. Jacob Mathew's judgment was a weighty judgment with a large bench strength with greater consultative value in itself. Two questions of law took center stage. (1) Is there a difference in civil and criminal law on the concept of negligence? (2) Whether a different standard is applicable for recording a finding of negligence when a professional, in particular a doctor, is to be held guilty of negligence. The following observations were made:

Attributing criminal liability to a professional: The principle of negligence in criminal and civil law is the same, that is, the conduct fails to meet the reasonable standard.[6] While the amount of damages incurred determines liability in tort; in criminal law, it is the higher degree of negligence. Thus, it was observed that even though "gross" is not a requirement of section 304A of IPC, the factor of the grossness of degree does assume significance. Even the BNS Bill 2023 that was recently passed by both the houses in the Parliament, the amended clause 106(1) of BNS for medical negligence still does not feature the word "gross" to help differentiate civil and criminal liability. In such a scenario, we shall continue to fall back on these landmark judgments and on judicial interpretations.

Negligence by professionals: The principle of negligence when applied to professionals undergoes greater refinement as they possess special skills, education, knowledge, and training and are scrutinized by the Professional Regulatory Body before admitting them into the profession. A professional is liable if he does not possess the requisite skill professed to have possessed, or did not exercise the skill he possesses with reasonable competence.

Benchmark of negligence: Law requires to compare the actual alleged act to that of the expected reasonable act, as the benchmark to determine negligence. The reasonable standard is an average between the highest and the lowest standard or that of an ordinary competent person exercising ordinary skill in that profession. However, in dealing with professional negligence the reasonable standard is judged by the lowest standard that would be regarded as acceptable.

Therapeutic privilege: Genuine difference of opinion is not negligence as long as he is performing his duties to the best of his ability and with due care and caution.

The error of judgment: The higher the acuteness of an emergency, the higher its complications and the more the chances of errors. The Apex Court has repeatedly held that an error of judgment is no negligence unless reckless disregard is shown with greater deviation from the accepted practice.

Professional reputation: The SC observed that no sensible professional would intentionally commit an act or omission, which would result in loss or injury to the patient as the professional reputation of the person is also at stake.

Professional versus ordinary men of skill: The SC opined that professional and ordinary men of skill are not intended to be treated equally by the framers of IPC and held that the word "gross" is to be suffixed in Section 304A of IPC in the case of medical professionals to criminally implicate a medical practitioner. However, no such change is seen in the recent BNS 2023 act. It remains to be seen how the amended clause 106(1) of the BNS 2023 qualifies the rash and negligent act in cases of death due to medical negligence, for invoking criminal liability is interpreted. However, it is necessary that the death should have been the direct result of a rash and negligent act of the accused which must be the proximate and efficient cause without the intervention of another's negligence.[1]

DEFENSES AVAILABLE IN CRIMINAL CASES TO MEDICAL PRACTITIONER

Certain IPC sections that protect doctors from allegations of negligence are:

- *Section 80 (Section 18 BNS):* It provides for accidents without any criminal intention while performing a lawful act in a lawful manner by lawful means with proper care and caution.
- *Section 81 (Section 19 BNS):* It provides for acts likely to cause harm, but done without any criminal intent, in good faith, to prevent other harms. For example, amputating a gangrenous body part.
- *Section 87, 88 (Section 25, 26 BNS):* It provides for acts not intended to cause death, done by consent, in good faith for the person's benefit. For example, a surgeon undertaking a risky operation.
- *Section 89 (Section 27 BNS):* It provides for acts intended in good faith for the benefit of a child or insane person done after obtaining consent from the lawful guardians.
- *Section 92 (Section 30 BNS):* It provides for acts done in good faith (in an emergency) for the benefit of a person without consent.
- *Section 93 (Section 31 BNS):* It provides for communication made in good faith for the benefit of the person if any harm is to occur to such a person.

LEGAL PROVISIONS

The legal provisions related to Medical Professionals through relevant Sections of IPC with corresponding BNS sections are:

- Section 29 (Section 2(8) BNS) defines "Document".
- Section 52 (Section 2(11) BNS) for "Good faith".
- Section 90 (Section 28 BNS) for consent given under fear/misconception of facts.
- Section 269-270 (Sections 271-272 BNS) for Negligent and Malignant Act likely to spread infection.
- Section 271 (Section 273 BNS) for disobedience to quarantine rule.
- Sections 272-276 (Sections 274-278 BNS) for adulteration and sale of food, drink, and drugs.
- Section 304 (Section 105 BNS) for causing death by a rash or negligent act with intention to cause death not amounting to culpable homicide.
- Section 304A (Section 106(1) BNS) for causing death by rash or negligent act not amounting to culpable homicide. Proposed to be applicable for death due to medical negligence with imprisonment up to 2 years.
- Sections 306-308 (Sections 108-110 BNS) are related to the abetment of suicide.
- Section 309 for attempt to commit suicide has been repealed in BNSS.
- Sections 312-314 (Sections 88-90 BNS) are related to MTP.
- Sections 315-316 (Sections 91-92 BNS) are related to feticide/infanticide.
- Section 491 (Section 357 BNS) to Breach of Contract.
- Sections 141-143 (Sections 189-190 BNS) for unlawful assembly (forceful entry into the hospital).
- Sections 319, 321 (Sections 114, 115 BNS) for hurt.
- Sections 320, 322 (Sections 116, 117 BNS) for grievous hurt.
- Sections 332-333 (Section 121 BNS) for voluntarily causing hurt/grievous hurt to a public servant.
- Sections 336-338 (Section 125 BNS) for causing hurt by rash or negligent act.

- Section 339–342 (Section 126–127 BNS) for wrongful restraint and wrongful confinement.
- Sections 352–353 (Sections 131–132 BNS) for assault or criminal force on a public servant.
- Section 427 (Section 324 BNS) for mischief causing damage (damage to property and equipment).
- Section 499 (Section 356 BNS) for defamation.
- Section 503 (Section 351 BNS) for criminal intimidation (threat to duty doctor).
- Section 504, 506 (Section 352 BNS) for intentional insult and provocation (use of abusive language, misbehavior with doctor/nurse/staff) and punishment for criminal intimidation.

BAIL PROVISIONS

Before detailing the bail provisions, it is prudent to understand a few legal terminologies.
- *Cognizable offences:* Offences for which the police are empowered to arrest without a warrant.
- *Noncognizable offences:* Offences for which prior permission of the court is required for an arrest.
- *Bailable offence:* Relatively less serious offences listed as bailable in the first schedule of CrPC for which bail is granted by the police or court that are generally punishable with imprisonment for or less than 3 years.
- *Nonbailable offence:* Serious offences not listed as bailable with higher quantum of punishment for which bail is granted only on the discretion of the court.
- *Bail:* The police is bound by subsection (1) of Section 50 CrPC (Section 47 BNSS) to inform the accused doctor of the reasons for arrest and by its subsection (2) to the legal right to be released on bail. Under Section 57 CrPC (Section 58 BNSS) and 167 CrPC (Section 187 BNSS), the police are bound to present the accused doctor before the nearest magistrate within 24 hours of his arrest.[7]
- *Anticipatory bail:* Section 438(1) of CrPC (clause 482 BNSS) empowers the High Court and Sessions Court to grant anticipatory bail on reasonable apprehensions of being arrested on charges of a nonbailable offence.[8] However, it does not apply to crimes that cannot be erased with bail.

SUMMARY

During the Lok Sabha debate on December 20, 2023, the Home Minister addressed the passage of three bills: The Bharatiya Nyaya Sanhita, Bharatiya Nagarik Suraksha Sanhita, and Bharatiya Sakshya Sanhita 2023. In this session, the Home Minister discussed the government's plan to introduce an amendment that would exclude doctors from criminal prosecution in cases of death caused by medical negligence, responding to a request from the Indian Medical Association. However, upon examining the BNS II Bill, which had already been passed by both houses, no such exemption was found.

Instead, an amended clause was eventually added to subsection 1 of clause 106 of the BNS II Bill. To understand the distinction between the existing archaic law, as represented by Section 304A of the IPC, 1860, which had been in effect until this point for deaths due to medical negligence, and the new amended section 106(1) of BNS 2023, which specifically addresses medical negligence, it is essential to closely examine these laws:

- *Section 304A IPC, 1860:* This section deals with causing death by negligence. It states that whoever causes the death of any person by engaging in a reckless or negligent act, which does not amount to culpable homicide, may be punished with imprisonment for up to 2 years, a fine, or both.
- *BNS Section 106(1):* This clause addresses cases where a person causes the death of another through a rash or negligent act that does not amount to culpable homicide. It prescribes imprisonment for a term of up to 5 years and the imposition of a fine. Notably, if such an act is committed by a registered medical practitioner while performing a medical procedure, the imprisonment term is reduced to 2 years, *and* a fine may still be imposed.

An analysis:

- Subsection 2 of section 106 BNS deals with aggravated punishment for rash and negligent driving of a vehicle, explicitly excluding medical negligence.
- The latter part of subsection 1 of section 106 BNS specifically mentions rash and negligent acts committed by registered medical practitioners, leaving no room for ambiguity.
- Section 106(1) BNS, however, does not specify the degree or "grossness" of medical negligence required to attract criminal liability, leaving this aspect open to interpretation.
- While clause 106(1) BNS reduces the imprisonment term for registered medical practitioners to 2 years compared to 5 years for other acts of rash or negligence causing death, it is important to note that a doctor's conviction under this clause results in the permanent termination of their medical license or registration, as outlined in Section 7.5 of the Code of Medical Ethics 2002. This not only affects their professional standing but also their livelihood, which is a fundamental right as Indian citizens.
- Section 106(1) BNS specifically mentions rash and negligent acts committed by registered medical practitioners "while performing a medical procedure", which remains ambiguous concerning cases of death due to medical negligence outside of medical procedures, leaving room for judicial interpretation.
- Section 106(1) BNS further specifies applicability of the reduced term of 2 years to "Registered Medical Practitioners". A registered medical practitioner is a medical practitioner who possesses any medical qualification recognized under the National Medical Commission Act, 2019 and whose name has been entered in the National Medical Register or a State Medical Register under the Act. Thus, in general understanding, excluding practitioners of alternative systems of medicine (AYUSH) from its purview.
- A comparison between the relevant sections of the outgoing IPC Section 304A and the new Section 106(1) of BNS, 2023, regarding deaths caused by medical negligence, reveals that, on the surface, the imprisonment term appears to be reduced from 5 years to 2 years. However, it is essential to note that the imprisonment term in the outgoing IPC Section 304A was always 2 years as alternative to fine. In effect, the period of imprisonment remains the same. Ironically, the punishment under

Section 106(1) BNS is harsher than that of Section 304A of IPC, as there is no option for a fine alone; instead, it stipulates both imprisonment and a fine. One more thing is uncertain. Is it only for "registered medical practitioners performing medical *procedures*" then what about physicians?

Meanwhile, it is crucial to emphasize that doctors must continue to carry out their duties with due care and diligence. They are protected by several Sections of the IPC, 1860 retained in BNS, 2023. It is important to recognize that the reasonable standard of care for medical professionals is judged by the lowest acceptable standard, and an error of judgment does not necessarily constitute negligence.

■ LEARNING KEY POINTS

- Three new bills have been passed by the Parliament to replace the existing archaic ones. BNS 2023 replaces IPC, 1860. BNSS replaces CrPC, 1973, and BSS replaces The Indian Evidence Act, 1972 as on date.
- The new law does not decriminalize Medical Negligence. Instead, it recognizes and introduces an explicit mention of medical negligence causing death.
- The relevant section assigning criminal liability for medical negligence finds mention in clause 106(1) of BNS, 2023.
- The new law instead of resolving the issue plaguing the medical fraternity since long seems to have opened several gray areas that remain ambiguous.
- Two things are uncertain. One, is it only for "registered medical practitioners performing medical *procedures*" then what about physicians? Second "... will face a maximum 2-year imprisonment *and* fine upon causing death through negligence". Meaning the option of fine only is removed and now imprisonment and fine both shall be slapped.
- The applicability of the new law awaits judicial interpretation to resolve the ambiguity and set a judicial precedence.
- The landmark judgments in the subject thus far shall also be under a scanner with respect to the applicability on the new law.

■ TAKE-HOME MESSAGES

Causing death by medical negligence now invokes a punishment for a term up to 2 years of imprisonment. The mantra of fearless practice is to follow ethical practice, refrain from unlawful activity like issuing false certificates, and perform duty with care and caution without digressing from one's area of specialization and training.

■ FREQUENTLY ASKED QUESTIONS

Q.1. What to do in case of unexplained death?

In case of unexplained death, postmortem should be advised.

Q.2. What is that one habit that can act as a safeguard against medical negligence?

Impeccable documentation is the habit that acts as a good defense in medical negligence litigation.

■ MEDICAL NEGLIGENCE PEARL

Stay calm and composed. Remember only "gross" negligence holds you criminally liable.

■ MUST AVOID THINGS

- Avoid haste. Avoid rushing through a surgical procedure.

- Avoid covering up postoperative complications or failure of operation. Take corrective measures.
- Avoid managing critical patients single handedly. Involve colleagues of other specialties as required.

DO NOT DO
- Do not hold the body for clearance of the bill.
- Do not accept or retain patients requiring ICU care in centers ill-equipped to handle them.
- Do not panic at death on the operation table. Inform the police.

WARNINGS
Practice beyond the scope of your qualification and training at your own peril.

MESSAGES WHICH THE READER MUST BE AWARE
Exercise due diligence and competence in your practice and restraint from being overzealous and over-adventurous.

MUST DO THING
- Follow established protocols wherever possible.
- Suggest second opinion in difficult cases or apparently dissatisfied patients or their relatives.
- Document refusal to follow instructions and take negative consent.

ONLY ONE FACT TO REMEMBER
A higher degree of negligence and greater deviation from ordinary practice needs to be established to prove criminal negligence under Section 304A, which is now clause 106(1) of BNS 2023. The medical fraternity awaits the final Act!

REFERENCES
1. Agarwal A. Medical negligence: Indian legal perspective. Ann Indian Acad Neurol. 2016;19(Suppl 1):S9-14.
2. Tiwari SK, Baldwa M. Doctors and criminal law. Indian Pediatr. 2002;39:1119-25.
3. SCC Online. (2023). [Medical Negligence] FIR cannot be registered on complaint guided by unsubstantiated assumptions only to satisfy discontentment with the treatment of child; Tis Hazari Court sets aside Trial Court's direction. [online] Available from: https://www.scconline.com/blog/post/2023/02/15/fir-cannot-be-registered-on-complaint-guided-by-unsubstantiated-assumptions-only-to-satisfy-discontentment-with-treatment-of-child-tis-hazari-court-sets-aside-direction-to-register-fir-against-doctor/ [Last accessed December, 2023].
4. Abplive.com. (2022). Rajasthan News: Now there will be no FIR on doctor-medical workers without investigation, guideline issued. [online] Available from: https://www.abplive.com/states/rajasthan/rajasthan-news-without-investigation-doctors-will-not-be-arrested-now-home-department-has-issued-new-sop-ann-2134896. [Last accessed December, 2023].
5. Kanoon. (2005). Jacob Mathew vs State Of Punjab & Anr on 5 August, 2005. [online] Available from: https://indiankanoon.org/doc/871062/ [Last accessed December, 2023].
6. Nandimath OV, Thomas A, Arpitha HC. Health Law and Ethics: Critical Reflections. Toronto, Canada: Thomson Reuters; 2022. pp. 215-20.
7. CoverYou. Bail and Anticipatory Bail. [online] Available from: https://www.coveryou.in/bail-and-anticipatory [Last accessed December, 2023].
8. Id.

CHAPTER 10

Dealing with Civil Pre-Litigation and Litigation Process

Mahesh Baldwa, Varsha Baldwa, Namita Padvi, Vijay Arora

The best way to defend yourself is to preempt prosecuting you in court of law.

Keywords: Affidavits, Arguments, CC: Complaint copy, Evidence, Expert witness, Legal notice, Outside court settlement, Written statement

Aim: How to defend alleged medical negligence case in pre-litigation and litigation phase in consumer court by pleading facts, circumstances along with pleading locus standii, maintainability, law of limitation, contributory negligence of patient party. Criminal court defenses are covered in Chapter 9 of this book. Pre-litigation out of court settlement are covered in Chapter 25 of this book.

Objective: What are defenses available to doctors in pre-litigation and litigation phase when faced with threat of case in consumer court, viz. proving duty of care, caution with due diligence supported by medical literature, expert witness, and eyewitness.

INTRODUCTION

The Supreme Court's major decision in Indian Medical Association versus V.P. Shantha (1995 SCC (6) 651)[1] brought all medical services under the jurisdiction of the Consumer Protection Act (CPA), same is upheld by Supreme Court in 2022 under MLAG versus UOI.[2]

Following questions and answers are made to understand simplified way civil and consumer alleged medical negligence cases be dealt

In most cases, multiple defendant medical providers are named when the plaintiff employs the "shotgun" approach, in which the plaintiff names any and all potential individuals, institutions, or business entities that may or may not have played a direct or indirect role in the patient's care at the time of the alleged injury.

OUTSIDE COURT SETTLEMENT PRIOR TO RECEIVING NOTICE

Q.1. Should doctor yield to patient or his relatives demand of asking money for alleged negligence when you feel that you were not at all negligent?

Ans. No. This will just postpone a problem. Reason being such patient's is more likely to take you through legal process once you pay them.

**Q.2. Should doctor yield to patient or his relatives demand of asking money for alleged negligence if you feel that you were negligent.

Ans. Depends upon facts and circumstance of attitude of relatives. If attitude is perceived to be favorable then get a "memorandum of out of court settlement for accord and satisfaction" be drafted and signed by following a proper procedure. Take lawyers or medicolegal advisor's help in drafting and executing the procedure. It is not recommended for bad attitude patient's relatives. Read Chapter 25 on outside court settlement of this book.

RECEIVING LEGAL NOTICE AND REPLYING IT

Q.3. Should one receive a legal notice sent by lawyer?

Ans. Yes, as doctor has an opportunity to answer, can focus on planning future defense if case is filed in any court.

Q.4. Should one reply legal notice himself or through lawyer?

Ans. Yes, doctor should reply legal notice through lawyer in consultation with medicolegal advisor's mind.

Q.5. Why doctor should reply legal notice through lawyer in consultation with medicolegal advisor's mind?

Ans. Lawyer cannot differentiate and gives the required flavor that doctor gave treatment diligently, prudently with due care and caution. Lawyer's reply is mechanical denying alleged negligence. Lawyers usually have no detail knowledge of medicine. Lawyers are not able to explain inherent and unavoidable medical complications. Medical complications are ubiquitous. Lawyers cannot understand intricate mechanisms involved in body medical physiology and underlying medical pathology. This lands Lawyers to draw half-baked conclusions in cases of alleged medical negligence. Most Lawyers wish to depend upon procedural aspects of law restricting them to the law of limitation, law of alibi, and law of evidence. Lawyers hardly touch upon medical facts to defend the case. Lawyers land their doctor clients in an odious situation of presenting the case alien to medical fraternity. Lawyer working in tandem with medicolegal advisor can bring forth medical facts in legal notice reply facts circumstances which led to death, disability, transfer, or increased expenses or hardships to relatives more convincingly for which doctor was not responsible.

OUTSIDE COURT SETTLEMENT AFTER RECEIVING NOTICE BY NEGOTIATIONS

Q.6. Should doctor yield legal notice demand of asking money for alleged negligence by negotiations with patient's lawyer or your own lawyer?

Ans. Chances of success are remote yet explore the possibility. But guiding principles are same as described above for "outside court settlement". Pre-litigation out of court settlement are covered in Chapter 25 of this book.

POST NOTICE: SLEEP OVER THE MATTER OR BE PROACTIVE

Q.7. What is the usual advice of a Lawyer in post notice period?

Ans. Lawyers says that wait till the next legal move of the patient. Lawyers attitude is do not take till trouble actually troubles doctor then only take trouble in hurry to address the trouble leaves no time for doctor to gather the evidence which is vital to the alleged medical negligence case.

Q.8. Should one be proactive in preparing defense?

Ans. Medicolegal advice is "Yes", because a forewarned doctor is forearmed in gathering evidence. In medical negligence case, it is very time-consuming to collect required evidence. Hurriedly collected scientific medical literature and evidence of affidavits of eyewitness and expert witness are less useful if not corroborated with pleadings in written statement (WS), affidavit of evidence, and rejoinders.

■ NATURE OF EVIDENCE

Q.9. What is the nature of evidence courts require?

Ans. Courts require evidence for diligence, prudence, care, and caution in the alleged medical negligence case. Case papers explaining the process of disease, treatment and surgery, complications, and their timely treatment need to be properly explained as part of documentary evidence.

■ PRUDENCE

Q.10. What is the evidence of prudence of doctor?

Ans. To prove doctors prudence in the court, evidence showing doctors qualifications, experience, competence, and skills is required.

■ QUALIFICATIONS

Q.11. What is the evidence of qualifications?

Ans. To prove prudence based on doctors qualifications in court as evidence, only submit Ethics and Medical Registration Board of National Medical Council Act 2019 recognized qualifications and say on the basis of that you have treated the case.

Q.12. How to plead prudence when postgraduate qualification which is not recognized by Medical Council India or State Medical Council (SMC)?

Ans. To prove prudence when postgraduate qualification which are not recognized by Medical Council India or SMC, you have to prepare your evidence of prudence-based MBBS qualifications only. Avoid writing on your letterhead words Expert or specialist or "Daksha" or "Tagya" or "Visheshgya" so as to avoid negligence per se observation of court. Instead such doctors should safely plead and write on their letterheads words like "advisor" or "counselor" or "Trained" or "Experienced" "salahagar" or "Anubhavi". Never plead or claim that you are by virtue of qualification and expert or specialist or super specialist in the field if your degree is not National Medical Council (NMC) or SMC recognized. Claiming in court that your qualified postgraduate specialist/expert if your degree is not MCI recognized may put you in gross legal trouble. Practicing medicine in the field of that any specialty on the basis of experience and training is allowed but do not plead or claim to possess the unrecognized qualification in the court of law in medical negligence case. If possible attach MBBS, MD, DM, and Mch mark sheets and transcripts.

■ WHEN EXPERIENCE IS CONSIDERED SKILL

Q.13. What is the evidence of experience?

Ans. To prove prudence based on doctors experience in court as evidence, submit work experience certificates of medical colleges, medical institutes, and attendance of medical workshop certificates. Prepare a good biodata with number of surgeries/procedures done.

COMPETENCE

Q.14. What is the evidence of MBBS doctor's field of competence?

Ans. To prove prudence of field of competence of MBBS doctors in court as evidence, MBBS person should submit and I, II, and III years MBBS mark sheets from medical college showing study, knowledge, competence, and skill in conducting the treatment given in alleged medical negligence. MBBS person should submit transcript from medical college. Also prepare a good biodata with number of surgeries/procedures done. Submit attendance of medical workshop certificates. One has to say very clearly that on the basis MBBS qualifications, one has treated the case and one is not claiming to have treated the case in the capacity of qualified specialist/expert in that specialty.

Q.15. Can MBBS doctor plead that one is competent to do give care to any diseases belonging to medical specialty usually given by qualified specialist in field possessing postgraduate diploma or degree?

Ans. Yes, there is no legal bar in conducting the treatment if one is competent to conduct treatment in cases belonging to any medical specialty as long as one does not claim to be qualified specialist in that field of senility. MBBS should not claim through signboards and letterheads that he is qualified specialist in that medical field.

PRUDENCE OF SKILL

Q.16. How to plead prudence of skill?

Ans. The prudence of skill is combination of qualifications, work experience, and competence, which should be reflected in biodata of doctor and case paper showing conduct of treatment of case to be in a peer approved way. Collected scientific medical literature and evidence of affidavits of eyewitness and expert witness are less useful if not corroborated with pleadings in WS, affidavit of evidence and rejoinders. Attach a *work log book* of surgeries performed and anesthesia given for surgical and anesthesia specialist.

RECEIVE OR REFUSE NOTICE

Q.17. Should you receive or refuse notice from any courts?

Ans. Receive summons from any courts and never refuse summons. Not defending yourself/hospital/nursing home properly in a case of alleged negligence shall enable the court to pass ex parte order of negligence and compensation against you. That will send wrong message to other doctors, press, and media precedent that doctors are generally negligent and not law abiding. This will cause spiraling of premiums of professional indemnity insurance by insurance companies and the medical professionals resorting to defensive practice.

TIME GIVEN FOR FILING WRITTEN STATEMENT

Q.18. In how many days one should prepare and file to answer complaints?

Ans. Usually within 30 and if allowed 45 days or date is specified in the summons.

Q.19. What is the legal name for answer/reply to complaint?

Ans. Legal name for answer/reply of any complaint is written version or WS of opposite party (OP) or respondent.

STUDY OF COMPLAINT

Q.20. What is title of complaint and how to read title of complaint with a view to reply C?

Ans. Title of complaint contains name of court, place, name of complainant and OPs, and their addresses. While one reads complaint one will find that it starts with the name of court and place where it is situated. It should have the territorial jurisdiction over place where you practice. Under new CPA, 2019 (new CPA, 2019) the complainant can file anywhere, where he/she resides. Read the name of complainant whether he is patient himself, guardian, parent, any organization or legal heir. If it does not fall in that category then challenge. Then read name of OP or all OP's and see whether you are sued in your own name or in the name of hospital/nursing home. You have to see whether it is beneficial to reply separately or jointly. If you have, individual medical indemnity policy replies separately. If you have additional hospital/establishment error and omission policy then reply jointly. See whether insurance party is named as OP or not? If not then make an application to add insurance company as a party. Also see who else treated this patient and if possible and necessary make an application to add their names as OP.

Q.21. How to read typical initial six to eight of paragraphs of complaint with a view to reply complaint copy (CC)?

Ans. Paragraphs no. 1 of complaint usually describes the age, occupation, and income or earning capabilities of the patient. Paragraphs no. 2 of complaint usually describes what patient was suffering from and laymen diagnosis and in complainant's view what treatment was required to be given. Paragraphs no. 3 of complaint usually describes doctor's capabilities/in-capabilities of leaving mop while doing surgery, infrastructure, and promises made to patient. Paragraphs no. 4 of complaint usually describes what payment was made? Paragraphs no. 5 of complaint usually describes whether doctor issued receipts and for some he did not issue receipts. Paragraphs no. 6 of complaint usually makes a point blank blunt allegation of negligence in conducting treatment, diagnosis or investigations, anesthesia, operation, or procedure. Paragraphs no. 7 of complaint describes if patient is transferred to some other hospital then that event, those doctor's views and money spent here. Paragraphs no. 8 of complaint is about the nurses/staff/assistants or any such related issue.

Q.22. How to read typical middle six to eight of paragraphs of complaint with a view to reply complaint?

Ans. Paragraphs no. 9 to 12 of complaint will describe in laymen details about doctors capabilities/in-capabilities, infrastructure, promises made to patient by repeating same thing again and again irritatingly. Paragraphs no. 13 to 18 of complaint will describe in laymen details about alleged negligence in conducting treatment, diagnosis or investigations, anesthesia, and operation or procedure by repeating same thing again and again. Paragraphs no. 19 to 22 of complaint will describe in laymen details about transferred to some other hospital then that event, those doctor's views and money spent there, by repeating same thing again and again.

Q.23. How to read typical penultimate three to six of paragraphs of complaint with a view to reply complaint?

Ans. Paragraphs no. 22 to 25 of complaint will describe in laymen correlation between negligence and loss suffered in details

CHAPTER 10: Dealing with Civil Pre-Litigation and Litigation Process

by repeating same thing again and again Paragraphs no. 25 to 27 of complaint will describe jurisdiction, cause of action, and fees paid with petition under new CPA, 2019. Complainant can file complaint in any territorial jurisdiction where he/she says or works for gain.

Q.24. How to read typical prayer clause paragraphs of complaint with a view to reply complaint?

Ans. Summarize alleged negligence causing damages and financial hardships. If it is consumer courts they usually will asks compensation of 100 lakhs (now reduced to less than 50 lakhs from 30-12-2022) in District court. For more than 100 lakhs to 1000 lakhs (now reduced to 50 lakhs to 2 crores from 30-12-2022) in state commission. National commission pecuniary jurisdiction was 10 crores and above (now reduced to 2 crores and above from 30-12-2022).

SUMMARY AND CLASSIFICATION OF ALLEGATIONS

Q.25. How to classify the allegations in complaint with a view to reply complaint?

Ans. Usually allegations are related to mean that doctor is not qualified, there was inadequate infrastructure, nurses and staff members are not qualified, did not attend, doctor delayed in diagnosing or misdiagnosis, or delay in investigating or treating the patient. Doctor was not present during emergency. Consent was not obtained. There was overcharging. Transfer to higher center delayed. Plethoras of derogatory words are used against medical profession, doctors, nurses, and staff members. Sometimes allegations of unnecessary investigations and treatment are used. Excessive irrational compensation is asked in complaint.

WRITTEN STATEMENT UNDER NEW CONSUMER PROTECTION ACT, 2019 OR ANY OTHER COURT

Q.26. How to reply initial six to eight of paragraphs of complaint in WS of doctor/OP?

Ans. Reply to Paragraph no. 1 of complaint that patient did not inform/misinformed you about occupation and income or earning capabilities. Patient is not a consumer. Reply to Paragraph no. 2 of complaint ignoring what patient has described and what patient was suffering from as per his laymen diagnosis and treatment and write what you have written in your case paper. Reply to Paragraph no. 3 of complaint agreeing to your capabilities as per what degrees medical council registration shows and deny in-capabilities in qualification, knowledge, experience, skill, and infrastructure by attaching required certificates to prove the same. Deny any promises or guarantee and warranty with respect to the 100% success or end results of treatment made to patient party, as professionals do not guarantee cure. Make a note of hiding previous illnesses. Reply to Paragraph no. 4 of complaint, deny if payment made was less and describe actual payment made and ask complainant to produce receipts in the court. Reply to Paragraph 5 of complaint, deny not issuing receipts. Reply to Paragraph no. 6 of complaint, deny point-blank blunt all allegations of negligence in conducting treatment, diagnosis or investigations, anesthesia, operation or procedure and say it was conducted diligently, prudently with due care and caution. Reply to Paragraphs no. 7 of complaint that patient is transferred to some other hospital diligently and prudently with due care and caution and give reason for transfer. Deny if you do not agree with doctor's views or confirm it. Deny money spent there and say you are not responsible for same as you did everything diligently and prudently with due care and caution. Reply to Paragraph no. 8 of complaint about the staff/assistants that they worked under your direct supervision and directions and they are individual for any action/inactions as you were deciding authority on conduct of all aspects related to patient.

Q.27. How to reply to middle six to eight of paragraphs of complaint?

Ans. Reply by saying Paragraphs no. 9 to 12 of complaint is repetition of allegations doctors capabilities/in-capabilities, infrastructure, and promises made to patient by repeating same thing again and again irritatingly and same is already replied in earlier paragraphs. Reply to Paragraphs no. 13 to 18 of complaint by denying all allegations and saying it is laymen view and details about alleged negligence in conducting treatment, diagnosis or investigations, anesthesia, failed operation or procedure by repeating same thing again and again, which is replied earlier. Reply to Paragraphs no. 19 to 22 of complaint, deny allegations by saying it is laymen details about transfer and your conduct of transfer is described in earlier para. Deny all allegations based on other hospital doctor's views. Deny allegations about money spent there and say it is being unnecessarily repeated describing same wrong things again and again. Do not forget to include willingness for *mediation* and file separate application for same.

Q.28. How to reply to penultimate three to six of paragraphs of complaint?

Ans. Reply Paragraphs no. 22 to 25 of complaint by saying that it is laymen correlation between negligence and loss suffered and enclose scientific literature and affidavit of expert from other doctors supporting your view. Reply to Paragraphs no. 25 to 27 of complaint and say whether jurisdiction, cause of action, and fees paid with petition are correct or incorrect. In case it is incorrect then one has to move separate miscellaneous application to lodge objection to jurisdiction, cause of action.

Q.29. How to reply prayer clause paragraphs of complaint?

Ans. Deny alleged negligence causing damages and financial hardships point-blank. Deny having incurred any liability of paying anything to complaint. All you say that alleged negligence is wrong and denied since you did everything diligently and prudently with due care and caution which is evident from certificates of qualification, experience, skill and competence, photographs show infrastructure, scientific literature shows complications which can occur leading to death or disability. With reference to the contents of alleged prayer clause is based on mere allegations without any admissible evidence under the Indian Evidence Act. Say that this is highly inflated claim. Section 34 (1) of CPA 2019 clearly states that the complainant has right to claim only what is actually paid for goods or services rendered to complainant. One should be excluding mental and physical trauma, which are notional and cannot be quantified in terms of money.

SYNOPSIS OR HOW TO SUMMARIZE WRITTEN STATEMENT

Q.30. How to reply by classifying the allegations of complaint and replying in summary way?

Ans. Deny allegations are related to mean that doctor is not qualified, there was inadequate infrastructure by certificates of qualification, experience, skill and competence, photographs, deny staff members did not attend, supported by affidavit of eyewitness, deny that doctor conducted delayed in diagnosing or misdiagnosis or delay in investigating or treating the patient on the basis of case papers. Deny that Doctor was not present during emergency supported by affidavit of eyewitnesses. Deny Consent was not obtained by showing consent. Deny overcharging by enclosing carbon copy of actual bill. Transfer to higher center was delayed. Deny plethora of derogatory words that are used against medical profession, doctors, nurses, and staff members by threatening to take legal action separately for these remarks. Deny allegations of unnecessary investigations and treatment by scientific literature and affidavit of expert witness. Prove that compensation asked is excessive and irrational of complaint and in any case you are not liable as you conducted everything diligently and prudently with due care and caution as described earlier.

Q.31. What general precautions should one take to reply by classifying the allegations of complaint and replying in summary way?

Ans. First and foremost denying all allegations of negligence and deficiency in service needs to be emphasized. Whatever pleas in defense are raised they should be supported by evidence in the first instance of mentioning specifically in reply to the complaint. Subsequent new explanation/pleas during hearing of the case are liable to be rejected.

LEGAL TECHNICAL DEFENSES

Q.32. What is legal technical defenses for doctors/hospitals in preparing WS defense?

Ans. Legal technical defenses for doctors/hospitals are:
- Cause of action
- Pecuniary/territorial jurisdiction
- Nonjoinder or misjoinder of proper and necessary parties
- Free service given
- *No locus standi* as legal representative (LR)
- *Case subjudice* civil/criminal court
- The compensation claimed is highly inflated or exaggerated.
- The complaint is time-barred.
- The complaint is frivolous and vexatious.
- CC has complicated issues involved, requiring recording of evidence of experts, hence complaint case should be filed in a civil court.
- Doctor is dead, i.e., action *personalis moritur cum persona*
- In case, there is indemnity insurance or hospital error and omission policy make insurance company a party to suit. File miscellaneous application to add them to array of respondents.

BURDEN OF PROOF

The court has held the opinion that medical negligence has to be established and cannot be presumed. In cases of medical negligence, the patient must establish her/his claim against the doctor.

FACTUAL DEFENSE

Q.33. What is factual defense for doctors/hospitals in preparing WS defense?

Ans. Factual defense includes:
- Prepare factual matrix supported by case paper/discharge summary record of patient
- Detailed biodata of doctor supported by qualifications, experience, *training, experience, expertise,* and certificates/

appreciation certificates/awards/attendance at various updates, conferences, and workshops
- Photographs showing infrastructure of operation theater (OT), ICU, special state of art gadgetry
- Affidavit of eyewitness.

AFFIDAVITS OF EXPERT DOCTORS AND SCIENTIFIC LITERATURE

Q.34. What is defense by supplying affidavits of expert doctors and scientific literature in preparing WS defense?

Ans. Annex 5–10 affidavits of expert doctors to state that you conducted everything diligently and prudently with due care and caution. Also annex 5–10 scientific literature to show you conducted everything diligently and prudently with due care and caution as per standard textbook way. If available, in case of death, if medical board was set up by police then its favorable report or favorable postmortem report or favorable civil surgeon report is valuable. In case of death due to poisoning, favorable forensic laboratory report is valuable. In case of alleged disability is available then submit any favorable disability certificate or report. In case of transfer, next hospital case records and discharge card to be submitted if favorable.

OTHER RESIDUAL DEFENSES

Q.35. What are other residual defenses to be written in WS defense?

Ans. These are:
- The complainant did not arrive in the court with clean hands, i.e., he withheld crucial facts, such as prior illness, treatment, and so on.
- There are discrepancies between notices delivered directly or through a lawyer/consumer group and the complaint filed in court. Inconsistencies should be carefully highlighted.
- Special circumstances, such as an emergency, a lack of facilities (for example, in a distant location), no one to offer a history of the patient's illness, and so on.
- The burden of showing the duty of care, breach of that duty, cause, injury, and so on is on the complainant.
- A claim against a doctor/hospital usually fails if there is a break in the chain of causation (novus actus interveniens). This occurs when a third-party act supersedes the OP's/doctor's/defendant's original negligent act. The court must determine whether the original act of the defendant caused the damage or whether the intervening act establishes a novus actus interveniens, which means that the second act caused the damage. The intervening act could be conducted by a third party or by the claimant himself.
- Concurrent consultation/treatment received by the patient from other doctors/medical systems. This will attenuate/dilute the alleged negligence of the OP, because there are too many other causes of damage to target at the OP.
- Negligence on one's part: This defense, like all others, must be argued in the first instance, demonstrating how it contributed to the damage caused by alleged medical negligence.

BASICS OF RULES OF DRAFTING OF REPLY

Q.36. What are other usual basics of rules of drafting of reply/defense by or on behalf of the doctor/hospital?

Ans. The very purpose of defense drafting is to create a record, which makes part and parcel of proceedings in court and helpful even when case is lost and one needs to appeal. Since you cannot add/alter/amend or take a new plea in appeal court. Defense should be in writing, which should contain plea about the doctor's/hospital's denial/clarification/explaining cause and effect relationship in reply to the complaint.

It is necessary to reply the complaint para-wise and the allegations needs denial or explanation and your comments should be written down para-wise against each of the allegations narrated in complaint.

Defense (reply) is legal opportunity to narrate or state in written format to reply each of the allegations made by the complainant as well as provides one's own version of the matters under dispute. A basic legal and fundamental purpose of the defense is that, when read in tandem or conjunction with the complaint, it should make clear those disputed points on which parties are not in agreeing to.

The most important rule in drafting a defense is to ensure that *every* material allegation in the complaint is properly answered and dealt with supporting evidence as annexure.

DEALING WITH AN ALLEGATION AGAINST THE DOCTOR/HOSPITAL

Q.37. How to deal with an allegation against the doctor/hospital?

Ans. You have to *admit and reply on statement in your favor. You have to deny* all unfavorable statements and allegations with explanation with evidence to show defendant's side of the story is wrong, false, vexatious, and motivated to extract money.

Sometimes the defendant has no evidence to rebut the allegation with the help of medical record then look whether it can be supported by affidavit of eyewitness or affidavit of expert witness. Court takes it for granted that if any allegation, which is neither denied nor admitted in your answer, is deemed to have been admitted as evidence without proof. The best way to make sure that nothing is admitted by above said legal dictum of court presumption of guilt since allegation is neither denied nor admitted; deal with each of the complainant's allegations one by one in para-wise manner. The defendant's response to the allegations made by the complainant gives proper picture of whole event on larger canvass with respect to case. Court is prompted to works with broad framework of the defense with respect to complaint. It gives court not only fair idea about disputes between the parties. Whenever a single paragraph contains more than one allegation, each must be specifically admitted or denied. When the allegation is denied, there is need to give elaborate explanation with evidence in that paragraph.

In some cases, a paragraph may appear to consist of one allegation while in fact containing a central allegation and one or more subordinate allegations. Therefore, it is essential that while dealing with a paragraph of the complainant, subordinate allegations should not be given a pass or overlooked. Simply admitting allegations in the paragraph would therefore admit subordinate allegations that the defendant should deny or traverse it diligently.

The defendant should not deny and traverse any *indirect or implied allegations* in the complainant's paragraphs with specific reply with evidence.

But where a single paragraph of the complaint contains multiple and complicated allegations, the appropriate reply/answer or response may be a conclusion of admissions, non-admissions and/or denials or to traverse the paragraph by a combination of non-admissions and denials with proper evidence. It should also be particularly noted that in drafting the reply, the proper approach is to deny or traverse both the fact and statement or narrations causing damage and its extent since they are not supported by disability certificate or expert witness by complainant.

PLEADING ADDITIONAL FACTS BY DOCTOR/HOSPITAL

Q.38. What are pleading additional facts by doctor/hospital?

Ans. An important function of the defense is to plead additional facts, which fill gaps and explain and clarify or correct cause and effect relationship based on theory of percentage of complications or death occurring while treating the illness. All errors in the complainant's account of the events alleged to have given rise to a cause of action should be accepted/denied or explained. It should be in conformity with reply to notice received, all the allegations made therein should be rebutted in as short language as possible reserving therein the right to take further appropriate defense after the filing of complaint.

PROCEDURAL DEFENSES/ACTION TAKEN BY DOCTOR/HOSPITAL

Q.39. What are the procedural defenses/action to be taken *by* doctor/hospital?

Ans. As mentioned above once again take objection to the pecuniary, territorial jurisdiction of any court as also that the complaint raises complicated questions of fact and law and/or requires leading of voluminous evidence should be raised if applicable.

SWORN VERIFICATIONS REQUIRED FOR

Q.40. How a WS should be properly verified and sworn.

Ans. Written statement should be properly verified and sworn in front of notary or registrar of court concerned.

Q.41. How all affidavits of eye or expert witness are properly verified and sworn?

Ans. The affidavits of eye or expert witness should be properly verified and sworn in front of notary or registrar of court concerned. Expert witness on letterhead has less value and liable for cross-examination more often than sworn affidavit.

FILE OBJECTION FOR THE COMPLAINT WITHOUT AFFIDAVIT

Q.42. How to file objection for the complaint without affidavit and which has not been properly verified, sworn, or attested?

Ans. Move a miscellaneous application to file objection for the complaint without affidavit and which has not been properly verified, sworn, or attested by notary, and prayer clause should ask for dismissal with cost.

APPLICATION FOR CROSS-EXAMINATION OF THE WITNESSES

Q.43. How to file application for cross-examination of the witnesses/questionnaire in lieu of cross-examination, and re-butt the evidence of the complainant?

Ans. Move a separate miscellaneous application for cross-examination of the witnesses of the complaint, and prayer clause should ask for dismissal with cost if they do not arrange for cross examination. File questionnaire in lieu of cross-examination of the witnesses.

Q.44. How to file application objecting additional pleas to be raised after receipt of complaint in rejoinder?

Ans. Doctor has to file application objecting for additional pleas to be raised after receipt of complaint in rejoinder by complainant. Move a separate miscellaneous application for objecting to additional pleas to be raised after receipt of complainant's cross-objection in rejoinder, and then prayer clause should ask for dismissal with cost if they do not arrange for cross-examination.

AFFIDAVIT OF EVIDENCE

Q.45. How to file affidavit of evidence?

Ans. Submit affidavit of expert witness and file a list of expert witnesses with affidavit of evidence. Expert Evidence could be rebuttal of complainant's evidence in the form of affidavits by doctors willing to give evidence in defense. Also submit relevant medical literature appended to expert witness.

WRITTEN ARGUMENTS

Q.46. How to file written arguments?

Ans. Written arguments should classify disputed and undisputed points. Then put medical scientific explanation of complication, leading to disability and death supported by affidavits of expert witness, relevant literature, and case laws.

APPEAL

Q.47. How to file an appeal and review?

Ans. An appeal must be filed after a complaint is decided against a doctor/hospital within the time limit, within 45 days of passing of the order from District Commission to state Commission or from State Commission to National Commission within 30 days, from National Commission to Supreme Court within 30 days. Appeal from District to State is described under Sections 41 and 47, 51 and 58 of the CPA. Sections 40, 50, and 60 of the CPA deal with review by a District, State, or National Commission, which has the authority to review any order passed by it if there is an error visible on the face of the record, either on its own motion or on an application made by any of the parties within 30 days of such order.

CROSS APPEAL

Q.48. What is cross appeal?

Ans. When both the parties are dissatisfied with the lower court decision, so complainant and OP both can file appeal within the time limit, within 45 days of passing of the order from District Commission to State Commission or from State Commission to National Commission within 30 days or from National Commission to Supreme Court within 30 days, respectively. This is known as cross appeal and both the appeals are together.

REVIEW/REVISION PETITION

Q.49. What is review/revision petition?

Ans. Only review is allowed for order passed by same commission. Sections 40, 50, and 60 of the CPA deal with review by a District, State, or National Commission, which has the authority to review any order passed by it if there is an error visible on the face of the record, either on its own motion or on an application made by any of the parties within 30 days of such order. Under the new CPA, 2019, revision applications are not permitted. Instead of a revision petition, only appeals are permitted.

EXECUTION PETITION

Q.50. What is execution petition?

Ans. Usually, if the order is not complied by OP then complainant can file an execution petition in the consumer courts. This enforcement is known as execution petition. Proceedings are separately taken up and both the parties have to attend the hearing on appointed day and time. Only way to halt execution proceedings is obtain stay of higher court on the lower court order.

■ MISCELLANEOUS APPLICATION

Q.51. What is miscellaneous application?

Ans. Matters related to errors in name of parties, not with in proper jurisdiction, not with in limitation period of 2 years under CPA 2019, Section 69, execution of orders, grant of stay on orders of lower court, interim relief's, removal of name from array of OP or adding name of extra OP or insurance company. All the matters, which are not covered above, need a miscellaneous application.

Application for set aside ex parte orders—Section 61 of CPA 2019: When the National Commission issues an ex parte order, the aggrieved party may file petition to the Commission to vacate the order.

Application for case transfer—Section 62 of the CPA 2019: The National Commission may, at any stage of the proceeding, transfer any complaint pending before a District Commission of one State to a District Commission of another State or from one State Commission to another State Commission on the application of the complainant or on its own motion, in the interest of justice.

■ DURATION OF PROCEEDINGS

Q.52. How much time for disposal of case in the consumer courts is prescribed?

Ans. Prescribed time limit is 90 days in cases of allegations of deficiency in service and 5 months where goods require testing in appropriate laboratory. File an application to decide within 90 days. That CPA 2019, Section 38 and subsection (7) states that every complaint before District Commission shall be disposed of as expeditiously as possible and endeavor shall be made to decide the complaint within a period of 3 months from the date of receipt of notice by OP where the complaint does not require analysis or testing of commodities and within 5 months if it requires analysis or testing of commodities; hence, as per Section 38 (7) if any compensation is granted against OP, he shall not be liable to pay any interest beyond the period of 3 months for the procedure and laxity in the judicial proceeding by way of adjournments after adjournments. That three Judges bench of Supreme Court under Article 141 of Constitution of India in Dr J.J. Merchant & Ors. versus Shrinath Chaturvedi (2002) 6 SCC 635[3] supports section.

Q.53. Are fees prescribed for filing complaint and appeal?

Ans. 50% of award o lower court needs to be deposited before filing appeal.

■ COURT FEES

Q.54. How much fee for complaint in court and how much for appeal is prescribed?

Ans. No fees up to claim for ₹5 lakhs, rest of the amount up to ₹2 crores have slabs of minimal amount of money in few thousand for complainant for filing appeals; for complainants no fees but respondent has to deposit half of decretal amount meaning for example if ₹10 lakhs are awarded, for appeal one has to deposit ₹5 lakhs (50%) amount. This may change, so kindly enquire form commission where one is filing case.

■ INFORM INSURANCE COMPANY

Q.55. How to inform insurance company?

Ans. In case there is an indemnity or hospital error and omission insurance policy in existence, the doctor/hospital should inform the insurance company in writing immediately on a complaint being lodged by a patient with a copy of the complaint and notice received from the court.

HOW TO AVOID LITIGATION
Factual Defenses
- A doctor's qualifications, training, experience, and expertise, among other things, must be mentioned. Documentation to back up your claim.
- The doctor should highlight his clinic/hospital's infrastructure, specific facilities, and document backup assistance.
- Written documentation of the patient's/relative's/attendant's consent to the assumption of inherent and particular risks in the therapy.
- Any evidence that the complainant has not gone to court with clean hands, i.e., he has omitted material facts, such as previous illness, treatment, and so on.
- Inconsistence between notices sent directly or through consumer groups and the complaint made in the court.
- Case circumstances, such as an emergency scenario, a lack of facilities (e.g., in a remote region), no responsible person accompanying the patient, no one to provide a history of the patient's sickness, and so on.
- The complaint bears the burden of proving: (1) Duty of care, (2) breach of that duty, (3) causation, (4) injury, and so on.
- Evidence that the treating doctor/hospital have adequate knowledge, ability, care, and infrastructure (refer to/quote standard textbooks with confirmed photocopies).
- Evidence that the patient sought advice/treatment from another doctor/system of medicine at the same time.
- Any other reasons/more than one reason/for occurrence of damage.
- Any proof of contributory negligence, i.e., patient was brought late, in critical condition, complication existed beforehand, treatment was not adhered to, was lost to follow up, etc.

Technical Defenses
- Proof that the medical service rendered was free of charge (now, this is applicable in certain situations only).
- Concurrent adjudication in another court.
- If the court does not have pecuniary/territorial jurisdiction.
- If the complaint is time-barred.
- A plea that since complicated issues are involved, which require recording of evidence of experts, hence case should be relegated to a civil court. But such a plea must be used at the beginning of the trial.
- Inform your insurance company in writing with a copy of the complaint.

PREVENTION BY PROFESSIONAL INDEMNITY

Insurance cover is important otherwise doctors in small towns will become bankrupt. The compensation amount awarded are in crores, highest being plus 11.5 crores till now. Profession indemnity insurance is a must for every practicing doctor, because it not only covers the claims of compensation awarded against doctor/hospital but also provides a sense of security to doctors that even if some negligence is proved the insurance company will take care of it. Doctors in small towns will become bankrupt. Hence for survival and continuity of practice, indemnity has become mandatory. Get clarification in detail about different premium rates of insurance in case of individual insurance, doctor/nursing home/hospital with qualified staff and unqualified but trained staff, because when the insurance company is paying the compensation it usually makes such enquiries. The insurance companies not only pay the compensation to other party but also arrange for the legal help from advocates. But please beware; there are reports that they sometimes join hand with other party for monetary gains justifying themselves that it is the insurance company and not the doctor who has to pay the compensation. Here we must understand that only the money paid as compensation is not everything, because our reputation and financial standing is also at stake. Indemnity insurance is covered in different Chapter 25 of this book.

What can be the Role of Professional Association Like Indian Academy of Pediatrics and Indian Medical Association?

These bodies can play a major role in resumption of harmonious relations between doctor community and patients. With the help of media they can arrange seminars inviting doctors and common public where public can discuss their grievances and doubts with the doctors. This will establish an atmosphere of transparency and will improve trust and faith of the patients for doctors; they can establish their own grievances cell where complaints of patients can be addressed and if the concerned doctors have really erred then some sort of out of court settlement can be arranged. They can arrange TV shows and talk shows to discuss various issues, which confuse public hence leading to mistrust and anger. The Indian academy of pediatrics and Indian Medical Association (IMA) keeps informing parents about various medical issues through its website. These efforts will go a long way in improving doctor–patient relationship.

Avoid Medical Malpractice Stress Syndrome

Medical malpractice lawsuits take time. It could take years after years, event after incident, for a malpractice case to be settled in court. Malpractice lawsuits must go through a lengthy process that includes a WS, proof, paperwork, consent, medical literature, expert witness discovery, and the finding of new evidence. While dealing with a malpractice lawsuit, it is critical to maintain attention on other aspects of your life. To live is to live. Continue regardless of the case against you. The support system of friends and family must be activated, and obsessing over the case must be avoided.

Medical malpractice stress syndrome (MMSS) exists. It is felt to some extent by all physicians who are sued. Anxiety, powerlessness, and embarrassment are some of the potential adverse effects of being labeled a malpractice defendant. Given the recriminations and cognitive dissonance that are frequently connected with malpractice litigation, a strongly emotional response is natural and understandable. Malpractice claims can take years to resolve; it is a marathon, not a sprint. Mentally prepare yourself for a lengthy, slow-moving procedure.

■ SUMMARY

Doctors should neither injure nor aggravate preexisting ailments or illnesses. And if they do, court wants them to explain what bad repercussions can occur. Simultaneously, good doctors should not be punished for doing nothing wrong. While these ideas appear simple, they are more challenging in practice. There are several defenses available to medical professionals accused of malpractice. The doctor may claim that his treatment was in conformity with medical standards or that the patient's injuries were not caused by a medical error.

Medical doctors cannot be blamed for injury due to negligence. If a medical professional can demonstrate that the damage would not have occurred if the patient had not been careless, he or she may have a legitimate defense against a malpractice claim.

Respectable Minority principle: In order to treat a patient efficiently, medical specialists may opt to pursue a novel or more radical type of treatment. While the doctor's decision may position him or her outside the medical mainstream, if a respectable minority of medical professionals supports the course of treatment was logical, reasonable, he or she may have a strong defense against a medical malpractice claim.

Of course, the doctor must first inform the patient about the risks. (Failing to fully notify a patient about potential dangers can lead to a lack of informed consent charge.). This is referred to as Bolam's law. If a doctor helps someone in an emergency, he or she is immune from civil liability if something goes wrong during the rescue. In principle, a medical professional who voluntarily serves another person owes that person the same duty of care and treatment that a reasonably competent physician would under the same or similar circumstances.

With the exception of the "discovery rule", which holds that the statute of limitations period does not begin until a harm is actually discovered, the statute of limitations limits when an action for medical malpractice can be initiated, usually 2 years for consumer cases and 3 years for other cases from the cause of action. If the medical expert can demonstrate that the patient detected the harm at a specified moment and that the statute of limitations has since expired, the case may be dismissed.[4-6]

▮ LEARNING KEY POINTS

- Outside court settlement prior to receiving notice when you feel that you were not at all negligent.
- Reply to legal notice.
- One should discourage outside court settlement after receiving notice.
- Do not sleep over the matter after receiving legal notice.
- Courts require evidence for diligence, prudence, care, and caution in the alleged medical negligence case. Case papers explaining the process of disease, treatment and surgery, complications, and their timely treatment need to be properly explained as part of documentary evidence.
- Legal technical defenses for doctors/hospitals are:
  - Maintainability
  - Cause of action
  - Absence of proof of payment
  - Pecuniary/territorial jurisdiction
  - Nonjoinder or misjoinder of parties
  - Free service given
  - *No locus standi* as LR
  - *Case subjudice* civil/criminal court
  - The compensation claimed is inflated or exaggerated.
  - The complaint is time-barred.
  - The complaint is frivolous and vexatious.
  - Complaint has complicated issues involved, requiring recording of evidence of experts; hence, complaint case should be filed in a civil court.
  - Doctor is dead, i.e., action *personalis moritur cum persona*
  - In case, there is indemnity insurance or hospital error and omission policy, make insurance company a party to suit.

TAKE-HOME MESSAGES
Reply to legal notice.

MUST AVOID THINGS
Resist to avoid compensation claimed being inflated or exaggerated by patient party.

DO NOT DO
One should preferably discourage outside court settlement after receiving notice as it will send wrong message to patient party and in medical fraternity.

WARNINGS
Be aware and warned that in case, there is indemnity insurance or hospital error and omission policy make insurance company a party to suit right from reply to legal notice stage by disclosing insurance details. This might give edge to patient party but not the less essential.

MESSAGES WHICH THE READER MUST BE AWARE
Look for if the complaint is time-barred.

MUST DO THING
One can submit eye and expert witness without being asked by consumer court.

MEDICAL NEGLIGENCE PEARLS
Courts require evidence for diligence, prudence, care, and caution in the alleged medical negligence case. Medical degree, SMC registration, case papers explaining the process of disease, treatment and surgery, complications, and their timely treatment/referral need to be properly explained as part of documentary evidence.

ONLY ONE FACT TO REMEMBER
Avoid medical malpractice stress syndrome.

REFERENCES
1. Indian Medical Association vs. V.P. Shantha (1995 SCC (6) 651).
2. Supreme Court in 2022 under MLAG versus UOI.
3. Dr. J.J. Merchant & Ors. v/s Shrinath Chaturvedi (2002) 6 SCC 635.
4. Baldwa M, Baldwa V, Padvi N, Baldwa S (Eds). Legal Issues in Medical Practice, 2nd edition, 2 volume set. New Delhi, India: CBS Publishers & Distributors Pvt. Ltd.; 2023.
5. Baldwa M, Baldwa V, Padvi N, Baldwa S (Eds). Legal Issues in Critical Care. New Delhi, India: CBS Publishers & Distributors Pvt. Ltd.; 2022.
6. Baldwa M, Baldwa V, Padvi N, Baldwa S (Eds). Legal Issues in Dermatology, 2nd edition. New Delhi, India; CBS Publishers & Distributors Pvt. Ltd.; 2024.

CHAPTER 11

Limiting the Liability in Case of Alleged Medical Negligence

Jyoti Kumar Gupta, Shashikant Tripathi, Amrita Verma, Rajat Dubey

Adding just a more dimension of limiting the liability to case makes litigation without doubt, a lengthy demanding process that should exert its toll on agitating patient party.

Keywords: Calculation of compensation, Capping of compensation, Contract for hiring of medical services, Limitation, No-fault liability

Aim: Knowing the principles of pleading to limiting the liability in medical negligence case.

Objective: To equip doctor about defending the alleged medical negligence along with not forgetting principles of pleading to limiting the liability in case of alleged medical negligence in court of law altogether. It is often seen doctors forget to limit liability available as defenses to plead are not used forcefully.

INTRODUCTION

Liability in common parlance implies responsibility for an act or omission. It is apparent exposedness to the sanction of law. Breach of legal rights and duties is called a wrong and one who has committed a wrong is said to be liable for it. Salmond says that liability is a bond of necessity that exists between the wrong door and the remedy of wrong. As per Austin, liability consists in those things which a wrongdoer must do or suffer. In cases where the remedy is civil one, the party who has suffered has right to demand the redress allowed by law and one who has committed the wrong is bound to comply with this demand. Civil liability arises in breach of contract or act of tort. When duty of care is dependent on agreement as in case of contract, liability is limited but when duty of care is imposed by law, it is unlimited and is covered in law of torts. Medical negligence traditionally has been understood as a tortuous liability and, therefore, unlimited liability is imposed on doctors and hospitals in consumer suits. The liberty of imposing unlimited liability in the name of tortuous act is now apparently being misused by courts and this unlimited liability has crossed the limit of financial capacity of medical practitioner or hospital and rendered them apparently bank corrupt. So, it becomes imperative to search for the measures that may limit the liability on medical professionals.

Why there is need to limit the liability?

In year 2014, Supreme Court in *Balram Prasad versus Kunal Saha*[1] case awarded a record ₹5.96 crores compensation for medical negligence to a US-based NRI doctor, Kunal Saha, who fought a 15-year battle to fasten the charge of gross medical negligence on four doctors and Kolkata's AMRI hospital for the death of his wife Anuradha in 1998. Supreme Court enhanced by over 400% the initial ₹1.73 crores compensation awarded to Saha by the National Consumer Disputes Redressal Commission (NCDRC). The court held three doctors Dr Balram Prasad, Dr Sukumar Mukherjee, and Dr Baidyanath Haldar, guilty of negligence in treating Anuradha, who had contracted a toxic epidermal necrolysis. The Apex Court awarded 5.96 crores compensation with interest of 6% on the amount from the date of filing of claim totaling >11 crores which is the maximum in any case. In ROP cases, Apex Court has awarded huge compensations; it was 1.8 crores compensation in V Krishnakumar versus State of Tamil Nadu and Ors.[2] and 1.2 crores in Shikhar Chand Jain (Dr) versus Dimple.[3] So, it can be seen that in name of unliquified damages exorbitant compensation is being slapped on medical professionals. In NALSA guidelines 2018, about compensation for women victims of crime, the maximum compensation for heinous crime leading to death of women is not more than ₹10 lakhs, for face disfigurement due to acid attack is ₹8 lakhs, pregnancy due to rape is 4 lakhs, and grievous physical or mental injury requiring rehabilitation if just ₹2 lakhs, indicates doctors are treated worse than rapist and murderers.

HUGE PECUNIARY LIABILITY IS AKIN TO FOLLOWING HAMMURABI CODE[4]

In 2030 BC, the code of Hammurabi, the king of Babylon, was to chop off a doctor's hand for making a mistake. This approach may prevent future mistakes but after some time few doctors would be left with hands to operate. India's current legal position on medical negligence is not vastly different from Hammurabi's code. 84% of hospitals in India have fewer than 30 beds, and they are where >60% of our children are born. Most of these "nursing homes" do not even have a medical records department to protect them in case of litigation. However sincere the effort to save the life of a patient may be, incomplete documentation may hamper a successful defense in a court of law. In case of award in crores, these small nursing homes and doctors will have to sell all their asset and still they may not arrange money to compensate. Deterrent effect conceptualized by these mammoth compensations is more apparent on kids of medical professionals and brilliant scholars in the fact that they are hesitant now to opt medical profession as career. Doctors are forced to follow defensive medical practice with bypassing serious cases and going for unnecessary investigations just to maintain documentation of clinical condition in spite of prevailing clinical sense.

JURISPRUDENCE BASIS OF HIGH LIABILITY IN MEDICAL NEGLIGENCE

The Fourth Jural Postulates propounded by famous Jurist Roscoe Pond says that People must be able to assume that other people will act with due care not to create unreasonable risk of injury to others. Failure to show due care in creating unreasonable injury in treating a patient is the crux of medical negligence. The basis of computing compensation under common law lies in the principle of *"restitutio in integrum"* which, when translated, refers to ensuring that the person seeking damages due to a wrong committed to him/her is in the position that he/she would have been had the wrong not been committed.

This implies that the victim needs to be compensated for financial loss caused by the doctor's/hospital's negligence, future medical expenses, and any pain and suffering endured by the victim. India, unlike the USA, does not have a jury system that determines culpability or quantum of compensation. In India, the judge in the consumer court, or the civil court, has complete discretion over the compensation amount and hence is bound to consider the impact of the judgment because he/she sets a precedent even in the manner and quantum of damages awarded.

REASONS OF HIGH LIABILITY IN MEDICAL NEGLIGENCE

The manner in which medical negligence compensation is calculated depends not just on the injury sustained or the death caused but is also contingent on the victim's income and standard of living. This system, therefore, perpetuates inequity by providing greater compensation to the rich, for the same injury or wrongful death claim, which prompts the question, how does one assess how much a life is worth? The argument of inequity also applies to the paying capability of the doctors concerned as the earning capacity of a doctor varies substantially across specialty, geographical location, and nature of practice. Hence, there is a need to assess and take into account the earning and paying capability of a practitioner, working condition, qualification, and experience before the compensation is awarded.

Methodology of Calculation of Compensation

The defendants in most medical negligence cases assert that the method of determining compensation ought to be the "Multiplier Method". The "multiplier method" was created to facilitate awarding compensation in relation to motor vehicle accidents to calculate "no fault" liability. Therefore, it accounts for the loss of income of the victim only. This sum is calculated by taking into account the "multiplicand," that is, the victim's salary minus the amount he spends on himself, and the "multiplier," that is, the total number of years that the victim would have earned his salary. The usual formula utilized in calculating compensation is [(70 − age) × annual income + 30% for inflation − 1/3 for expenses].

Defendants assert that this is the figure that will adequately calculate the loss incurred, and therefore it should be utilized in cases of medical negligence. However, compensation that is solely based on the income of the victim would imply that medical negligence causing death or injury to a wealthy individual is worth more than medical negligence that impacts an unemployed individual or homemaker or a child or senior citizen. The Supreme Court has, therefore, refused to restrict compensation to the multiplier method in the case of medical negligence.[5] Further, the Supreme Court has added other dimensions to the calculation of compensation such as the medical costs incurred by the victim during the litigation, cost of future medical expenses, compensation toward mental agony and physical pain, and compensation toward loss of consortium and cost of litigation. This has led to large compensation.

Discretionary Power to Award Compensation

The judge in medical negligence litigation has complete and absolute discretion in awarding compensation, therefore unless evidentiary proof of the expenses incurred, or proposed expenses, is provided, the judge may in his/her own capacity determine the claim to be excessive or not reflective of prevalent costs. The practice of placing complete reliance on a judge may result in inappropriate compensation. In *ESI Hospital versus Ram Kishan Yadav (2012)*[6] case, the lower court awarded compensation on a humanitarian basis in spite of clearly establishing that there was no negligence from the medical practitioners, thereby sending wrong signals to the community at large. These kinds of humanitarian judgments and awarding compensation may encourage the public at large to approach the court for every negative outcome.

In *Sarla Verma versus Delhi Transport Corporation (2009) 6 SCC 121,* Supreme Court noted that "The lack of uniformity and consistency in awarding compensation has been a matter of grave concern... If different tribunals calculate compensation differently on the same facts, the claimant, the litigant, the common man will be confused, perplexed, and bewildered. If there is significant divergence among tribunals in determining the quantum of compensation on similar facts, it will lead to dissatisfaction and distrust in the system".

Delay in Adjudication of Cases

The case of Balram Prasad versus Kunal Saha saw 15 years of litigation, with varying reasoning across different tribunals, before it finally reached the Supreme Court. Immeasurable delays in court and incessant appeals effectively deny justice to the victims of medical negligence in India. Considering the pace of justice delivery in India, uncertainty regarding their culpability can cause significant mental trauma to doctors; furthermore, damage to a doctor's reputation is immediate, but acquittal may take a decade or more. For instance, in the Kunal Saha case, one of the respondents had died by the time the Supreme Court made a ruling, and a second doctor claimed inability to pay on the grounds of ill health and unemployment. Most of the time, delay in adjudication is unrelated to act of defendants. Courts give longer dates due to large pendency of case, absence of councils, or judges are other reasons for adjourning date and all the delay culminates in punishment on defendant in form of interest.

Ignoring Working Environment and Capability of Doctor

Doctors working in small town and small healthcare setting are having suboptimal working conditions. They lack in infrastructure, human resources (both medical and nonmedical), poor referral, and expert backup and facing other issues such as overcrowding of patients, nonavailability of essential drugs and investigations, irregular/erratic supply of medicines, poor quality of supplied medicines, deplorable state of maintenance of medical equipment, and administrative work. In light of the above, it is worth asking whether a medical practitioner can be held liable for medical negligence arising from an inability to diagnose due to the absence of required investigative facilities, poor quality of supplied medicines, or nonmaintenance of equipment and poor infrastructure. Hence, the court should take into account the exact circumstances the practitioners working and the specific situations that led to the negative outcome so that justice is served. Similarly, doctors with plain graduate or PG diploma cannot be equated with postgraduate and superspecialists working in tertiary care set up in metros.

TORTUOUS NATURE OF LIABILITY IN MEDICAL NEGLIGENCE CLAIM IS THE MAIN CULPRIT OF HUGE COMPENSATION

Expectations of a patient are twofold: doctors and hospitals are expected to provide medical treatment with all the knowledge and skill at their command and secondly they will not do anything to harm the patient in any manner either because of their negligence, carelessness, or reckless attitude of their staff. Failure of a doctor and hospital to discharge this obligation is essentially a tortious liability. A tort is a civil wrong (*right in rem*) as against a contractual obligation (*right in personam*)—a breach that attracts judicial intervention by way of awarding damages. Thus, a patient's right to receive medical attention from doctors and hospitals is essentially a civil right.

In law of tort, liability is unlimited while in contract it is limited. The aim of tort damages is to restore the claimant, in so far as money can do so, to his or her pre-incident position, and this purpose underlies the assessment of damages. Tort compensates both for tangible losses and for factors which are enormously difficult to quantify, such as loss of amenity and pain and suffering, nervous shock, and other intangible losses. Tort damages are therefore said to be "unliquidated". The claimant is not claiming a fixed amount of compensation. The aim of the award of damages in contract is to place the claimant in the position he or she would have been in if the contract had been performed. Thus, tort is concerned with restoring the status quo, while contract is concerned with loss of expectation.[7]

With regard to the quantum of compensation payable to an injured patient, the Supreme Court observed in the case of IMA versus VP Shanta and Ors. III (1995) CPJ I (SC), as follows: *"A patient who has been injured by an act of medical negligence has suffered in a way which is recognized by the law—and by the public at large as deserving compensation. This loss may be continuing and what may seem like an unduly large award may be little more than that sum which is required to compensate him for such matters as loss of future earnings and the future cost of medical or nursing care. To deny a legitimate claim or to restrict arbitrarily, the size of an award would amount to substantial injustice".*

ELEMENTS THAT MUST BE ESTABLISHED IN NEGLIGENCE CLAIM

Negligence suits have historically been analyzed in stages, called elements, similar to the analysis of crimes. Elements that must be established in every negligence case are—duty, breach, causation, and damages. Negligence can be conceived of as having just three elements—conduct, causation, and damages. More often, it is said to have four (duty, breach, causation, and pecuniary damages) or five (duty, breach, actual cause, proximate cause, and damages).

Duty of Care

In England *Caparo versus Dickman* (1990) introduced a "threefold test" for a duty of care. Harm must be—(1) reasonably foreseeable, (2) there must be a relationship of proximity between the plaintiff and defendant, and (3) it must be "fair, just and reasonable" to impose liability. In the case of *Dr Laxman Balkrishna Joshi versus Dr Trimbark Babu Godbole and Anr, AIR 1969 SC 128* and *AS Mittal versus State of UP, AIR 1989 SC 1570*, it was laid down that when a doctor is consulted by a patient, the doctor owes to his patient certain duties which are: (1) duty of care in deciding whether to undertake the case, (2) duty of care in deciding what treatment to give, and (3) duty of care in the administration of that treatment. A breach of any of the above duties may give a cause of action for negligence and the patient may on that basis recover damages from his doctor. Every doctor who enters into the medical profession has a duty to act with a reasonable degree of care and skill. This is what is known as "implied undertaking" by a member of the medical profession that he would use a fair, reasonable, and competent degree of skill.

Breach of Duty of "Standard of Care"

The second element, breach of duty, is synonymous with the "standard of care." Once it is established that the defendant owed a duty to the plaintiff/claimant, the matter of whether or not that duty was breached must be settled. The test is both subjective and objective. The defendant who knowingly (subjective) exposes the plaintiff/claimant to a substantial risk of loss breaches that duty. The defendant who fails to realize the substantial risk of loss to the plaintiff/claimant, which any reasonable person (objective) in the same situation would clearly have realized, also breaches that duty.

Factual Causation (Direct Cause)

For a defendant to be held liable, it must be shown that the particular acts or omissions were the cause of the loss or damage sustained. The basic test is to ask whether the injury would have occurred but for, or without, the accused party's breach of the duty owed to the injured party.

Harm

Even though there is breach of duty, and the cause of some injury to the defendant, a plaintiff may not recover unless he can prove that the defendant's breach caused a pecuniary injury. As a general rule, a plaintiff can only rely on a legal remedy to the point that he proves that he suffered a loss. It means something more than pecuniary loss is a necessary element of the plaintiff's case in negligence.

Damages

Damages place a monetary value on the harm done, following the principle of *restitutio in integrum* (Latin for "restoration to the original condition"). Thus, for most purposes connected with the quantification of damages, the degree of culpability in the breach of the duty of care is irrelevant. Once the breach of the duty is established, the only requirement is to compensate the victim.

GENERAL MEASURES FOR LIMITING THE LIABILITY BEFORE ANY LITIGATION

At the Time of Establishing Doctor–Patient Relationships

Traditional formula utilized in calculating compensation has been [(70 – age) × annual income + 30% for inflation – 1/3 for expenses]. Although Supreme Court has added other dimensions also in calculation of compensation such as the medical costs incurred by the victim during the litigation, cost of future medical expenses, compensation toward mental agony and physical pain, and compensation toward loss of consortium and cost of litigation. Still the age and annual income are main determining factors in determining quantum of award. So, it is highly recommended for medical professionals that declaration regarding annual income of patient must be taken before starting treatment by the way of self-declaration proforma from the patient. In self-declaration proforma, other important history may be taken as declaration regarding past history of any significant illness, drug allergy, vaccination, previous treating doctor, referring doctor, etc.

Augmentation of Informed Consent as "Contract for Hiring of Medical Services"

Damages in torts are compensated by civil court as unliquidated while damages in breach of contracts are decided as per terms and conditions of contract defined as liquidated damages. Consumer and Civil court usually decide one of the following aspects in malpractice suits:

- Deficiency in medical service
- Was there unfair trade practice?
- Was there medical negligence?

One should defend forcefully against alleged medical negligence and try to convert all the allegations of negligence into deficiency of service under law of contract with liquidated damages. Once damages are defined and liquidated within the confines of contracted terms and conditions of contract in inform consent, civil court has to decide it as per law of contract. Primary aim should be to convert all allegation of negligence to deficiency of service domain so as to align court granting liquidated compensation as per contract terms and conditions.

Inform consent has usually many components of contract and inform consent can be augmented by its transformation into *"Contract for hiring of medical services"*. It can be done by following incorporation in consent taking process:

- An offer (in form of proposed surgery/treatment)
- Acceptance by patient party by obtaining valid consent
- Clearly defined terms and conditions (about complications, disabilities, guarantee, warrantee, warnings, and disclaimers)
- Consideration (defined in terms of money and payment schedules)
- Intention to create legal relations (doctor–patient relationship)
- Capacity of the parties (competent to contract)
- Legality of purpose (standard surgery/treatment)
- Description of liquidated damages in case of breach of contract.

MEASURES FOR LIMITING THE LIABILITY AT LITIGATION PHASE

At the time of defending any medical negligence claim, there can be many precautionary steps which may prove game changer in determining the damages and at time absolving the defendant. These measures should be adopted ab initio at the stage of written argument and should be a part of argument. These measures ought to be adopted at the appellate stage also.

Duty of Care: Highlight the Duties of Care which were Successfully Accomplished

Duty of care is one of the essential components of tortuous liability. It is not an isolated one but a bunch of duties that is expected to be performed from a person under duty of care. Most of the time breach of duty is an isolated event. One had performed so many duties during management of patients like managing critical life-threatening event like managing shock, managing sepsis, managing complications, taking care of other aspect of duty of care, etc. So, at the time of refuting allegation of negligence, defendant should highlight other aspects of duty of care which were duly performed by him diligently and resulted in saving patient from other complications which might have occurred in absence of this duty of care.

Standard of Care

Negligence, in general, is legally defined as "the standard of conduct to which one must conform... (and) is that of a reasonable man under like circumstances".[8] So, deviation from standard of conduct is breach of duty of care. In *Hall versus Hilbun*,[9] CJ Robertson stated:

"*Medical malpractice is a legal fault by a physician or surgeon. It arises from the failure of a physician to provide the quality of care required by law. When a physician undertakes to treat a patient, he takes on an obligation enforceable at law to use minimally sound medical judgment and render minimally competent care in the course of services he provides. A physician does not guarantee recovery... A competent physician is not liable per se for a mere error of judgment, mistaken diagnosis or the occurrence of an undesirable result*".

The standard of care is a legal term, not a medical term. Basically, it refers to the degree of care a prudent and reasonable person would exercise under the circumstances. Statutes, Regulations, Administrative agencies, Court opinions, Authoritative clinical guidelines, Accreditation standards, Facility policies and procedures, and Policies and guidelines from professional organizations define the legal degree of care required, so the exact legal standard varies by state. The standard of care is not optimal care. Rather, it is a continuum, with barely acceptable care at one end, and the ultimate in care at the other end. Physicians should aim in the direction of optimal care and should document their clinical judgment and decision-making so that their treatment can be understood. Standard of care has basic two elements which must conform in establishing negligence:

- To be done by prudent and reasonable person
- Under like circumstances

Figure out yourself in reasonable man norms of the standard care: As standard of care refers to the degree of care, a prudent and reasonable person would exercise under the circumstances, figuring out yourself in reasonable man norm is very important. There cannot be same standard of care for a graduate, postgraduate, or PG diploma doctors, beginner or senior person, private practitioner or government/medical college faculty. Figuring our self as very senior, experienced with best capabilities and facilities may sometimes can go against, as reasonable man standard goes high. Awareness or success rate data of particular condition in particular setting or particular class of professionals may prove useful in defense under standard care norms. In the *Bolam's case*,[10] McNair, J summed up the law as the following:

"*In the case of a medical man, negligence means failure to act in accordance with the standards of reasonably competent medical men at the time. There may be one or more perfectly proper standards, and if he confirms with one of these proper standards, then he is not negligent*".

Standard of care with reference to working environment: A doctor in our country generally works in an atmosphere replete with constraints such as poor infrastructure, overcrowding of patients, lack of human resources (both medical and nonmedical), violence against medical personnel, nonavailability of essential drugs and investigations, irregular/erratic supply of medicines, poor quality of supplied medicines, deplorable state of maintenance of medical equipment, administrative work, deadlines and targets to increase the patient turnover, all while receiving inadequate remuneration for their demanding work. In the case of *McCourt versus Abernathy*,[11] court held:

"Negligence may not be inferred from a bad result. Our law says that a physician is not an insurer of health, and a physician is not required to guarantee results. He undertakes only to meet the standard of skill possessed generally by others practicing in his field under similar circumstances".

In light of the above, it is worth asking whether a medical practitioner can be held liable for medical negligence arising from an inability to diagnose due to the absence of required investigative facilities, poor quality of supplied medicines, or nonmaintenance of equipment and poor infrastructure. Hence, the court should be persuaded to take into account, the exact circumstances the practitioners working and the specific situations that led to the negative outcome so that justice is served.

Challenge the Damages Claimed by Evaluating Harm Sustained

Alleged harm is crucial part of malpractice suit in claiming damages. So claim for damages must be refuted at earliest opportunity at written statement stage itself. Harm sustained must be evaluated as per standard legal norms and damages must be refuted as wrongly claimed with false facts in inflated manner. There is tendency to exaggerate the damages and make the claim highly inflated. It should be denied in preliminary objection and court must be realized of inflated and exaggerated claims. Documentary proof of physical harm claimed must be asked. The basis of computing compensation under common law lies in the principle of *"restitutio in integrum"* which, when translated, refers to ensuring that the person seeking damages due to a wrong committed to him/her is in the position that he/she would have been had the wrong not been committed. So, harms must be evaluated with condition of the patient at the start of treatment and not at as absolute physical health of a person.

Issue of Limitation and Other Technical Defense must be Raised in Preliminary Objection

Supreme Court in State Bank of India versus M/S BS Agricultural[12] has said that *"The expression, 'shall not admit a complaint' occurring in Section 24A is sort of a legislative command to the consumer forum to examine on its own whether the complaint has been filed within limitation period prescribed thereunder".* Still complaints are admitted in wrongful manner. Issue of limitation must be issued at earliest opportunity and its disposal must be stressed at foremost priority. Law of limitation has been mentioned in section 24A of CPA 1986 and section 69 of CPA 2019 as:

1. The Commission shall not admit a complaint unless it is filed within 2 years from the date on which the cause of action has arisen.
2. Complaint may be entertained after the period specified in sub-section (1), if complainant satisfies the Commission that he had sufficient cause for not filing the complaint within such period.

The principle of determination of accrual of cause of action has been propounded by Supreme Court in VN Shrikhande versus Anita Sena Fernandes[13] as:
- If the effect of negligence is PATENT, the cause of action will be deemed to have arisen on the date when the act of negligence was done.
- If, on the other hand, the effect of negligence is LATENT—then the cause of action will arise:
  1. On the date when the patient/complainant discovers the harm/injury caused due to such act
  2. Or the date when the patient or his representative-complainant could have, by exercise of reasonable diligence discovered the act constituting negligence.

So, accrual of cause of action is the crucial event and it is to be determined as per principal propounded by Supreme Court as above. Supreme Court in VN Shrikhande versus Anita Sena Fernandes has mentioned that: *If the complaint is per se barred by time and the complainant does not seek condonation of delay under Section 24A(2), the consumer forums will have no option but to dismiss the same.* "Supreme Court in State Bank of India versus M/S BS Agricultural 2009 has said: *If the complaint is barred by time and yet, the consumer forum decides the complaint on merits, the forum would be committing an illegality and, therefore, the aggrieved party would be entitled to have such order set aside*." "Supreme Court in Gannmani Anasuya versus Parvatini Amarendra Chowdhary (2007) has said that: *Since the complaint is barred by time and liable to be dismissed on that count, it would be unnecessary to examine the other grounds of challenge*".

Challenging the Interest

It has been seen in many occasions that litigation process stretches for years without any causative role from defendants, still huge amount of interest is slapped in arbitrary manner by the courts. In Balram Prasad versus Kunal Saha case, supreme court awarded 5.6 crore compensation but real monetary compensation goes beyond 11 crores which was due to the fact that case stretched for 15 years and 6% interest was slapped in addition.

Section 13-3A of CPA 1986 and Section 38(7) of CPA 2019 say that "Every complaint shall be disposed of as expeditiously as possible and endeavor shall be made to decide the complaint within a period of 3 months from the date of receipt of notice by opposite party where the complaint does not require analysis or testing of commodities and within 5 months if it requires analysis or testing of commodities". Five judge bench of Supreme Court in *New India Assurance Co. Ltd. versus Hilli Multipurpose Cold Storage (P) Ltd*[14] has stressed that statutory provisions of CPA of CPA 1986 like section 13, 15, 19, 24A should be followed strictly.

In Consumer Protection Act, there is no provision of imposing interest on compensation award, it is opted out by consumer courts from Section 34 of THE CODE OF CIVIL PROCEDURE, 1908 which provisions for imposing interest in pecuniary awards. Honorable Supreme Court in *Savita Garg versus The Director, National Heart Institute Civil Appeal No. 4024 of 2003* has said that: "Therefore, as far as the Commission is concerned, the provisions of the Code of Civil Procedure are applicable to the limited extent and not all the provisions of the Code of Civil Procedure are made applicable to the proceedings to the National Forum". Application of civil procedure code is limited to section 13(4) of CPA 1986 or section 38(9) of CPA 2019 whereby Forums have been vested same powers as are vested in a civil court under the Code of Civil Procedure, 1908 (5 of 1908) while trying a suit in respect of the following matters, namely summoning and enforcing the attendance of any defendant or witness, discovery and production of any document or other material object, reception of evidence on affidavits, requisitioning of the report of the concerned analysis or test from the appropriate laboratory or from any other relevant source, issuing of any commission for the examination of any witness and any other matter which may be prescribed.

Challenging Ex-Gratia Compensation

Supreme Court in *State of Punjab versus Shiv Ram and Ors., IV (2005) CPJ 14 (SC)* held that medical men and hospitals should not be saddled with damages unless they are found negligent. The apex court felt that awarding ex gratia compensation against doctors and hospitals without any findings on negligence is not proper. The court further held that there is a need for developing a welfare fund or insurance scheme. This judgment makes very pragmatic observations in the midst of several verdicts against medical professionals and hospitals especially when an award is made based on sympathetic considerations.

OTHER MEASURES FOR LIMITING THE LIABILITY

Tort Reform in Medical Negligence Litigation

In the United States of America, increasing medical malpractice litigation and compensation toward victims prompted healthcare personals to demand caps on damages that can be awarded. States in the USA have therefore imposed caps on total damages awarded or on noneconomic damages, or they impose restrictions on damages based on whether a wrongful death occurred, or if the hospital where the victim was treated was a public or private hospital.

Several states of the USA have adopted apology and mandatory disclosure legislations to provide victims with alternative remedies. These legislations encourage doctors to admit to their faults and apologize for the same, provided their apologies are not treated as admissions of legal liability in the court. However, the impact of such apology laws has been minimal because of the narrow scope of the definition of apology under the legislations. Such tort reforms attempt to address the need for transparency within the health sector.[15]

Capping on Compensation

Eleven crore rupees compensation in Dr Balram Prasad versus Dr Kunal Saha case created a roar in medical fraternity for capping of compensation on medical negligence claim in India. Capping on compensation is established phenomenon practiced in many countries. In the US, about 26 states have passed effective legislations for imposing capping on noneconomic damages to cover pain, suffering, and other nonpecuniary injuries varying from state to state in the range of USD 250,000 up to USD 500,000. In California, noneconomic damages awarded in medical malpractice actions are capped at $250,000, Michigan has a cap of $280,000 for "noneconomic loss", and in West Virginia, noneconomic damages are capped at $500,000. In a study published in 2005 in the Journal of the American Medical

Association, 93% of physicians surveyed reported practicing defensive medicine, or (altering) clinical behavior because of the threat of malpractice liability.[16] In view of that former American President George W Bush proposed a nationwide $250,000 cap in medical malpractice cases.[17]

Indian Medical Association (IMA) has written a letter to PM Narendra Modi demanding a law for Capping on Compensation in medical negligence claim in our country also as prevalent worldwide.[18] IMA has pleaded that in India also there is a capping on the compensation being given to victims of natural calamity which is approximately ₹4 lakh being given by the Union Government, in death following sterilization in hospital compensation is ₹2 lakh, in death following sterilization compensation is ₹50,000 and according to Article 21 of the Montreal Convention, in case of death of passengers, the airline is liable to pay up to $174,000. But still government of India has not given ear to this genuine demand and more stern movement is needed regarding this.

No-fault Liability in Medical Negligence Litigation

No-fault liability in medical negligence exists in New Zealand, Denmark, and Sweden. An unconditional, minimum, fixed financial support to the victims of alleged medical negligence resulting in permanent disability or death at the commencement of any trial before any court without any finding(s) or bearing on the ultimate merits of the case. This compensation can be paid either by the defendant/hospital/insurance or by the state itself.[19]

The basis for no-fault liability is that medical errors are an expected phenomenon that are compensated for through specially instituted tribunals which assess the compensation payable to the victim purely on the presence of a medical error, without having to determine fault—that is actual negligence on the part of a specific party. The no-fault liability system attempts to encourage reporting of medical negligence, and equity in relation to compensation by ensuring all victims get some degree of compensation although it may be substantially lesser. This acts in the favor of minorities, and the poor who cannot afford to bring their claims to court.[20] World Health Organization has introduced a "no-fault compensation" program on COVID-19 vaccines. In this program, compensation is available to eligible individuals in 92 low- and middle-income countries without the need to resort to law courts. India, too, falls in this bracket. The COVAX no-fault compensation program is operationalized through its web portal (www.covaxclaims.com).[21]

Alternative Dispute Resolution in Medical Negligence Litigation

Mediation and arbitration in medical negligence cases have brought to light the different forms of remedies that victims or patients can seek, in addition to compensation, as well as the limited time it takes.[22] The flexibility of alternative dispute resolution measures allows for the variety of remedies, including (1) admission of negligence on the part of the doctor, (2) institution of training programs to prevent avoidable faults, and (3) emergency training to hospital staff which by their own admission, have provided great satisfaction to the victims. In our country also, alternative dispute resolution system is working by the way of Lok Adalat and Mediation in Consumer Protect Act but it is not available in medical negligence suits widely due to barring condition in mediation and ADR clause. As per Notification GSR 450(E) July 15th 2020, Matters not to be referred to mediation are matters relating to proceedings in respect of medical negligence resulting in grievous injury or death; cases involving allegations of fraud, fabrication of documents, forgery, impersonation, coercion; cases relating to prosecution for criminal and noncompoundable offences; cases which involve public interest.

SUMMARY

Jeremy Bentham's Utilitarian theory entails that the greatest happiness for the greatest number of people should be the guiding principle of actions and policies. Medical professionals who are giving maximum happiness to maximum number of people by their dedication toward patients and society should not be punished with so much of pecuniary punishment that may cause their financial death and make them bank corrupt. Giving such drastic payment in the name of restorative justice is being denied worldwide. Global Tort Reforms with reference to medical negligence like Capping on Compensation and No-Fault Insurance become more relevant in our country as most medical professionals are forced to serve community in suboptimal condition with miniature fees structure and most victims do not have mean to fight litigation for years.

Indian Medical Association has written a letter to the Prime Minister for capping on compensation for malpractice suits. Indeed compensating a family by ₹2 crore instead of ₹20 lakh will not revive the lost life. But it can wreck the doctor's family and close down small nursing homes in rural areas, putting the lives of thousands of people at risk. It is well accepted that negligent doctors should be punished financially but this should not result in bankruptcy. Serious financial hardship caused by mammoth compensation award is encouraging doctors to practice defensive medicine and discourage young people from choosing the profession. Similarly, No-fault Insurance can be answer for restorative justice enlarge without putting much burden on medical professionals. Our associations should bat high for getting these much-awaited global tort reforms for medical negligence.

LEARNING KEY POINTS

- Augmented informed consent may convert tortuous liability of medical negligence into deficiency of services which will cost liquidated damages of contract that is less bitter pill in comparison to unliquidated damages of tort.
- While defending consumer litigation, limitation ground, alleged harm, quantum of compensation must be refuted in preliminary objection in written statement.
- Always mention in reply in written statement and argument your working environment and limitation of clinical settings even if they are not relevant.
- Figure out yourself in reasonable man norms of the standard care with reference to working environment.
- Always take professional indemnity insurance of at least one crores.

TAKE-HOME MESSAGES

- Main culprit for huge compensation is tortuous nature of liability in medical negligence cases which attract unliquidated damages.
- Judicial discretion and imposing interest on pecuniary compensation for undue delay without any fault of defendant are other main causes of mammoth compensation.

- Augmented informed consent may convert tortuous liability of medical negligence into deficiency of services which will cost liquidated damages of contract that is less bitter pill in comparison to unliquidated damages of tort.
- Aggressive "Batting for Capping on compensation and No-Fault Insurance" from our professional associations is the need of the hour as these are well established concepts worldwide and may be granted by Governments in future by continuous persuasion.

MUST AVOID THINGS— DO NOT DO

- Never boast your academic and clinical capabilities.
- Never forget to take declaration from patient about his annual income and social status.
- Never forget to mention in reply in written statement and argument your working environment and limitation of clinical settings even if they are not relevant.

MUST DO THINGS

- While defending consumer litigation, limitation ground, alleged harm, and quantum of compensation must be refuted in preliminary objection in written statement.
- One should augment the informed consent as "Contract for hiring of medical services".
- Slapping of interest on pecuniary compensation must be challenged in appeal.

MESSAGES WHICH THE READERS MUST BE AWARE

Methodology of calculation of compensation always takes age and annual income of the patient into account so patient of lower age and high income will cost higher compensation.

WARNINGS

Issue of limitation and other technical defense must be raised in preliminary objection.

MEDICAL NEGLIGENCE PEARLS

- Highlight the duties of care which were successfully accomplished.
- Figure out yourself in reasonable man norms of the standard care with reference to working environment.

ONLY ONE FACT TO REMEMBER

Always take professional indemnity insurance of at least 1 crores.

MCQs

Choose one correct answer

1. As per Notification GSR 450(E) July 15th 2020, matters not to be referred to mediation are matters relating to proceedings in respect of medical negligence resulting in:
   a. Cases involving allegations of fraud, fabrication of documents, forgery, impersonation, coercion
   b. Cases which involve public interest
   c. Cases relating to prosecution for criminal and noncompoundable offences
   d. All of the above
2. Honorable Supreme Court in VN Shrikhande versus Anita Sena Fernandes case has propounded the principle for determination of:
   a. Accrual of cause of action
   b. Quantum of punishment
   c. Arrest in criminal negligence
   d. Medical board formation
3. In which case Honorable Supreme Court held that medical men and hospitals

should not be saddled with damages unless they are found negligent?
   a. State of Punjab vs. Shiv Ram and Ors., IV (2005) CPJ 14 (SC)
   b. Balram Prasad v Kunal Saha (2014) 1 SCC 384
   c. Martin F D'Souza versus Mohd Ahfaq 2009
   d. None of the above
4. Cause of mammoth compensation in medical negligence is:
   a. Unliquidated liability of tort in medical negligence
   b. Interest on pecuniary compensation awarded in undue delayed litigation
   c. Inappropriate use of discretion by judiciary in determining compensation
   d. All of the above

Answers

1. d   2. a   3. a   4. d

REFERENCES

1. (2014) 1 SCC 384.
2. Civil Appeal No. 8065 of 2009, with Civil Appeal No.5402 of 2010.
3. 2016 SCC OnLine MP 4247, 01-09-2016.
4. History.com editors. (2009). Code of Hammurabi. [online] Available from: https://www.history.com/topics/ancient-middle-east/hammurabi. [Last accessed December, 2023].
5. Balram Prasad vs. Kunal Saha, (2014) 1 SCC 384 & Nizam's Institute of Medical Sciences vs. Prashant S. Dhanaka, (2009) 6 SCC 1.
6. In the court of Shri Dig Vinaysingh, addl. district judge-04: Central Delhi, In re: RCA no. 27/11. date of judgment 4th December 2012.
7. Burrows A. Understanding the Law of Obligations: Essays on Contract, Tort and Restitution. Oxford: Hart Publishing; 2000.
8. Restatement of Torts, Second. Section 283.
9. Hall v. Hilburn, 466 So. 2d 856 (Miss. 1985).
10. Bolam V. Friern Hospital Management Committee, (1957) 2 All ER 118.
11. McCourt v Abernathy, 457 S.E.2d 603 (S.C. 1995).
12. CIVIL APPEAL NO. 2067 OF 2002, Decided On, 20 March 2009.
13. (2010) INSC 883, (2011) 1 SCC 53.
14. (2020) 5 SCC 757: (2020) 3 SCC (Civ) 338].
15. Mastroianni AC, Mello MM, Sommer S, Hardy M, Gallagher TH. The flaws in state "apology" and "disclosure" laws dilute their intended impact on malpractice suits. Health Aff (Millwood). 2010;29:1611-9.
16. Studdert DM, Mello MM, Sage WM, DesRoches CM, Peugh J, Zapert K, et al. Defensive medicine among high-risk specialist physicians in a volatile malpractice environment (abstract). JAMA. 2005;293:2609-17.
17. Cnn.com. "Bush outlines medical liability reform". [online] Available from: https://edition.cnn.com/2003/ALLPOLITICS/01/16/bush.malpractice/. [Last accessed December, 2023].
18. Indian Medical Association. Letter to PM by Indian Medical Association. [online] Available from https://www.ima-india.org/ima/left-side-bar.php?pid=588. [Last accessed December, 2023].
19. Pandya SK. Compensation by state: Eliminating legislation against doctors. Issues Med Ethics. 1993;1:4.
20. Mello MM, Kachalia A, Studdert DM. Administrative compensation for medical injuries: Lessons from three foreign systems. Issue Brief (Commonw Fund). 2011;14:1-18.
21. Datta J. (2021). Covid vaccines, WHO introduces 'no-fault compensation programme'. [online] Available from: https://www.thehindubusinessline.com/news/national/who-introduces-no-fault-compensation-programme/article33915375.ece. [Last accessed December, 2023].
22. Sohn DH, Bal BS. Medical malpractice reform: The role of alternative dispute resolution. Clin Orthop Relat Res. 2012;470:1370-8.

SUGGESTED READING

1. Baldwa M, Baldwa V, Padvi N, Baldwa S. Legal Issues in Critical Care. New Delhi: CBS Publishers; 2022.
2. Baldwa M, Baldwa V, Padvi N, Baldwa S. Legal Issues in Medical Practice, 2nd edition. New Delhi: CBS Publishers; 2023.

CHAPTER 12

Outdoor and Indoor Practice Giving Rise to Legal Liabilities in Medical Practice

Ishita Banerji

In law, a man is liable if one violates the rights of others.

Keywords: Advertisements, DAMA, Discharge summary, Emergency, IPD, Liabilities, OPD

Aim: If the court finds doctor liable under tort, then comes up requirement to compensate the patient party. So learn preventive aspects of liability to avoid payment of claims.

Objective: Causation is the connection between the breach of duty of care and the damage/injury that a person suffers. Unless the casual connection can be drawn between the two, a person cannot maintain a claim for damages.

INTRODUCTION

The first dream of every graduating doctor is to start his or her own outdoor and indoor practice. With the advent of the era of medico legally safe medical practice, it has become obligatory to understand the intricacies involved.

ELEMENTS OF IDEAL OPD PRACTICE

The purpose of the pediatric outpatient department (OPD) is to provide standardized attention and care to children who attend the hospital on an ambulatory basis.[1] It is a contact point for early diagnosis and initiation of treatment. *The registration counter* should display the names of consulting pediatricians with their qualifications, registration numbers, and OPD timings. The *waiting area* as per the patient load with an electronic display and an announcement system should have an enclosed area earmarked as a *feeding area*.

Pediatric Consultations

Every child needs to be *weighed* with complete *anthropometry measurements* done as well. An outdoor prescription should carry the *details of the doctor* along with qualifications, affiliations, OPD timings, and contact details. *The demographic profile of the child* with names of parents, address, contact number, age, weight, and gender needs to be specified. The prescription should carry a *summary of the child's overall health*. Besides the chief complaint and history of present illness, taking a detailed perinatal history is vital. Past medical history, family history, and social history are important to unravel any familial disease and to understand the child's social milieu. Development history gives an insight into the attainment of milestones and delays if any and nutritional history gives an opportunity to correct faulty feeding practices. Immunization history and further guidance according to the schedule are also needed. *Examination findings* must be noted as the prescription is a legal document and what is not documented is assumed as not done in the court of law. *A provisional diagnosis* must be made and noted before the investigations and treatment plan is charted. A note regarding refusal of admission if so was required should be made and the signature of the accompanying parent or guardian may be taken. *Digitalization of prescriptions* is a way of keeping the prescription legible besides keeping a record of it. If not typed, it is advisable to write legibly in capital letters and retaining a copy of it is a good practice though not a legal requirement.

Emergency Setup at OPD

An ideal OPD practice requires the availability of an emergency setup with basic facilities to help tide over a medical crisis. An oxygen supply, nebulizer, glucometer, pulse oximeter, BP instrument, and facility for IV access should also be available. It is not uncommon to have a medical emergency come unannounced as a cyanotic spell or syncope, seizure, or a sudden post-vaccination anaphylactic reaction to name a few. It is ideal to have a resuscitation tray ready with an Ambu bag and mask, a laryngoscope with an extra pair of batteries, ET tubes of different sizes, a suction machine, a suction catheter, emergency medicines, etc.

Publicizing: Sign Boards and Advertisements

Clause 6.1.1 of Code of Medical Ethics IMC 2002 prohibits soliciting patients or adopting any advertising or publicity measure that would ordinarily result in his self-aggrandizement. *Clause 6.1.2* considers any material for publicity as self-advertisement and unethical conduct. *Clause 7.11* prevents a physician from contributing articles and giving interviews that may reflect self-advertising or soliciting practices. *Clause 7.12* directs advertisements to contain only the name of the institution, the type of patients admitted, the type of training, and other facilities offered, and the fees. *Clause 7.13* prohibits the use of unusually large signboards.

LIMITED RESOURCE SETTINGS OF OPD: RURAL VERSUS URBAN VERSUS METROPOLITAN

The healthcare system in India is vast but not uniform. Healthcare remains polarized and huge disparities exist regarding accessibility and affordability to quality healthcare in rural areas that are still dependent on the local quacks and unqualified personnel, with a concentration of tertiary-level public and private healthcare in the metropolis. Under the stewardship of the Child Health Division of the Ministry of Health and Family Welfare, Government of India, the operational guideline for strengthening of pediatric health services has been brought about for planning and implementation in district hospitals.[2] It is a welcome step in the direction of setting standards for pediatric facilities and service delivery whereby, district hospitals as referral health facilities would be able to address the most common causes of morbidity and mortality in children and especially those due to diarrhea and pneumonia, which are the leading causes of under-five mortality.

HOW TO HANDLE OPD LOAD?

Managing the OPD load can be very challenging. Methods may be devised to streamline the process and reduce the waiting time for patients. Most hospitals with large OPD loads follow an online appointment system and multiple registration windows to ease the initial obstacle. A study was successfully conducted by Nishant D Goyal et al. on "OPD TRIAGE"—a novel concept for better patient management in heavily loaded orthopedic OPDs in government-run tertiary care centers.[3] Along similar lines, pediatric OPD triaging with multiple screening and consultation stations could be created as the first point of contact manned by junior doctors to help screen out a large number of patients requiring symptomatic treatment, feeding advice, and counseling which can be effectively handled by the junior doctors themselves. Unnecessary investigations must be avoided. The level 2 station would receive patients referred from level 1 only and not directly and those requiring expert opinion of the consultant would then be referred to level 3.

RIGHT OF A DOCTOR TO CHOOSE HIS PATIENT IN EMERGENCY VERSUS NONEMERGENCY

Clause 2.1.1 of the Code of Medical Ethics IMC 2002 declares that barring an emergency, a doctor has the right to choose his patient which translates to the corollary that a doctor has the right to refuse to treat a patient. *Clause 2.4* of the IMC 2002 states that though a physician is free to choose whom he will serve, he should, however, respond to any request for his assistance in an emergency. In the landmark judgment on *Parmanand Katara versus Union of India*, the Apex Court removed all ambiguity and laid down the guidelines for all doctors to follow in an emergency. The Court held that the preservation of life is of paramount importance that every doctor must extend his services to protect lives and that this obligation upon the medical profession is total, absolute, and paramount.

What is an emergency and who decides emergency—patient or doctor?

A medical emergency is usually interpreted as a life-threatening condition with an immediate risk of mortality or long-term serious morbidity. While a medical practitioner is the best judge of what is an emergency, the apprehensions of parents cannot be ignored either. It would be a good policy to triage patients in the OPD itself.

INDOOR PEDIATRIC PRESCRIPTIONS

Indoor documents comprise case sheets including initial assessment forms, progress notes, daily nursing assessment forms, nursing charts, laboratory and other investigation reports, treatment sheets, all consents, etc. Every page of the case sheet should carry the name of the patient with the unique identification number. Daily progress notes are required to be duly written down legibly, dated, and timed with the signature and name of the doctor, such that when read chronologically reveals the course of the ailment during the hospital stay. In case of any procedure or surgery being carried out, preprocedural/preoperative notes, procedural/operative notes, and postprocedural/postoperative notes should be duly entered into the file. These documents are the property of the hospital. However, if asked for by the patient party, a copy of it needs to be handed out to them within 72 hours after having numbered the sheets and taken a receiving. If duplicate copies are asked for, citing loss of documents mark "Duplicate" on the second copy to avoid misuse of the same.

Discharge summary needs to be detailed with the date of admission, date of discharge, date of procedure/surgery if any, diagnosis, presentation, investigation reports, the course in hospital, treatment given, condition at discharge, treatment advised on discharge, instructions for diet and activity, precautions to be taken and abstinence that need to be observed, date of next follow-up, probable side effects or complications to watch out for and details of emergency contact persons and numbers. It should be signed by the doctor preparing the discharge summary and countersigned by the consultant in charge. A copy of it should be tagged to the case file. A similar detailed discharge summary needs to be given in LAMA (Left Against Medical Advice) or DAMA (Discharged Against Medical Advice) patients as well, mentioning the proposed course of action and that they understand its ramifications yet refuse on their own volition with signatures from the relatives. Similarly, in case of transfer or referral to another hospital, the ongoing treatment should be mentioned along with the reason for such transfer/referral.

RETENTION PERIOD

Record keeping is a vital aspect. The National Medical Council (NMC) requires IPD records to be preserved for 3 years and OPD records for 2 years. The Consumer Protection Act (CPA Act) prescribes maintenance of records for 3 years; however, it is not uncommon for cases to be filed beyond the said period and condoned for delayed filing. Poor records mean poor defense and no records mean no defense. Hence, it is only in the interest of the medical practitioners and hospitals that records are retained for a sufficient period. Section 29 of the PCPNDT Act requires all documents to be maintained for a period of 2 years. The MTP Act mandates a period of 5 years from the end of the calendar year it relates to for retention of documents. The retention of pediatric files is not treated separately by MCI. Income Tax Act requires books and records to be maintained for 6 years from the last date of filing of the annual return (31st December) for that year. The records of medicolegal cases should be retained until the final disposal of the case. However, if an assessment has been reopened then the records need to be maintained till the assessment is closed. Death files have to be retained forever.

How to Destroy Old Records?

It is required by the hospital to first notify by a public notice in the newspapers its intent to destroy old case sheets of a specified period stating therein that a copy of their documents if required may be collected within a designated time, beyond which the documents would not be obtainable anymore. Manual records should be shredded and disposed of so that information is not retrievable.

MEDICAL NEGLIGENCE DUE TO FAULTY PRESCRIPTIONS

Most of the litigations arising out of faulty prescriptions or errors in administration are due to unqualified, untrained, or inexperienced staff carrying out orders. An illegible prescription or a misunderstood verbal or telephonic order sets the stage for error. The basics of avoiding medication error are to follow the six "Rs"—*right patient, right document, right drug, right dose, right route, and right time interval*. Extra precaution is required in children, particularly for intravenous administration of drugs, drug dilution, and rate of IV injection emphasizing prior sensitivity tests. Medical negligence may arise due to a lack of caution in prescribing and administering medication as is evident from the landmark judgment of *M/S Spring Meadows Hospital versus Harjot Ahluwalia through KS Ahluwalia and another* wherein the nurse and the resident doctor were found negligent and held liable for administering a high dose of Lariago via the intravenous route and the hospital held vicariously liable for employing unqualified people as nurses.

SUMMARY

It was not too long back when a doctor armed with just a stethoscope was good to consult. Today, without paraphernalia a doctor finds himself medico legally wanting. While the importance of documentation cannot be overemphasized, the demeanor of the doctor is no less important. Children are not half adults and neither are the pediatric dosages of medication half of the adult dosages! Common errors noted in an OPD prescription are the absence of the child's age, body weight, and provisional diagnosis, errors in drug doses, dosing interval, and duration besides necessary instructions for patients in an understandable language or form.

LEARNING KEY POINTS

- One must display one's name, NMC-recognized qualifications, and Registration number outside one's OPD chamber.
- An emergency setup with basic facilities must be available in the OPD to tide over medical crisis if any.
- Use of huge signboards is prohibited.
- Publicity or advertisements that indicate self-aggrandizementare prohibited.
- While a doctor has the right to choose his patient he is bound ethically and legally to attend emergency cases.
- Prescriptions should be legible and the direction of dosing understandable by the patients.
- Indoor case sheets should be complete with daily doctor's notes and detailed documentation.
- NMC requires IPD records to be preserved for 3 years and OPD records for 2 years.
- Follow procedure before destroying old records.

TAKE-HOME MESSAGE

Before one embarks on his or her professional journey, it is prudent to be aware of the law of the land, the statutory laws applicable, and the specific laws that govern one's field of practice. But most importantly, one must be conversant with the code of Medical Ethics.

FREQUENTLY ASKED QUESTIONS

Q.1. Who is a specialist?

Ans. Clause 7.20 IMC Regulations 2002 states that "a physician shall not claim to be a specialist unless he has a *special qualification* in that branch". Clause 1.42 of the IMC Regulations 2002 states that "Physicians shall display as suffix to their names only recognized medical degrees or such certificates/diplomas and memberships/honors which confer professional knowledge or recognizes any exemplary qualification/achievements". However, the recently amended NMC guidelines currently held in abeyance specify "only NMC recognized qualifications" may be displayed. The views of the courts are understood through the case of *Ms Shahla Imam versus Dr Nahid Fatima* wherein NCDRC set aside the complaint on specialty practice noting that the defendant a qualified surgeon (MS) and practicing obstetrics was competent to do deliveries and that no extraordinary expertise was required and neither was she transgressing in another field. In the case of *Sangeeta Dubey versus Dr Sunita Verma and others*, NCDRC opined that the doctor, a general surgeon with sufficient urology work experience could not be held liable for doing a urology surgery and a successful one at that, merely based on not being an urologist himself.

Q.2. What is Sudden death?

Ans. The World Health Organization has defined it as death, nonviolent, and not otherwise explained occurring <24 hours from the onset of symptoms.[4] All such deaths that occur within 24 hours of hospitalization without the establishment of a diagnosis must be informed to the police as per Section 39, CRPC. More than the suddenness, it is the unexpected and unexplained death that draws merit and a death certificate should not be issued.

MEDICOLEGAL PEARL

A doctor–patient relationship is established as soon as a patient walks into a doctor's chamber and the onus of nurturing this relationship lies with the doctor.

MUST AVOID THINGS

- Avoid transgressing specialty in one's daily practice.
- Avoid unholy nexus with practitioners of other "pathies"
- Avoid self-aggrandizement.

DO NOT DO

- Do not manipulate records.
- Do not give false assurances nor claim guaranteed results.
- Do not build unrealistic hopes and expectations.
- Do not delegate responsibility to untrained staff.

WARNINGS

Medical Jousting is a boomerang that comes back to one's own self someday.

MESSAGES WHICH THE READER MUST BE AWARE

It is a legal requirement to attend emergencies to the best of one's ability and ensure the safe transfer of the patient after stabilization with appropriate medical assistance to an appropriate facility.

MUST DO THING

Document all communications made related to the patient and communicate all that is documented.

ONLY ONE FACT TO REMEMBER

Practice within the scope of one's specialization and training.

REFERENCES

1. Quality Assurance Cell, Delhi State Health Mission, Department of Health and Family Welfare, Government of NCT of Delhi. (2016). Standard Operating Procedures (SOPs) for Pediatrics, 1st edition. [online] Available from: https://dshm.delhi.gov.in/pdf/QAC/SoPs/Pediatrics.pdf. [Last accessed December, 2023].
2. National Health Mission. (2015). Strengthening facility based Pediatric Care, Operational Guidelines for Planning and Implementation in District Hospitals. [online] Available from: https://nhm.gov.in/images/pdf/programmes/child-health/guidelines/Strenghtening_Facility_Based_Paediatric_Care-Operational_Guidelines.pdf. [Last accessed December, 2023].

3. Goyal ND, Chavan RK, Pahwa A, Gautam VK, Mishra N, Tripathi PK. "OPD Triage": a novel concept for better patient management in heavily loaded orthopedic OPDs. J Clin Orthop Trauma. 2020;11(Suppl 4):S472-8.
4. World Health Organization. International Classification of Diseases (ICD-10). Geneva: World Health Organization; 2005.

SUGGESTED READING

1. Baldwa M, Baldwa V, Padvi N, Baldwa S. Legal Issues in Critical Care. New Delhi: CBS Publishers; 2022.
2. Baldwa M, Baldwa V, Padvi N, Baldwa S. Legal Issues in Medical Practice, 2nd edition. New Delhi: CBS Publishers; 2023.

CHAPTER 13

Advance Deposit Before Admission and While Discharge Bill not Paid in Hospital

Hemant R Gangolia, Ramesh B Dampuri, Sanjio Borade

The love of money is the root of all kinds of evil.

Keywords: Advance deposit, Bill on discharge, Emergency, Sudden death

Aim: One of the primary reasons for non-deposit of advance and nonpayment of hospital bills is the financial burden faced by patients, especially those from lower socioeconomic backgrounds who in face of so-called "emergency medical condition" instead of going to government hospital get in private pay for service hospital. Hospital should anticipate and guide patients to government hospital instead treating in private set up to avoid such unpleasant scenarios.

Objective: In India, the practice of requiring advance deposits from patients before admission to a hospital is prevalent, particularly in private hospitals. This practice is often justified by hospitals as a means of ensuring to see affordability by potential patient. The amount of the deposit can vary depending on the hospital and the type of care being provided. In some cases, the deposit may cover the entire cost of treatment, while in others it may only cover a portion of the cost. While there is no legal justification for deliberately evading hospital dues, financial constraints and misunderstandings regarding treatment costs often lead to such situations.

INTRODUCTION

As said "Money is the root of all evil", the bills at the medical establishments are the main reason for the episodes of violence and litigations. The settlement and recovery of bills is a difficult situation and one needs more of social, managerial, manipulative, and tactful skills rather than medical knowledge. It is imbibed in the minds of society and people that medicine being a noble profession, the job of doctors is to serve the people without the expectations of remuneration even though it may be appropriate to the medical services offered. Hence, they do not realize the value of medical services offered to them in terms of remuneration as well they feel it is to be bargained.[1]

THE MONETARY ISSUES

Related to the medical practice can be seen at different levels of:
- OPD
- Day care procedures
- IPD
- Surgeries
- Emergencies
- Sudden death.

How to Solve?

The solution to any issue is possible if one learns to apply the six words in our practice to all the above stated scenarios. They are as follows:

- Anticipation of the likely expense, patient's psychology, value of medical service, etc.
- Communication of the estimated cost of treatment, consultation, and follow-up charges
- Documentation of the communication more so in IPD, surgeries, and day care services
- Limitations in terms of infrastructure and facilities availability at one's set ups
- Ethics in terms of four principles of the medical ethics, viz., respect (autonomy), do good (beneficence), do no harm (nonmaleficence), and equality (justice)
- Introspection in terms of our near and dear ones in the shoes of the patient.

Let us analyze the monetary issues at different levels:

- OPD:
  - The rates of the medical services available as per the facilities and infrastructure should be displayed at appropriate place in waiting room such as:
    - Consultation
    - Follow-ups
    - Injections
    - Dressings
    - BP checkup/diabetes sugar checkup
    - Emergency fees
    - Home visit, etc., as per the medical services offered at the OPD
  - The stated rates as bills can be collected in advance before the consultation or after the consultations as per the setup of OPD at individual or group or corporate practice
  - No free business at the OPD as Doctors are always considerate while charging their fees throughout their medical practice. Still if there is unaffordable patient, one should charge to minimum by giving concession to maximum possible. By offering free services, one should not devalue oneself moreover by providing free services is not a defense in court of law if any litigation gets filed later on.

  Clinical Establishment Act endorses the display of rates in the states where it is implemented and will in other states too after it get implemented there.

- *Day care procedures/surgeries:*
  - After the explanation of the procedure, its complications, consent, the estimated cost of the procedure to be explained, the communication of which to be documented as well the possibility of percentage rise in the cost in view of any anticipated explained complications.
  - It is advisable to collect the estimated cost as a deposit with the settlement of the bill accordingly after the procedure as one cannot predict the worst mishap even possible with minor procedures/surgeries. Depending on the setting of the practice, one may opt for the part advance payment and final settlement of bill on discharge but that carries the risk of bill recovery in case of mishap.
  - Usually there is an issue of so-called discount/concession as an Indian has the habit of bargaining, hence by keeping this issue at the back of the mind, one can have bill on higher side and so-called concession offered

gets appreciated by the patient. But once done, same trend sets in, hence advisable to avoid it or otherwise at an individual call.

- *IPD:*
  - On admission, the important job is the preparation of indoor paper, filling of consent forms, and the explanation of the estimated cost of indoor treatment particulars and category wise for which the decision makers of patient should be very well defined. The documented communication of the estimated indoor treatment cost with the decision makers is the important aspect. Here again, the various charges as bed, nursing, doctor, etc. can be displayed at appropriate place or as a leaflet with the indoor papers.
  - It is advisable to have the dedicated personnel for that and after the admission to do the counseling of the decision makers on day-to-day basis making them to pay the advances appropriately. The daily review is important and at the same time, one should be a good listener to the grievances of patient as well of decision makers.
  - It has to be clearly explained and documented the payment modes in terms of deposit, advances, day-to-day payments, concessions if any, receipts as well the options of cash, cheques, DD, online, and card payments. Any issue regarding the amount to be sorted out immediately and if need arises to be intervened by the in-charge of the setup. In raising the bills, the facilities and infrastructure have to be taken into consideration.
- *Surgeries:* The same principles applies to the elective surgeries with regards to the documented communication of the estimated cost with the payment mode options in terms of deposits, advances, and settlement bills.
- *Emergencies:* The emergencies may be per se the emergency brought to the medical establishment or the emergency surgery arising out of the hospitalized patient. As per the Parmanand Katra versus Union of India[2] case law, the patient has right to get treated in emergency state that is Doctor does not have the right to choose the patient in an emergency state but has the right to choose the patient in a non-emergency state as per Regulation 2.1 of the Ethics of the MCI. Hence, in emergency, there is huge issue of deposit and advance payment though if properly communicated can have the sufficient deposit by anticipating the probable outcome of the emergency state management?

  The major issue arises in case of nonaffordability of the patient where in spite of explaining the estimated cost one has to provide emergency care to the best of one's limitations and ability as per above case law and treat it. Try to stabilize and in depending on the infrastructure to transfer the emergency by appropriate ambulance accompanied by appropriate personnel and to settle with whatever payment has received. It is advisable to issue the complete bill of the emergency management and to document the pending balance payment on the receipt after deducting the received amount.
- *Sudden death:* This is the most important, dicey, tricky situation very difficult to handle and the raised bill is most of the time the reason for assaults and litigation.

Two scenarios arise:
1. In case of sudden death of stable patient on admission which is unexpected to both relatives of patient and doctor, the issue has to be handled tactfully with the appropriate communication
2. In case of death of the serious or gasping patient on or after admission, the communication of the advance must be apt and reasonably placed.

In both situations, the deposit is very important in view of the death as anticipated outcome, hence advisable to advance paid whatever is possible.

The last scenario is whether the medical establishment can withheld the release of the dead body against the pending bill payment. There are interesting case laws over the period when for the first time the above issue of not releasing the dead body in view of nonpayment of the settlement bill went to Tamil Nadu State Commission where the decision went in favor of doctor. Any judgment comes with the reasoning. The reasoning being as there is contractual relationship between patient and doctor, both have equal rights as per Consumer Protection Act in terms of doctor as service provider and patient to pay the fees for it. In this case, the service was provided by doctor but the relatives of the patient have not paid the bill, hence the breach of the contract thereby the withholding the dead body against the pending bill was appropriate and justified.

In view of the similar case known as Hiranandani Hospital Mumbai case law, Mumbai High Court gave the judgment in favor of patient thereby the order to release the dead body with following reasoning. The reasoning being that there are three wrongs involved, viz., legal, ethical, and moral. Legally speaking the dead body can be held in view of contractual relationship, ethically cannot withheld as an alternate remedy available as well morally sentiments attached to the death in the family. Hence, dead body cannot be withheld in view of alternate remedy available which being to file a civil suit for the recovery of the bills but then it requires advocate, court fees, and long waiting period therefore not advisable. But in such cases though the settlement bill has been refused, the bill to be stamped as pending and issued.

Hence in such cases, it is better to forget the bill thereby the most important aspect is the advance collection with appropriate counseling, documented communication with introspection and ethical considerations in raising such bills with the limitations of the medical establishment.

SUMMARY

Ultimately, all these difficult situations are going to stay and we have to learn to live with them, tackle them, as nicely as possible and reduce the stress. In the light of basic legal knowledge, let dispel these unfounded legal fears and do the right things in right directions.

LEARNING KEY POINTS

- Display of the rates of medical services available at medical/clinical establishment.
- Documented communication of the estimated cost of the medical services.
- Well anticipated smartly executed hospital deposit/advance collection plan.
- Dedicated personnel to counsel for regular advance deposit on day-to-day basis with an ear to their grievances.
- To be watchful for deposits in emergency/serious/surgical cases.
- Forget the bill in case of death if pending bill is refused in spite of counseling.

CHAPTER 13: Advance Deposit Before Admission and While Discharge Bill not Paid in Hospital

TAKE-HOME MESSAGES
Display of the rates.

MUST AVOID THINGS
Physically and verbally fighting for the unpaid bill.

DO NOT DO
Never get you bill collected by strongmen using force.

WARNINGS
Never ever keep patient indoors if bill is not paid.

MESSAGES WHICH THE READER MUST BE AWARE
Documented communication of the estimated cost of the medical services.

MUST DO THING
One can submit eye and expert witness without being asked by consumer court.

MEDICAL NEGLIGENCE PEARLS
Forget the bill in case of death if pending bill is refused in spite of counseling.

ONLY ONE FACT TO REMEMBER
Dedicated personnel to counsel for regular advance deposit on day-to-day basis with an ear to their grievances.

REFERENCES
1. Tiwari S. Textbook on Medicolegal Issues, 2nd edition. New Delhi: Jaypee Brothers Medical Publisher; 2018.
2. Rangnath M. (1989). Pt. Parmanand Katara vs Union Of India & Ors on 28 August, 1989. [online] Available from: https://indiankanoon.org/doc/498126/. [Last accessed December, 2023].

SUGGESTED READING
1. Baldwa M, Baldwa V, Padvi N, Baldwa S. Legal Issues in Critical Care. New Delhi: CBS Publishers; 2022.
2. Baldwa M, Baldwa V, Padvi N, Baldwa S. Legal Issues in Medical Practice, 2nd edition. New Delhi: CBS Publishers; 2023.

CHAPTER 14

Landmark Supreme Court Judgments and Their Importance in Medicolegal Litigations

Jyoti Kumar Gupta, Ashish Jain, AB Jaiswal, Jitendra Pratap Singh Chauhan

*A lawsuit is to ordinary life what war is to peacetime.
In a lawsuit, everybody on the other side is bad.*

Keywords: Contempt of court, Judicial impropriety, Judicial precedents, Obiter dicta, Ratio decidendi, Stare decisis

Aim: A doctor should use landmark Supreme Court judgments as preventive tools for medicolegal litigations.

Objective: In India the purpose of a lawsuit is to harass doctors by patient as they know it well that doctor did not do anything intentionally. The law can be used very easily to harass, and enough harassment on somebody who is simply on the thin edge anyway, will generally be sufficient to cause his "professional death" or "professional disability" due to hanging litigation and that will ruin him utterly. Most doctors will suffer from medical malpractice stress syndrome (MMSS). Going through landmark Supreme Court judgments shall give courage to doctor and avoid MMSS.

INTRODUCTION

The Honorable Supreme Court has enacted various principles and law medical negligence suits through its landmark judgments. Precedents set by the Supreme Court in its judgments are the leading source of declared law in field of Medical Negligence. These Judicial Precedents of Supreme Court are binding on all on the subordinate courts and cannot be challenged in subordinate courts. The concept of law of precedents evolved in England, and was later adopted in Indian law as well. It was integral part of the Government of India Act, 1935 by way of Section 212 and when the Constitution of India was enacted, the law makers made certain provisions to give binding effect of judicial precedents of higher judiciary on subordinate courts. It is important for us to know about law of precedent and principles propounded by Supreme Court through its landmark judgments in medical malpractice suits and their binding value in the light of mandate of Indian constitution.

DOCTRINE OF PRECEDENTS: STARE DECISIS

Principle of precedents emanates from the Legal doctrine of *stare decisis et non quieta movere,* which means "to stand by decisions and not to disturb what is settled binds the courts to follow legal precedents set by previous decisions. This doctrine makes it abundantly clear that legal precedents play a pivotal role in deciding an issue having identical facts and questions of law. This doctrine is an integral part of Common Law. Precedents are considered an important

CHAPTER 14: Landmark Supreme Court Judgments and Their Importance in Medicolegal Litigations

source of law. Keeton defines judicial precedents as *"judicial decisions to which authority in some measure has been attached"*. The court's policy of adhering to precedents is known as stare decisis. It simply means "to stand by the decided matters", i.e., stick to a decision. The principle and concept of stare decisis is embodied in Article 141 of the Constitution of India. It states that the law declared by the Supreme Court shall be binding on all courts within the territory of India.

RATIO DECIDENDI

According to Salmond, a precedent is a judicial decision that contains a principle. This principle has authority, or the force of law, which will bind the Courts in their subsequent judgements. So, this authoritative principle in a judicial decision is called the ratio decidendi. The entire judgement as a whole binds the parties to the case completely, but the "Principle", which constitutes the ratio decidendi of the judgement alone, has force of law vis-a-vis the world at large. Ratio decidendi literally translates to *"reason for deciding"*. In the case of *Shailyamanyu Singh versus the State of Maharashtra (2023)*, Bombay High Court clarified that neither the finding of the facts by the court nor the reasons given for deciding on granting specific relief can be considered precedent. Only the statement of law applied to the legal issue raised on the facts based on which the case is decided forms the ratio decidendi, which constitutes a binding precedent.

OBITER DICTA

"Obiter dicta" means *"things said by the way"*. Obiter dicta, much in contrast to ratio decidendi, are those statements, discussions, legal opinions, or remarks given by the judges that do not directly play a role in how the decision or judgement of the case turns out. These are miscellaneous statements that constitute the major portions of the judgement; however, they are not legally binding like a precedent. They provide insights into the thought process of the judges and gain their views and opinions on a certain legal point. In Indian legal system, certain cases have reiterated the binding capacity of obiter dicta of the Supreme Court over the High Courts and other subordinate courts. In *Hiralal Gnaeshmal Jain versus State of Maharashtra (1992)*,[1] the judges observed that even the obiter dicta of the Supreme Court will be binding on them.

CONSTITUTIONAL MANDATE ON BINDING EFFECT OF JUDICIAL PRECEDENTS OF SUPREME COURT

Articles 141, 142, and 144 of the Indian Constitution pertain to the law declared by the Supreme Court of India. Article 141 states that "The law declared by the Supreme Court shall be binding on all courts within the territory of India". This means that the decisions of the Supreme Court are considered binding precedent for all other courts in India. Article 142 pertains to the powers of the Supreme Court to pass such decrees or make such orders as may be necessary for doing complete justice in any cause or matter pending before it. Article 144 mandates that civil and judicial authorities to act in aid of the Supreme Court; all authorities, civil and judicial, in the territory of India shall act in aid of the Supreme Court.

Supreme Court in *Director of Settlements, Andhra Pradesh versus M.R Apparao and Anr*[2] *case* has emphasized the power of declaring law by way of precedents by mentioning that *Article 141 of the Constitution unequivocally* mentions that the decisions of the Supreme Court are binding on all the subordinate courts. The aforesaid article empowers the Supreme Court to declare the law".

Supreme Court in *Dr Shah Faesal and Others versus Union of India and another*[3] case has made it clear that *"It is only the principle laid down in the judgment that is binding law under Article 141 of the Constitution* and in *State of Punjab and others versus Surinder Kumar and others*[4] that a *"decision is available as a precedent only if it decides a question of law".*

In *Islamic Academy of Education and Another versus State of Karnataka and Others*[5] case, the Supreme Court observed that *"The ratio decidendi of a judgment has to be found out only on reading the entire judgment. In fact, the ratio of the Judgement is what is set out in the Judgement itself. The answer to the question would necessarily have to be read in the context of what is set out in the Judgement and not in isolation. In case of any doubt as regards any observations, reasons and principles, the other part of the Judgement has to be looked into. By reading a line here and there from the judgment, one cannot find out the entire ratio decidendi of the judgment".*

Article 141 states that only the ratio decidendi which is the determining point which becomes the base for judgement of a case is binding not the obiter dicta and the mere facts of the cases. Therefore, while applying the decision of Supreme Court by other courts, what is required is to understand the true principle laid down by the previous decision. The judgment has to be read as a whole and at the same time, the observation from the judgment has to be determined in the light of the questions presented before the court. The judicial precedents passed by the Supreme Court are not binding on them as they can depart from its earlier judgements.

IMPORTANCE OF PRECEDENTS SET BY SUPREME COURT JUDGMENTS

As per Article 141, the law declared by Supreme Court to be binding on all courts and tribunals within the territory of India. Apex court has said in *Suganthi Suresh Kumar versus Jagdeeshan*[6] case that *"It is impermissible for the High Court to overrule the decision of the Apex Court on the ground that Supreme Court laid down the legal position without considering any other point. It is not only a matter of discipline for the High Courts in India, it is mandate of the Constitution as provided in article 141 that the law declared by the Supreme Court shall be binding on all courts within the territory of India".* In *State of Himachal Pradesh versus Paras Ram*[7] case also, the Supreme Court has emphasized that *"The judicial discipline to abide by Supreme Court decision cannot be forsaken under any pretext by any authority or court, be it even High Court".*

So, at one end in Article 141 all subordinate courts and tribunals are under obligation to abide by the law and principle declared by the Supreme Court; at another end in Article 144 all civil and judicial authorities are under obligation to act in aid of Supreme Court to follow the law and principles declared by it in the territory of India. It means that police and other public authorities are under obligation to follow the principles and directions given in Supreme Court judgments. No police and public authority can deny following the direction and principle enunciated in Supreme Court judgments.

VIOLATION OF SUPREME COURT JUDICIAL PRECEDENTS

Contempt of Court

Article 129 of Constitution of India says that "The Supreme Court shall be a court of record and shall have all the powers of such a court including the power to punish for contempt of itself".

Supreme Court in *Vinay Chandra Mishra, In re, (1995) 2 SCC 584* has defined contempt of court in following terms: *"Under the common law definition, 'contempt of Court' is defined as an act or omission calculated to interfere with the due administration of justice. This covers criminal contempt (that is acts which so threaten the administration of justice that they require punishment) and civil contempt (disobedience of an order made in a civil cause)".*

Supreme Court in *B. Mishra versus B Dixit, AIR 1972 SC 2466, 2468* has said that *"Contempt of Court is disobedience to the Court, by acting in opposition to the authority, justice and dignity thereof. It signifies a wilful disregard or disobedience of Court's order; it also signifies such conduct as tends to bring the authority of the Court and the administration of the law into disrepute".*

So any person including public authority and police showing wilful disregard to direction given by Supreme Court or violating law or principle declared by Supreme Court in judicial precedents may attract contempt proceeding under Article 129 of Constitution of India.

Judicial Impropriety

"Wilful judicial impropriety" occurs if the Bench ventures to interpret the matter when it has judicial notice when similar with the same issue is already decided higher court in hierarchy.

In *Dwarikesh Sugar Industries Ltd. versus Prem Heavy Engineering Works (P) Ltd. and another 1997 (6) SCC 450* the Hon'ble Supreme Court has held: *"When a position, in law, is well settled as a result of judicial pronouncement of this Court, it would amount to judicial impropriety to say the least, for the subordinate courts including the High Courts to ignore the settled decisions and then to pass a judicial order which is clearly contrary to the settled legal position. Such judicial adventurism cannot be permitted and we strongly deprecate the tendency of the subordinate courts in not applying the settled principles and in passing whimsical orders which necessarily has the effect of granting wrongful and unwarranted relief to one of the parties. It is time that this tendency stops".*

Again, in *M/s D. Navinchandra and Co., Bombay versus Union of India and others, 1987 (3) SCC 66* case, Apex Court stated the law in the following terms: *"Generally legal positions laid down by the court would be binding on all concerned even though some of them have not been made parties nor were served normally notice of such proceedings".*

In *Markio Tado versus Takam Sorang (SC), 2013(3) SCC (Cri) 597: 2013(3) R.C.R. (Civil) 274* case, Supreme Court has again mentioned that *"Before we conclude, we may state that it is unfortunate that such acts of judicial impropriety are repeated in spite of clear judgments of this court on the significance of Article 141 of the Constitution. Thus, in a judgment by a bench of three judges in Dwarikesh Sugar Industries Ltd. v. Prem Heavy Engineering Works (P) Ltd. and Anr., reported in (1997) 6 SCC 450, this court observed. When a position, in law, is well settled as a result of judicial pronouncement of this Court, it would amount to judicial impropriety to say the* least, for the subordinate courts including the High Courts to ignore the settled decisions and then to pass a judicial order which is clearly contrary to the settled legal position. Such judicial adventurism cannot be permitted and we strongly deprecate the tendency of the subordinate courts in not applying the settled principles and in passing whimsical orders which necessarily has the effect of granting wrongful and unwarranted relief to one of the parties. It is time that this tendency stops".

MEANINGFUL SUPREME COURT JUDGMENTS

Law Related to Medical Emergencies

Parmanand Katara versus Union of India 1989 AIR 2039, SCR (3) 997

The Apex Court observed that when accidents occur and the victims are taken to hospitals or to a medical practitioner, they are not taken care of for giving emergency medical treatment on the ground that the case is a medicolegal case and the injured person should go to a Government Hospital. The SC emphasized the need for making it obligatory for hospitals and medical practitioners to provide emergency medical care. Based on the petition, the Supreme Court held that:

- Preservation of human life is of paramount importance.
- Every doctor, at a government hospital or otherwise, has the professional obligation to extend his/her services to protect life. No law or State action can intervene to avoid/delay the discharge of the paramount obligation cast upon members of the medical profession. The obligation being total, absolute and paramount, laws of procedure whether in statutes or otherwise which would interfere with the discharge of this obligation cannot be sustained and must, therefore, give way.
- There should be no doubt that the effort to save the person should receive top priority. This applies not only to the legal profession, but also to the police and other citizen's part of the matter.

Apex Court also held that:

- A man in the medical profession should not be unnecessarily harassed for the purposes of interrogation or for any other formality and should not be dragged during investigations at the police station and it should be avoided as far as possible. We also hope and trust that our law courts will not summon a medical professional to give evidence unless the evidence is necessary and even if he is summoned, attempt should be made to see that the men in this profession are not made to wait and waste time unnecessarily and it is known that our law courts always have respect for the men in the medical profession and they are called to give evidence when necessary and attempts are made so that they may not have to wait for long.
- We have no hesitation in saying that it is expected of the members of the legal profession which is the other honorable profession to honor the persons in the medical profession and see that they are not called to give evidence so long as it is not necessary. Where the facts are so clear it is expected that necessary harassment of the members of the medical profession either by way of requests for adjournments or by cross examination should be avoided.

Paschim Banga Khet Mazdoor Samity versus State of West Bengal and ANR

The petitioner sustained multiple injuries falling off from a train. He got denial for admission into six successive state hospitals either with an excuse of not having required equipment or having no vacant bed.

The Apex Court declared that "the right to life enshrined in the Indian Constitution (Article 21) imposes an obligation on the State to safeguard the right to life of every person and that preservation of human life is of paramount importance. This obligation on the State stands irrespective of constraints in financial resources. The Court stated that denial of timely medical treatment necessary to preserve human life in government-owned hospitals is a violation of this right. The Court asked the Government of West Bengal to pay the petitioner compensation for the loss suffered. It also directed the Government to formulate a blue print for primary health care with particular reference to treatment of patients during an emergency".

Definition of Consumer Vendor Includes Medical Services

Three judge bench Indian Medical Association versus V.P. Shantha, 1996 AIR 550[8]

CPA made applicable to doctors by Supreme Court of India—not over-ruled
As there were increasing cases relating to doctor (Medical) negligence, and it was ambiguous that whether medical services are services under COPRA, 1986 or not and whether hospital or doctor or medical practitioner is in the ambit of COPRA, 1986 or not, a PIL was filed in Supreme Court under Article 32 of Constitution of India, to decide upon Scope and Jurisdiction of the Consumer Protection Act, 1986.

Issue:
- Whether and, if so, in what circumstances, a medical practitioner can be regarded as rendering "service" under Section 2(1)(o) of the Consumer Protection Act, 1986.
- Whether the service rendered at a hospital/nursing home can be regarded as "service" under Section 2(1) (o) of the Act.

Cases referred for deciding:
- Bolam versus Friern Hospital Management Committee [1957] 1 W.L.R. 582
- Dharangdhara Chemical Works Ltd. versus State of Saurashtra, AIR 1957 SC 264
- Lucknow Development Authority versus M.K. Gupta, 1994 AIR787.

Judgment:
- Medical Services are treated as in ambit of "services" under Section 2(1)(o) of the Act.
  - It is not contract of personal service as there is absence of master–servant relationship.
  - Contract of service in Section 2(1)(o) cannot be confined to contracts for employment of domestic servants only. The services rendered to employer are not covered under the Act.
- Medical Services rendered by hospital/ nursing home free of charge are not in the purview of Section 2(1)(o) of the Act.
- Medical Services rendered by independent doctor free of charge are under Section 2(1)(o) of the jurisdiction of the Act.
- Medical Services rendered against payment of consideration are in the scope of the Act.
- A medical service where payment of consideration is paid by third party is treated as in the ambit of the Act.

- Hospital in which some person are charged and some are exempted from charging because of their inability of affording such services will be treated as consumer under of Section 2(1)(d) of the Act.

It was opined by Hon'ble Judge that since patients, who are availing services free of charge, belonging to third category are beneficiary as patients who are paying consideration in that category are, actually, paying for nonpaying patients too. So, being beneficiary they are under scope of the Act. Hence are treated as consumer under Section 2(1)(d) of the Act.

Critical analysis:
- This case gave effect to consumers who were suffering from medical negligence and including medical services in the ambit of Consumer Protection Act, 1986 enabled consumer to get more speedy and cheap justice. As this is the main aim of the Act.
- This case also differentiated contract for service and contract of service, in respect of medical practice and profession.
- System of liability which it established is not appropriate in case where patients are not treated as consumer even in government hospital availing services free of charge. It is question of common conscience and equity as person who are availing services in government hospital are not economically sound that is why they are availing services in government hospital. It is point of reconsideration.
- Hospital rendering services free of charge are outside the purview of the Consumer Protection Act, 1986. As some charitable trust do not have profit motive they can be sued in either civil case but not in Consumer court.

Definition on of Negligence

1968—three judge bench of Supreme Court of India defines what medical negligence is?— not over-ruled

Long major bone fracture set right without anesthesia—death was due to negligence

Laxman Balkrishna Joshi, Dr versus Dr Trimbak Bapu Godbole, (SC) three judge bench, Civil Appeal No. 547 of 1965. D/d. 2.5.1968.

Trial Court accepted the eyewitness account given by respondent 1 and came to the conclusion notwithstanding the denial by the appellant that the appellant had performed reduction of the fracture; that in doing so he applied excessive force with the help of three of his attendants, that such reduction was done without giving anesthetic, that the said treatment resulted in cerebral embolism or shock which was the proximate cause of the boy's death. The trial court disbelieved the appellant's case that he had decided to postpone reduction of the fracture or that his treatment consisted of immobilization with only light traction with plaster splints. The trial Judge was of the view that this defense was an afterthought and was contrary to the evidence and the circumstances of the case. On these findings, he held the appellant guilty of negligence and wrongful acts which resulted in the death of Ananda and awarded general damages in the man of ₹3,000/-.

High Court agreed with the trial court. The injury was a simple fracture. The reasons given by the appellant for his decision to delay the reduction were that (1) there was swelling on the thigh, (2) that 2 days had elapsed since the accident, (3) that there was no urgency for reduction, and (4) that the boy was exhausted on account of the long journey. The High Court observed that there could not have been swelling at that time for neither the clinical notes, nor the case paper, mentioned swelling or any other symptom which called for delayed reduction. Merely mentioned one morphia injection, one X-ray photograph, and putting the leg in plaster of Paris.

Supreme Court observed that death was due to shock, resulting from reduction of the fracture attempted by the appellant without taking the elementary caution of giving anesthetic to the patient. The trial court and the High Court were, therefore, right in holding that the appellant was guilty of negligence and wrongful acts toward the patient and was liable for damages.

Negligence of surgeon towards his patient—Question of liability of surgeon—

Duties of doctor toward his patient:
- *Person who holds himself out ready to give medical advice and treatment impliedly skill undertakes that he possessed of skill and knowledge for the purpose.*
- *Practitioner must bring to his task a reasonable degree of skill and knowledge and must exercise a reasonable degree of care.*

Held, on facts that High Court was right in its conclusions that death of patient was due to negligence of doctor.

RES IPSA Loquitur

1979—two judge bench of Supreme Court

Supreme Court on 25 July, 1979 in a judgment reported as Syad Akbar versus State of Karnataka.

Equivalent citations: 1979 AIR 1848, 1980 SCR (1) 25 explained the principle of res ipsa loquitur in a criminal trial as under:

"As a rule, mere proof that an event has happened or an accident has occurred, the cause of which is unknown, is not evidence of negligence. But the peculiar circumstances constituting the event or accident, in a particular case, may themselves proclaim in concordant, clear and unambiguous voices the negligence of somebody as the cause of the event or accident. It is to such cases that the maxim res ipsa loquitur may apply, if the cause of the accident is unknown and no reasonable explanation as to the cause is coming forth from the defendant. To emphasize the point, it may be reiterated that in such cases, the event or accident must be of a kind which does not happen in the ordinary course of things if those who have the management and control use due care. But, according to some decisions, satisfaction of this condition alone is not sufficient for res ipsa to come into play and it has to be further satisfied that the event, which caused the accident, was within the defendant's control. The reason for this second requirement is that where the defendant has control of the thing which caused the injury, he is in a better position than the plaintiff to explain how the accident occurred. Instances of such special kind of accidents which "tell their own story" of being offsprings of negligence, are furnished by cases, such as where a motor vehicle mounts or projects over a pavement and hurts somebody there or traveling in the vehicle; one car ramming another from behind, or even a head on collision on the wrong side of the road".

Vicariously Responsibility

1989—two judge bench of Supreme Court of India—state held vicariously responsible

Medical misadventure causing irreversible damage to eyes of the 88 patients out of 108 patients—negligence

A.S. Mittal versus State of U.P., (SC) two judge bench, Writ Petition. No. 1247 of 1986. D/d. 12.5.1989.[9]

"Eye Camp"—conducted—several people operated for cataract—many becoming totally blind in operated eyes—social organization filed Public Interest Litigation espousing the cause of unfortunate victims and prosecuting it with diligence—victims granted monetary relief payment on humanitarian considerations ordered by Court—necessity for strict compliance with guidelines issued by Government for conduct of eye camps—emphasized on suggestion to the Union to incorporate some recommendations noted in the judgment made by Expert Subcommittee of the Indian Medical Council in the Revised Guidelines—State Government directed to pay costs to the organization.

Supreme Court observed eye camps—guidelines issued on 9-2-88 by Union Government on holding of eye camps are quite comprehensive—Supreme Court further directed the Union Government to consider incorporation of these guidelines.

Eye camp—medical misadventure causing irreversible damage to eyes of the patients—State held vicariously responsible. On humanitarian considerations, the Supreme Court directed the States to pay ₹12,500/- to each of the victims in addition to interim relief already paid.

RES IPSA Loquitur and Vicarious Liability

1996—two judge bench of Supreme Court of India—mop left—res ipsa loquitur—State held vicariously responsible

Achutrao Haribhau Khodwa versus State of Maharashtra, (SC) two judge bench, Civil Appeal No. 3318 of 1979. D/d. 20.2.1996.[10]

Operation of patient in Government Medical Hospital—mop left in the body of the patient—formation of pus, eventually leading to death of patient—negligence in the hospital established—vicarious liability of Government—Doctrine of res ipsa loquitur clearly applies—State is clearly liable to pay damages.

Supreme Court held that *"State must be held to be vicariously liable for the negligent acts of its employees working in the said hospital. The claim of the appellants cannot be defeated merely because it may not have been conclusively proved as to which of the doctors employed by the State in the hospital or other staff acted negligently which caused the death of Chandrikabai. Once death by negligence in the hospital is established, as in the case here, the State would be liable to pay the damages".*

Sure Shot Negligence, RES IPSA and Vicarious Liability

1998—two judge bench of Supreme Court

Wrong route or bolus injection can be hazardous

In Spring Meadows Hospital & Another versus Harjot Ahluwalia (through K.S. Ahluwalia) & Another, 1998 (3) CPR I (SC): 1998 (1) CPJ I: JT 1998 (2) SC 620.

On 30.12.1993 Miss BM, nurse of the Spring Meadows Hospital, New Delhi, on advice of the senior consultant pediatrician, Dr PB, asked the father of the minor patient to get injection Lariago. The father of the child purchased the medicine, which was written down by the nurse and gave it to her. The nurse injected the same intravenously to the child, upon which the child collapsed, had cardiac arrest, and consequently suffered brain damage and continues to survive in a vegetative state. The nurse pleaded that as the child was already taking Chloroquine syrup and when the doctor advised that injection should be given, she thought that the same drug Chloroquine was to be given as an intravenous (IV) injection. In fact, Dr PB had asked for injection IV Chloramphenicol to be given for typhoid. It was the duty of the Resident doctor who was on the round to write, give the injection, and take all care. *The Supreme Court held that a consultant could be negligent where he delegates the responsibilities to his junior with the knowledge that the junior was incapable of carrying out his duties properly.* The insurance company, with whom the hospital was insured, pleaded that they cannot be made liable because the nurse Ms BM was not a qualified nurse nor registered with the nursing council of any State. As the present condition of the child was on account of the negligence of an unqualified nurse, they could not be made liable. But the court held that since both the nurse and the resident doctor were negligent the insurance co. was liable to indemnify the amount of ₹12.375 lakhs as per the terms of the policy as the case was fully covered under the indemnity insurance. The remaining amount was to be paid by the hospital as it was held vicariously liable. The court held that the hospital is responsible for the negligence of the employees and is also liable for its consequences. The court concurred with the findings of the National Commission that the hospital was negligent in employing unqualified people as nurse and in entrusting a minor child to her care. There had been considerable delay in reviving the heart of the child, and this delay damaged the brain.

In this landmark judgement the Apex Court decided on three questions of law:
1. Whether the parents of the child could be held as consumers to claim compensation under the provisions of the Consumer Protection Act.
2. Is the commission entitled to award compensation to parents for mental agony, in view of the powers of the commission under Section 14 of the Act?
3. Whether compensation can be awarded to both consumers, considering parents also come under the definition of "consumer", or can it be awarded only to the beneficiary?

Answering the questions of Law the Apex Court opined:
1. That Clause (ii) of Section 2(1)(d) of the CPA 1986 that defines the word "consumer" is wide enough to include not only the person who hires the services (parents) but also the beneficiary of such services (child) in which beneficiary is other than the person who hires the services, thereby concluding that both the parents as well as the child will be consumers and can claim compensation under the Act.
2. That the Commission is fully justified in awarding compensation to both the child and in addition to the parents for the injury sustained by each of them, the child for the vegetative life ahead, and the parents for mental agony and lifelong care to be given to the child.
3. That the agony of the parents would remain so long as they remain alive and the so-called humanitarian approach of the hospital authorities in no way can be considered to be a factor in denying compensation for mental agony suffered by parents.

Gangrene—Amputation—Compensation Enhanced by Supreme Court

2014—two judge bench of Supreme Court

Right arm of a baby girl had to be amputated due to negligence of hospital staff—Compensation to ₹20 lakhs awarded

Alfred Benddict versus M/s. Manipal Hospital, Bangalore (2JJ, SC) Civil Appeal No. 7620 of 2014 (Arising out of S.L.P. (C) No. 35632 of 2013). D/d. 11.8.2014.

A 2-year-old baby got admission in M/s. Manipal Hospital, Bangalore in pediatric intensive care unit for pneumonia. She was given intravenous fluids by inserting needle on the dorsal aspect of right wrist. The baby developed gangrene initially in the finger tips, which spread to the portion of the hand below writs joint, due to blockage of blood supply. The baby girl developed gangrene in the portion of hand due to negligence of hospital staff. Allegation was that needles were wrongly inserted into artery instead of vein due to which blood supply was blocked—her right arm had to be amputated.

National Commission awarded a compensation of ₹5 lakhs only. Compensation enhanced by Supreme Court to ₹20 lakhs. Apex court held that "We agree that complainant suffered mental agony and spent more than ₹110,000/- for the treatment of the child as bills produced. Considering the facts that the child has to spend the entire life without her right forearm, we feel that interest of justice requires that compensation of ₹500,000/-, in the least, has to be granted in favor of the complainant. We therefore, agree with the order of State Commission and up hold the same".

Failure of Treatment is Not Negligence

Tubectomy—operated for right tube and not for left tube—negligence

State of Haryana versus Smt. Santra, (2JJ, SC), Civil Appeal No. 2897 of 2000 (Arising out of S.L.P. (Civil) No. 18827 of 1999). D/d. 24.4.2000.

A poor laborer woman, who already had many children and had opted for sterilization, developed pregnancy and ultimately gave birth to a female child in spite of sterilization operation which, obviously, had failed. Smt Santra, the victim of the medical negligence, filed a suit for recovery of ₹2 lakhs as damages for medical negligence, which was decreed for a sum of ₹54,000/- with interest at the rate of 12% per annum from the date of institution of the suit till the payment of the decretal amount. Two appeals were filed against this decree in the court of District Judge, Gurgaon, which were disposed of by Additional District Judge, Gurgaon by a common judgment dated 10.5.1999. Both the appeals—one filed by the State of Haryana and the other by Smt Santra were dismissed. The second appeal filed by the State of Haryana was summarily dismissed by the Punjab & Haryana High Court on 3.8.1999. It is in these circumstances that the present Special Leave Petition has been filed in this court.

The Apex Court held that "we are positively of the view that in a country where the population is increasing by the tick of every second on the clock and the Government had taken up the family planning as an important program for the implementation of which it had created mass awakening for the use of various devices including sterilization operation, the doctor as also the State must be held responsible in damages if the sterilization operation performed by him is a failure on account of his negligence, which is directly responsible for another birth in the family, creating additional economic burden on the person who had chosen to be operated upon for sterilization. The unwanted child (girl) born to her has created additional burden for her on account of the negligence of the doctor who performed sterilization operation upon her, and therefore, she is clearly entitled to claim full damages from the State Government to enable her to bring up the child at least till she attains puberty".

Average Standard of Care

2001—two judge bench of Supreme Court of India—Bolam upheld

Negligence of doctor—if the doctor adopted the proper practice as recommended by a responsible body of medical skill then merely because the other group of experts takes a contrary view the doctor cannot be said to be negligent.

Smt Vinitha Ashok versus Lakshmi Hospital, (SC) two judges bench, Civil Appeal No. 2977 of 1992. D/d. 25.9.2001.

Removal of uterus of a woman due to negligent diagnose for cervical pregnancy. Use of laminaria test in dilatation of carvix is one of the accepted standard procedures and it cannot be stated that the use of that procedure constitute a negligent act of doctor; whatever was done by the doctor was part of general practice available in the area. The patient had no history from which presence of cervical pregnancy could have been suspected. Hysterectomy was the only solution on account of profuse bleeding or severe vaginal or peritoneal bleeding. Doctor used traditional method of procuring first trimester abortion by suction evacuation. Even if there is difference of opinion amongst the experts on the procedure adopted by a doctor, but a procedure which is commonly in practice in an area if adopted by a doctor, it cannot be said that there is negligence on his part. The test is whether the act performed conforms to the standard of reasonable care demanded by the law and that is for the Court to decide and that cannot be delegated to any profession or group of community.

Medical Termination of Pregnancy Act, 1971, Regulation 4—Operation—Consent forms—Content forms signed by the parent are supposed to be in the custody of the doctor and is a secret document. If the same are found in the custody of the patient and not on the treatment file, the presumption is that the patient or his agent took away the record.

Removal of uterus—allegation of failure to send the uterus for histopathological examination. Case of the patient was one of a normal trophoblast getting implanted in the uppermost part of cervix. In such cases, the question of having carcinoma could not raise. It cannot be said that failure of doctor to send the uterus and the products of conception after surgery for histopathological examination resulted in any negligence on his part.

In the present case, though large amount of medical literature had been placed and expert evidence had been put forth before the Commission to indicate that ultrasonography would not have established ectopic pregnancy. Some textbooks indicate that it was possible to identify such problem. But when two views even if possible, the general practice in the area in which the respondents practiced such procedure was not followed, and therefore, no negligence can be attributed to the respondents on that ground.

Expert opinion—not binding on the Court—whether performance conforms to the standards of reasonable care demanded by the law is the question to be decided by the Court and cannot be delegated to any profession or group in the community.

Expert Witness Mandatory for Criminal Prosecution

2005—three judge bench of Supreme Court—Medical Board opinion required before prosecuting doctor under criminal law—not over-ruled

Jacob Mathew versus State of Punjab Judgment

In this case a patient was admitted to CMC Hospital, Ludhiana. He felt difficulty in breathing. No doctor turned up for about 20-25 minutes. Later two doctors—Dr Jacob Mathew and Dr Allen Joseph—came and an oxygen cylinder was brought and connected to the mouth of the patient. Surprisingly, the breathing problem increased further. The patient tried to get up. The medical staff asked him to remain in bed. Unfortunately, the oxygen cylinder was found to be empty. Another cylinder was brought. However, by that time the patient had died. The matter against doctors, hospital staff, and hospital went up to the Supreme Court of India. The court discussed the matter in great detail and analyzed the aspect of negligence from different perspectives—civil, criminal, torts, by professionals, etc. It was held that there was no case of criminal rashness or negligence. On August 5, 2005, Supreme Court three judge bench of Chief Justice RC Lahoti, Justice GP Mathur, and Justice PK Balasubramanyan while pronouncing its judgement came to the rescue of doctors accused of medical negligence and criminal action. This judgment has been followed in many subsequent cases of similar nature.

The liability of the doctor shall be civil or criminal or both. One of the essential elements in criminal law is mens rea—the guilty mind or an evil intention. The question arises as to whether in cases of medical negligence—whether slight, ordinary, or gross—is there any criminal liability? As mens rea is essential, it is difficult to argue that the doctor had a guilty mind and was negligent intentionally. This has been the main argument in most of the cases in which the decision was to decide about the criminal liability. For instance, in Jacob Mathew, neither the doctor nor any other hospital staff intentionally connected the empty cylinder. Similarly, in Bolam, the doctors or the hospital did not want to do something wrong intentionally. At no point of time, they had a guilty mind.

In the judgement, the apex court observed: "A medical practitioner faced with an emergency ordinarily tries his best to redeem the patient out of his suffering. He does not gain anything by acting with negligence or by omitting to do an act ... A surgeon with shaky hands under fear of legal action cannot perform a successful operation and a quivering physician cannot administer an end-dose to his patients ... Blame is a powerful weapon. Its inappropriate use distorts tolerant and constructive relations between people".

The court's observations can be summed up as following:
- Negligence is the breach of a duty caused by omission to do something which a reasonable man guided by those considerations which ordinarily regulate the conduct of human affairs would do, or doing something which a prudent and reasonable man would not do. The definition of negligence as given in Law of Torts, the essential components of negligence are three: "duty", "breach", and "resulting damage".
- Negligence in the context of medical profession necessarily calls for a treatment with a difference. To infer rashness or negligence on the part of a professional, in particular a doctor, additional considerations apply. A case of occupational negligence is different from one of professional negligence. A simple lack of care, an error of judgment or an accident is not proof of negligence on the part of a

medical professional. So long as a doctor follows a practice acceptable to the medical profession of that day, he cannot be held liable for negligence merely because a better alternative course or method of treatment was also available or simply because a more skilled doctor would not have chosen to follow or resort to that practice or procedure which the accused followed. When it comes to the failure of taking precautions what has to be seen is whether those precautions were taken which the ordinary experience of men has found to be sufficient; a failure to use special or extraordinary precautions which might have prevented the particular happening cannot be the standard for judging the alleged negligence. So also, the standard of care, while assessing the practice as adopted, is judged in the light of knowledge available at the time of the incident, and not at the date of trial. Similarly, when the charge of negligence arises out of failure to use some particular equipment, the charge would fail if the equipment was not generally available at that particular time (that is, the time of the incident) at which it is suggested it should have been used.

- A professional may be held liable for negligence on one of the two findings: either he was not possessed of the requisite skill which he professed to have possessed, or, he did not exercise, with reasonable competence in the given case, the skill which he did possess. The standard to be applied for judging, whether the person charged has been negligent or not, would be that of an ordinary competent person exercising ordinary skill in that profession. It is not possible for every professional to possess the highest level of expertise or skills in that branch which he practices. A highly skilled professional may be possessed of better qualities, but that cannot be made the basis or the yardstick for judging the performance of the professional proceeded against on indictment of negligence.
- The test for determining medical negligence as laid down in Bolam's case [1957] 1 WLR 582, supra, holds good in its applicability in India.
- The jurisprudential concept of negligence differs in civil and criminal law. What may be negligence in civil law may not necessarily be negligence in criminal law. For negligence to amount to an offence, the element of mens rea (guilty mind/intention) must be shown to exist. For an act to amount to criminal negligence, the degree of negligence should be much higher, i.e., gross or of a very high degree. Negligence which is neither gross nor of a higher degree may provide a ground for action in civil law but cannot form the basis for prosecution.
- The word "gross" has not been used in Section 304A of Indian Penal Code (IPC), yet it is settled that in criminal law negligence or recklessness, to be so held, must be of such a high degree as to be "gross". The expression "rash or negligent act" as occurring in Section 304A of the IPC has to be read as qualified by the word "grossly".
- To prosecute a medical professional for negligence under criminal law, it must be shown that the accused did something or failed to do something which in the given facts and circumstances no medical professional in his ordinary senses and prudence would have done or failed to do. The hazard taken by the accused doctor

should be of such a nature that the injury, which resulted, was most likely imminent.
- Res ipsa loquitur (an act speaks for itself) is only a rule of evidence and operates in the domain of civil law, especially in cases of torts and helps in determining the onus of proof in actions relating to negligence. It cannot be pressed in service for determining per se the liability for negligence within the domain of criminal law. Res ipsa loquitur has, if at all, a limited application in trial on a charge of criminal negligence.

Guideline for Arresting Doctors in Case of Criminal Action

A private complaint may not be entertained unless the complainant has produced prima facie evidence before the Court in the form of a credible opinion given by another competent doctor to support the charge of rashness or negligence on the part of the accused doctor. The investigating officer should, before proceeding against the doctor accused of rash or negligent act or omission, obtain an independent and competent medical opinion preferably from a doctor in government service qualified in that branch of medical practice, who can normally be expected to give an impartial and unbiased opinion applying Bolam's test to the facts collected in the investigation. A doctor accused of rashness or negligence may not be arrested in a routine manner (simply because a charge has been levelled against him). Unless his arrest is necessary for furthering the investigation or for collecting evidence or unless the investigation officer feels satisfied that the doctor proceeded against would not make himself available to face the prosecution unless arrested, the arrest may be withheld.

Martin D'Souza's Case

Martin F. D'Souza versus Mohd. Ishfaq, Supreme Court of India, 17 February 2009; Bench: Markandeya Katju and G.S. Singhvi, JJ.; the judgment was delivered by Katju J.; citation: AIR 2009 SC 2049.

In 1991, the patient who was suffering from chronic renal failure went to Nanavati Hospital, Mumbai for kidney transplant. He was undergoing hemodialysis twice a week. Later he got his kidney transplant done at Prince Aly Khan Hospital. During his treatment at Nanavati Hospital he did not complain of deafness. At Nanavati Hospital he was prescribed Amikacin of 500 mg twice a day for 14 days. Much later, the patient filed a complaint at the National Consumer Dispute Redressal Commission, New Delhi and claimed compensation of ₹12 lakhs as his hearing had been affected. He complained that the dosage of Amikacin was excessive and caused hearing loss. The matter finally went to the Supreme Court where it was held that the doctor and the hospital were not negligent.

This case very strongly defended the position of doctors vis-à-vis the patients. The court has made an interesting observation: "The law, like medicine, is an inexact science. One cannot predict with certainty an outcome of many cases. It depends on the particular facts and circumstances of the case, and also the personal notions of the Judge concerned who is hearing the case. However, the broad and general legal principles relating to medical negligence need to be understood".

Difficulties in application of Mathew Guidelines

The Supreme Court observed that there were difficulties in the application of principles as laid down in Jacob Mathew's case. For instance:

CHAPTER 14: Landmark Supreme Court Judgments and Their Importance in Medicolegal Litigations

- "The practitioner must bring to his task a reasonable degree of skill and knowledge, and must exercise a reasonable degree of care. Neither the very highest nor a very low degree of care and competence is what the law requires". *(as per Jacob Mathew's case)*. The court observed that it is a matter of individual understanding as to what is reasonable and what is unreasonable. Even experts may disagree on certain issues. They may also disagree on what is a high level of care and what is a low level of care.
- The Jacob Mathew's case said that "simple" negligence may result only in civil liability, but "gross" negligence or recklessness may result in criminal liability. Now, what is simple negligence and what is gross negligence may not be so easy to be determined. Experts may not agree on this because the dividing line between the two is quite thin.

Judges as Lay Men

Thus, Martin D'Souza judgment held that it was very difficult or rather impossible to understand, and therefore, define as to what is "reasonable" and what is "simple" and what is "gross". At one place, the court observed: Judges are not experts in medical science, rather they are lay men. This itself often makes it somewhat difficult for them to decide cases relating to medical negligence. In short, the Martin D'Souza judgment is like a confession by the judges that in cases of medical negligence, the judges are ill-equipped to make any decision and that too on the finer aspects of "simple" or "gross" negligence.

Referral to Committee of Doctors Whenever Complaint is Received by Court

Apex Court held that "We, therefore, direct that whenever a complaint is received against a doctor or hospital by the Consumer Fora (whether District, State or National) or by the Criminal Court then before issuing notice to the doctor or hospital against whom the complaint was made the Consumer Forum or Criminal Court should first refer the matter to a competent doctor or committee of doctors, specialized in the field relating to which the medical negligence is attributed, and only after that doctor or committee reports that there is a prima facie case of medical negligence should notice be then issued to the concerned doctor/hospital. This is necessary to avoid harassment to doctors who may not be ultimately found to be negligent".

Warning to Police not to Harass Doctors and Arrest in Routine Manner

Apex Court warned police officials in following words "We further warn the police officials not to arrest or harass doctors unless the facts clearly come within the parameters laid down in Jacob Mathew's case (supra), otherwise the policemen will themselves have to face legal action".

2010—two judge bench of Supreme Court in Kishan Rao's case—over-ruled Martin D'Souza as far medical board opinion required before prosecuting doctor under civil law. Expert witness is advisory in nature and not binding to court.

Kishan Rao's Case

Kishan Rao got his wife admitted to Nikhil Super Speciality Hospital in Hyderabad as she was suffering from fever and complaining of chill. She was not given any treatment for malaria. Instead she was being treated for typhoid. She did not respond to the treatment. In a very precarious condition, she was shifted to Yashoda hospital where she died due to cardiorespiratory arrest and malaria. Kishan Rao filed a case in the District Forum and sought compensation for the negligence of the Nikhil hospital. Finally, the District Forum decided in favor of Kishan Rao. Hospital appealed in the State Commission, which overturned the decision of the District forum on the ground that there was no expert opinion to the effect that the treatment given by the hospital was wrong or the hospital was negligent. National Commission upheld this decision. Kishan Rao appealed in the Supreme Court, which observed that the case was not complicated which required expert opinion as evidence. It was a simple case of wrong treatment. The patient complained of intermittent fever and chill and was being treated for typhoid instead of malaria.

Judgment was Per Incuriam

The court held that it was not bound by the earlier decision of the same court in Martin D'Souza's case as that judgment was *per incuriam* regarding the directions for expert opinion is concerned. The court held that it was not necessary in all cases to seek expert opinion before proceeding with the matter. For simple and obvious cases, the consumer courts were free to proceed without seeking expert opinion and the instant case fell in such a category.

In Martin D'Souza's case, the court did not follow the distinction, as laid down in Jacob Mathew's case, regarding criminal prosecution and seeking compensation under Consumer Protection Act. Thus, the guidelines, as laid down in Martin D'Souza, regarding expert opinion before proceeding with any case do not hold good in consumer protection cases and that too which are quite obvious and straightforward. Moreover, the consumer protection law has been enacted to expedite the entire process and the idea of expert opinion at the outset shall defeat the very purpose of the law. Hence the guidelines, as far as expert opinion before issuing notice, are concerned need not be followed. Supreme Court allowed the appeal and ordered Nikhil hospital to pay the amount to Kishan Rao as ordered by the District Forum.

Critique

This is a very bold judgment in which a bench (equivalent size to the bench of Martin D'Souza's case—both two judges, and one judge common) held that the abovementioned observations of Martin D'Souza's case were *per incuriam*. It was held in A.R. Antulay versus R.S. Nayak, reported in (1988) 2 SCC 602{36} that *per incuriam* are those decisions, which are made in ignorance or forgetfulness of some inconsistent statutory provision or of some authority binding on the court concerned, so that in such cases some part of the decision or some step in the reasoning on which it is based, is found on that count to be demonstrably wrong. The court held that it was not bound by the directions given in D'Souza's case and expert evidence from a committee was not required. This is really unfortunate that contradictory judgments are being pronounced by benches of equal size in the Supreme Court. Common man is unable to comprehend as to what is the interpretation of law. Which judgment should a person follow: The earlier judgment or the latter? In case he does not follow the earlier one, is he going to be punished for contempt of court and in case he follows the earlier judgment will it not be a mockery of the procedural and substantive law as laid down by the legislature. The matter should be decided by a larger bench of the Supreme Court so that

CHAPTER 14: Landmark Supreme Court Judgments and Their Importance in Medicolegal Litigations

there is certainty and the doctors as well as the patients are absolutely clear about the provisions of law.

Real Consent

2008—three Judge Bench of Supreme Court—real consent not informed consent

During a scheduled operation without prior consent of patient except in case where life of patient was in danger.

Samira Kohli versus Dr Prabha Manchanda, SC in three judge bench, in Civil Appeal No. 1949 of 2004. D/d. 16.1.2008.

The patient (unmarried woman) aged 44 years had serious menstrual problems. She got herself admitted for diagnostic and operative laparoscopy. Patient gave consent only for diagnostic operative laparoscopy, and laparotomy if needed. When patient was under general anesthesia Doctor took the consent of aged mother of patient and removed reproductive organs (uterus and ovaries). Patient filed claim of ₹25 lakhs before consumer forum. Doctor directed to pay ₹25,000/- as compensation and not to claim fee for surgery. The National Consumer Disputes Redressal Commission (NCDRC) dismissed the case. Then appeal filed at Supreme Court which set aside the order of the Commission and allows the appellant's claim in part.

In this case Supreme Court gave principles relating to consent as follows:

- A doctor has to seek and secure the consent of the patient before commencing a "treatment" (the term "treatment" includes surgery also). The consent so obtained should be real and valid, which means that: the patient should have the capacity and competence to consent; his consent should be voluntary; and his consent should be on the basis of adequate information concerning the nature of the treatment procedure, so that he knows what is consenting to.
- The "adequate information" to be furnished by the doctor (or a member of his team) who treats the patient, should enable the patient to make a balanced judgment as to whether he should submit himself to the particular treatment as to whether he should submit himself to the particular treatment or not. This means that the Doctor should disclose (1) nature and procedure of the treatment and its purpose, benefits, and effect; (2) alternatives if any available; (3) an outline of the substantial risks; and (4) adverse consequences of refusing treatment. But there is no need to explain remote or theoretical risks involved, which may frighten or confuse a patient and result in refusal of consent for the necessary treatment. Similarly, there is no need to explain the remote or theoretical risks of refusal to take treatment which may persuade a patient to undergo a fanciful or unnecessary treatment. A balance should be achieved between the need for disclosing necessary and adequate information and at the same time avoid the possibility of the patient being deterred from agreeing to a necessary treatment or offering to undergo an unnecessary treatment.
- Consent given only for a diagnostic procedure, cannot be considered as consent for therapeutic treatment. Consent given for a specific treatment procedure will not be valid for conducting some other treatment procedure. The fact that the unauthorized additional surgery is beneficial to the patient, or that it would save considerable time and expense to the patient, or would relieve the patient

from pain and suffering in future, are not grounds of defense in an action in tort for negligence or assault and battery. The only exception to this rule is where the additional procedure though unauthorized is necessary in order to save the life or preserve the health of the patient and it would be unreasonable to delay such unauthorized procedure until patient regains consciousness and takes a decision.
- There can be a common consent for diagnostic and operative procedures where they are contemplated. There can also be a common consent for a particular surgical procedure and an additional or further procedure that may become necessary during the course of surgery.
- The nature and extent of information to be furnished by the doctor to the patient to secure the consent need not be of the stringent and high degree mentioned in Canterbury but should be of the extent, which is accepted as normal and proper by a body of medical men skilled and experienced in the particular field. It will depend upon the physical and mental condition of the patient, the nature of treatment, and the risk and consequences attached to the treatment.

11 GUIDELINES FOR MEDICAL NEGLIGENCE

2010—two judge bench of Supreme Court in Kusum Sharma & Others versus Batra Hospital &Med. Research gave 11 point guidelines for medical negligence.

On 18.3.1990, the deceased Shri R.K. Sharma admitted in Batra Hospital, Delhi with complaints of general edema and hypertension. He was advised surgery for removal of "left adrenal tumor" which was the cause of his aliments. On tests, the tumor was found to be malignant. The surgery was carried out on 2.4.1990 by Opposite Party No. 3, Dr Kapil Kumar. During the surgery, the body of the pancreas was damaged, which was treated and a drain was fixed to drain out the fluids. Since the flow of fluids did not stop, thereby causing pain, inconvenience, and anxiety to the deceased and the complainants, after another expert consultation with Dr T.K. Bose, Opposite Party No. 4, a second surgery was carried out on 23.5.1990 in Batra Hospital by Dr Bose assisted by Dr Kapil Kumar. The surgery was successful. The deceased was fitted with two bags and drain the fluids and in due course, wounds were to heal inside and fluid to stop. The patient was discharged on 26.6.1990 carrying two bags in his body, with an advice to follow-up and change in dressing. The deceased next showed up in Batra Hospital only on 31.8.90 and that too to obtain a Medical Certificate from Opposite Party No. 2, Dr Mani, which was given. Next time the deceased came to Batra Hospital on 9.10.1990 after vomiting at home and when arrangements for bringing him by the Hospital's ambulance were made by Opposite Party No. 2, Dr Man, Shri Sharma died in the Hospital on 11.10.1990 on account of "pyogenic meningitis".

Apex Court held that the National Commission was justified in dismissing the complaint of the appellants. No interference is called for. The appeal being devoid of any merit is dismissed. In view of the peculiar facts and circumstances of this case, the parties are directed to bear their own costs. Apex Court promulgated that while deciding whether the medical professional is guilty of medical negligence, following well-known principles must be kept in view:

1. Negligence is the breach of a duty exercised by omission to do something which a reasonable man, guided by those considerations which ordinarily regulate the conduct of human affairs, would do, or doing something which a prudent and reasonable man would not do.
2. Negligence is an essential ingredient of the offence. The negligence to be established by the prosecution must be culpable or gross and not the negligence merely based upon an error of judgment.
3. The medical professional is expected to bring a reasonable degree of skill and knowledge and must exercise a reasonable degree of care. Neither the very highest nor a very low degree of care and competence judged in the light of the particular circumstances of each case, is what the law requires.
4. A medical practitioner would be liable only where his conduct fell below that of the standards of a reasonably competent practitioner in his field.
5. In the realm of diagnosis and treatment, there is scope for genuine difference of opinion and one professional doctor is clearly not negligent merely because his conclusion differs from that of other professional doctor.
6. The medical professional is often called upon to adopt a procedure, which involves higher element of risk, but which he honestly believes as providing greater chances of success for the patient rather than a procedure involving lesser risk but higher chances of failure. Just because a professional looking to the gravity of illness has taken higher element of risk to redeem the patient out of his/her suffering which did not yield the desired result may not amount to negligence.
7. Negligence cannot be attributed to a doctor so long as he performs his duties with reasonable skill and competence. Merely because the doctor chooses one course of action in preference to the other one available, he would not be liable if the course of action chosen by him was acceptable to the medical profession.
8. It would not be conducive to the efficiency of the medical profession if no Doctor could administer medicine without a halter round his neck.
9. It is our bounden duty and obligation of the civil society to ensure that the medical professionals are not unnecessary harassed or humiliated so that they can perform their professional duties without fear and apprehension.
10. The medical practitioners at times also have to be saved from such a class of complainants who use criminal process as a tool for pressurizing the medical professionals/hospitals particularly private hospitals or clinics for extracting uncalled for compensation. Such malicious proceedings deserve to be discarded against the medical practitioners.
11. The medical professionals are entitled to get protection so long as they perform their duties with reasonable skill and competence and in the interest of the patients. The interest and welfare of the patients have to be paramount for the medical professionals.

LAW OF LIMITATION

2010—two judge bench of Supreme Court in V.N. Shrikhande versus Anita Sena Fernandes,[11] *Civil Appeal No. 8983 of 2010. Arising out of SLP (C) No. 5479 of 2009. D/d. 20.10.2010 gave the principle for determining accrual of cause of action for deciding limitation.*

Respondent was having stones in gall bladder. Appellant (Doctor) performed surgery in November 1993. After surgery she was constantly having pain in abdomen off and on for which he took pain killers. She again underwent surgery in the year 2002 and gauze pieces were found in the abdomen which were left in the abdomen at the time of first surgery. Respondent claimed compensation from the Appellant. Appellant contended that there was no negligence on his part and he had performed thousands of operation in past 50 years. Respondent filed complaint before Consumer Forum in the year 2004 claiming compensation on account of pain and sufferings for 9 years and also cost of second operation. It was held that complaint was barred by limitation. Cause of action arose in the year 1993 and not in the year 2002.

The Apex Court gave following principle for determination of accrual of cause of action for deciding bar on limitation. "If the effect of negligence on the doctor's part or any person associated with him is patent, the cause of action will be deemed to have arisen on the date when the act of negligence was done. If, on the other hand, the effect of negligence is latent, then the cause of action will arise on the date when the patient or his representative-complainant, discovers the harm/injury caused due to such act or the date when the patient or his representative-complainant could have, by exercise of reasonable diligence, discovered the act constituting negligence".

2009—three judge bench of Supreme Court—Cardiothoracic surgeon and institute found negligent or not referring to neurosurgeon.

In Nizam's Institute of Medical Sciences versus Prasanth S. Dhananka and Others (2009) 6 SCC 1 relied upon by the learned counsel for the respondent, broad principles under which the medical negligence as a tort have to be evaluated is taken note, as have been laid down in the case of Jacob Mathew. The ultimate conclusion reached in the case of Nizam's Institute relating to the lack of care and caution and the negligence on the part of the attending doctors was with reference to the medical report, which was available on record, which indicated the existence of tumor located at left upper chest and in that circumstance the presence of neurosurgeon was essential and the said procedure not being adopted, a case of negligence or indifference on the part of the attending doctors had been proved. Cardiothoracic surgeon and institute found negligent or not referring to neurosurgeon. The court awarded 1 crores.

■ HIGHEST EVER COMPENSATION

2013—two judge bench of Supreme Court—highest award in case of "TEN" treated with high doses of steroids—death—5.6 crore plus interest builds up more than 11.5 crores.

In Dr Balram Prasad versus Dr Kunal Saha, 2013(4) RCR (Civil) 946: 2013(6) Recent Apex Judgments (R.A.J.) 165: (2013) 13 SCALE 1.

Anuradha Saha suffered with rashes in May 1998 at the age of 36 years, her skin sloughed off all over her body, except for her skull. Her husband Dr Kunal Saha consulted Dr Sukumar Mukherjee. Dr Mukherjee prescribed Depo-Medrol to be injected into Mrs Saha's muscles so that the long-acting glucocorticoid could suppress her immune system's inflammatory response, which was presumably causing her rash. Depo-Medrol's chemical structure ensures it stays in the blood for a long time. The maximum dosage recommended by the drug's Indian manufacturer, Pharmacia India Ltd., is

40–120 mg once a week. Dr Mukherjee prescribed two injections of Depo-Medrol at 80 mg every day. Patient's immunity had been compromised after receiving a high dosage of steroids. Mrs Saha's rashes and fever worsened, and she was admitted to the AMRI Hospital in Kolkata. Dr Mukherjee examined her there and prescribed Depo-Medrol again before leaving on a trip to the United States. A dermatologist later diagnosed her with toxic epidermal necrolysis (TEN), which is as painful as it sounds. By May 12, 1998, large sheets of Mrs Saha's skin had separated from her back and limbs. The Supreme Court noted in its 2009 judgment that she had lesions on her tongue and mouth, which made it difficult to eat or drink. Yet the nursing staff at AMRI hospital did not set up a feeding tube, nor did they give her any painkillers. The next day, Dr Mukherjee left for the United States, and Dr Balram Prasad and Dr Baidyanath Halder continued her treatment. The core medical team did not pause to question why Mrs Saha was getting worse despite all the steroids. On May 17, 1998, Dr Saha evacuated his wife by a private plane to one of Mumbai's top hospitals. On arrival, doctors noticed a dark green patch on her back, an unpropitious sign of an infection that claimed her life on May 28. For the past 15 years, her husband, Dr Kunal Saha, has pushed Indian courts to hold at least five doctors and the hospital responsible. Though the lower courts rejected his cases, Dr Saha persisted, appealing all the way to the Supreme Court, which found the doctors and AMRI Hospital (Advanced Medicare & Research Institute Ltd.) in Kolkata guilty of negligence in 2009. It took another 4 years for the Supreme Court to award Dr Saha an unprecedented amount in a medical negligence case in India— 60.8 million rupees, plus 6% annual interest for each of the 15 years that Dr Saha has been fighting his legal battle totaling to ₹11 crores plus.

DNR—RIGHT TO DIE WITH DIGNITY

2018—five judge constitutional bench of Supreme Court—"Right to die with dignity" is a fundamental right—passive and active euthanasia, Do not resuscitate, Living will

Common Cause (A Regd. Society) versus Union of India, (SC) (Constitution Bench)

Dipak Misra, CJI, A.K. Sikri, A.M. Khanwilkar, D.Y. Chandrachud, Ashok Bhushan, JJ. Writ Petition (Civil) No. 215 of 2005. D/d. 9.3.2018.

Constitutional Bench held that: (1) The right to die with dignity as fundamental right has already been declared by the Constitution Bench judgment of this Court in Gian Kaur case (supra), which we reiterate. (2) We declare that an adult human being having mental capacity to take an informed decision has right to refuse medical treatment including withdrawal from lifesaving devices. (3) A person of competent mental faculty is entitled to execute an advance medical directive in accordance with safeguards as referred to above.

DEFENSIVE MEDICINE

2019—two judge bench of Supreme Court— treating doctor held liable for delay in treatment—practice of defensive medicine— Director of hospital and referring doctor— not liable for medical negligence—avoid a situation where doctors resort to "defensive medicine" to avoid claims of negligence.

Arun Kumar Manglik versus Chirayu Health and Medicare Private Limited and Anr., (2019) 7 SCC 401—case of dengue fever was treated defensively and that delayed vigorous treatment in spite of falling platelets, nothing was done much to save patient.

Delay in treatment—finding of Medical Council that treatment was administered to patient according to the guidelines but patient did not receive timely treatment. Patient had a prior medical history which included catheter ablation and paroxysmal supraventricular tachycardia, suggestive of cardiac complications thus fell in group of patients that require in-hospital management (Group B) under WHO guidelines. Patient was evidently suffering from abdominal discomfort and hospital authorities were required to closely monitor her condition which they failed to do so in a timely manner. Impugned order of National Commission reversing award and not holding respondents guilty of medical negligence was unsustainable and hence set aside. Case of medical negligence made out. Complainant lost his wife though she was not employed. It was held that contribution made by a nonworking spouse to welfare of family has economic equivalent. Appellant/husband entitled to receive amount of ₹15 Lakhs. Director of hospital and referring doctor are not liable for medical negligence.

Apex Court held that "In the practice of medicine, there could be varying approaches to treatment. There can be a genuine difference of opinion. However, while adopting a course of treatment, the medical professional must ensure that it is not unreasonable. The threshold to prove unreasonableness is set with due regard to the risks associated with medical treatment and the conditions under which medical professionals function. This is to avoid a situation where doctors resort to "defensive medicine" to avoid claims of negligence, often to the detriment of the patient. Hence, in a specific case where unreasonableness in professional conduct has been proven with regard to the circumstances of that case, a professional cannot escape liability for medical evidence merely by relying on a body of professional opinion".

DEGREE QUALIFICATION

Poonam Verma versus Ashwin Patel & Ors. on 10 May, 1996 Equivalent citations: 1996 AIR 2111, 1996 SCC (4) 332.

In July, 1992, Pramod Verma, treated by Respondent No. 1, Dr Ashwin Patel, who was homeopathy doctor, kept him on allopathic drugs for viral fever for 2 days, and thereafter, for typhoid fever. When condition of Pramod Verma deteriorated, he was shifted to Sanjeevani Maternity and General Nursing Home of Dr Rajeev Warty (Respondent No. 2) as an indoor patient. Thereafter he was transferred to the Hinduja Hospital in an unconscious state where, after about four and a half hour of admission, he died. Poonam Verma filed petition in NCDRC for compensation for negligence but forum dismissed.

Apex Court held in appeal that Respondent No. 1, having practiced in Allopathy, without being qualified in that system, was guilty of negligence per se, and therefore, the appeal against him has to be allowed.

PROPER INFRASTRUCTURE

Hysterectomy operation of the patient conducted in hospital having no ICU facility—death of patient. It is medical negligence. Also other observations for speedy disposal of consumer cases were made.

Bijoy Sinha Roy (D) versus Biswanath Das, (2 JJ,SC) Civil Appeal Nos. 4761 of 2009. D/d. 30.8.2017.

CHAPTER 14: Landmark Supreme Court Judgments and Their Importance in Medicolegal Litigations

The deceased had some menstrual problem in June, 1993. She consulted Dr Bishwanath Das, respondent No. 1, a gynecologist. It was found that she had multiple fibroids of varying sizes in uterus. She was advised to undergo hysterectomy. After about 5 months, she had severe bleeding and was advised emergency hysterectomy at Ashutosh Nursing Home. She was also suffering from high blood pressure and her hemoglobin was around 7 g%, which indicated that she was anemic. The treatment was given for the said problems but without much success. Finally, operation was conducted on 01.12.1993 at about 8.45 AM. She did not regain consciousness and since the Nursing Home did not have the ICU facility, she was shifted at 2.15 PM to repose Nursing Home and thereafter to SSKM Hospital where she died on 17th January, 1994.

The appellant filed a complaint before the State Commission on 16th June, 1994. The State Commission, vide order dated 19th September, 2005, held that there was medical negligence as surgery was conducted without controlling the blood pressure and hemoglobin. The complainant as well as the opposite parties preferred appeals. The National Commission reversed the above finding. On appeal, the Apex Court held that "We however, find that neither the State Commission nor the National Commission have examined the plea of the appellant that the operation should not have been performed at a nursing home which did not have the ICU when it could be reasonably foreseen that without ICU there was post-operative risk to the life of the patient … We consider it appropriate in the interests of justice to direct the opposite party No. 1 to pay a sum of ₹5 lakh to the heirs of the appellant without any interest".

LEARNING KEY POINTS

- Always keep copy of Jacob Mathews vs. State of Punjab, Martin F D'Souza vs. Mohd Ashfaq judgments.
- Jacob Mathews vs. State of Punjab, Martin F D'Souza vs. Mohd Ashfaq judgments are the shield against arrest provided by Apex Court to medical professionals.
- VN Shrikhande vs. Anita Sena Fernandes Supreme Court judgment gives the principle for determination of accrual of cause of action and is important tool in technical defense of bar on limitation.
- Supreme Court has issued guidelines for lower courts for determination of Medical Negligence in Kusum Sharma vs. Batra Hosiptal judgment.
- Do consult medicolegal adviser while dealing with medicolegal litigation as routine lawyer may not be aware of all important landmark judgments of Apex Court and NCDRC.

TAKE-HOME MESSAGES

- Precedents set by the Supreme Court in its judgments are the leading source of declared law in field of Medical Negligence.
- Authoritative principle in a judicial decision constitutes the ratio decidendi of the judgement has force of law vis-a-vis the world at large.
- Article 141 of the Constitution of India unequivocally mentions that the decisions of the Supreme Court are binding on all the subordinate courts. The aforesaid article empowers the Supreme Court to declare the law.
- Under Article 144 of the Constitution of India, all civil and judicial authorities are under obligation to act in aid of Supreme Court to follow the law and principles declared by it. Police and other public

authorities are under obligation to follow the principles and directions given in Supreme Court judgments.

MUST AVOID THINGS—DO NOT DO
- Never forget to quote landmark judgments in your favor in litigation or otherwise.
- Never hesitate to submit Jacob Mathew versus State of Punjab and Martin F D'Souza versus Mohd Ashfaq Judgment to police official in case of criminal negligence suit.

MUST DO THINGS
- Be aware of all landmark judgment pertaining to medical negligence.
- Always consult Medicolegal Consultants while facing medical malpractice lawsuits.

MESSAGES WHICH THE READER MUST BE AWARE

The Supreme Court judgments are binding on subordinate court and obligatory on civil and judicial authorities and police officials.

WARNINGS

One should be careful in following the principles of medical practice like Real and Valid Consent, Documentation, and Record Keeping laid down by Supreme Court.

MEDICAL NEGLIGENCE PEARLS

The Supreme Court Judgments are binding on subordinate courts and ignoring will be Judicial Impropriety. Violation by civil and police authorities will be Contempt of Court.

ONLY ONE FACT TO REMEMBER

Landmark judgments like Jacob Mathew versus State of Punjab, Martin F D'Souza versus Mohd Ashfaq, VN Shrikhande versus Anita Sena Fernandes, and Kusum Sharma versus Batra Hospital are the legal weapon for doctors facing medical negligence lawsuits.

MCQs

Choose one correct answer

1. Which landmark judgment held that medical professionals and hospitals are under ambit of Consumer Protection act 1986?
   a. IMA versus VP Shantha
   b. Jacob Mathew versus State of Punjab
   c. Parmanand Katara versus Union of India
   d. None of the above

2. Which Supreme Court judgment held that doctors cannot be arrested in routine manner?
   a. Dr Suresh Gupta versus Union of India
   b. Jacob Mathew versus State of Punjab
   c. Sameera Kohli versus Prabha Manchanda
   d. None of the above

3. In which case as landmark judgment, the Supreme Court held Emergency Medical Care for saving life and limb is obligatory on doctors and hospitals?
   a. Parmanand Katara versus Union of India
   b. IMA versus VP Shantha
   c. Jacob Mathew versus State of Punjab
   d. Paschim Banga Khet Mazdoor Samity versus State of West Bengal

4. In which case largest compensation 11.6 crores was awarded in medical negligence suit?
   a. Poonam Verma versus Ashwin
   b. Smt Vinitha Ashok versus Lakshmi Hospital
   c. Dr Balram Prasad versus Dr. Kunal Saha
   d. Alfred Benddict versus M/s. Manipal Hospital, Bangalore

CHAPTER 14: Landmark Supreme Court Judgments and Their Importance in Medicolegal Litigations

5. In which case principle of Real and Valid Consent was established by the Supreme Court?
   a. Poonam Verma versus Ashwin
   b. Smt Vinitha Ashok versus Lakshmi Hospital
   c. Sameera Kohli versus Prabha Manchanda
   d. Parmanand Katara versus Union of India
6. In which case referral to Committee of Doctors was mandated in medical malpractice lawsuits by the Supreme Court?
   a. Martin F. D'Souza versus Mohd. Ishfaq
   b. Dr Suresh Gupta versus Union of India
   c. Jacob Mathew versus State of Punjab
   d. Nikhil Super Speciality Hospital

Answers

1. a   2. b   3. a   4. c
5. c   6. a

REFERENCES

1. (1992) 94 BOMLR 128, 1993 CriLJ 1209.
2. Director of Settlements, Andhra Pradesh Vs M.R Apparao & Anr (AIR 2002 SC 598).
3. [(2020) 03 SC CK 0001].
4. [AIR 1992 SC 1593].
5. [(2003) 6 SCC 697].
6. (2002) 2 SCC 420.
7. AIR 2008 SC 930.
8. 1996 AIR 550 1995 SCC (6) 651, JT 1995 (8) 119 1995 SCALE (6)273.
9. 1989 AIR 1570, 1989 SCR (3) 241, 1989 SCC (3) 223, JT 1989 (2) 419, 1989 SCALE (1)1535.
10. 1996 SCC (2) 634 JT 1996 (2) 624, 1996 SCALE (2)328.
11. (2010) INSC 883.

SUGGESTED READING

1. Baldwa M, Baldwa V, Padvi N, Baldwa S. Legal Issues in Critical Care. New Delhi, India: CBS Publishers & Distributors Pvt Ltd.; 2022.
2. Baldwa M, Baldwa V, Padvi N, Baldwa S. Legal Issues in Medical Practice, 2nd edition, 2 volume set. New Delhi, India: CBS Publishers & Distributors Pvt Ltd.; 2023.

SECTION 3

Various Scenarios in Medical Negligence

- **Medicolegal Aspects of Difficult Situation of Unexpected Death**
  Mahesh Baldwa, Namita Padvi, Amit Padvi, Varsha Baldwa

- **Prevention of Violence Against Doctors**
  Hemant R Gangolia, Bela Amichandra Verma, Samik Basu, Rajakumar Marol

- **Medicolegal Issues in Pediatric Critical Care**
  Dnyanesh DK, Suma Dnyanesh

- **Medicolegal Aspects of Vaccinations**
  Jyoti Kumar Gupta, Vivek Saxena, Raj Tilak, Sanjay Niranjan

- **Medicolegal Aspects of Transferring the Acute Ill Patients, Transit Death, Inadvertent use of Expiry Drug**
  Jyoti Kumar Gupta, Anurag Mehrotra, Satish Sharma, Ambrish Gupta

- **Legalities in Developmental Pediatrics**
  Samir Hasan Dalwai, Atanu Bhadra, Abraham Paul, Pranjal Agarwal

- **Medicolegal Aspects for Pediatric Surgery**
  Mahesh Baldwa, Namita Padvi, Varsha Baldwa, Sushila Baldwa

- **Legalities in Neonatology**
  Anurag Pangrikar, Hemant R Gangolia, Jyoti Kumar Gupta, Mahesh Baldwa

- **Legal Hurdles of Police, RTI, Labor and Drug Inspectors, Fire NOC, Bio-Waste in Medical Practice etc.**
  Hemant R Gangolia, Satish Agrawal, Sameer Sadawarte, C Nirmala

15. Medicolegal Aspects of Difficult Situation of Unexpected Death

Mahesh Baldwa, Namita Padvi, Amit Padvi, Varsha Baldwa

Unfortunately, no matter how frivolous the lawsuit may be, yet one still, of course, has to pay lawyers to defend oneself even after saving a life.

Keywords: Consumer Protection Act-2019 (CPA), Critical care (CC), Emergency treatment (ET), Indian Penal Code (IPC), Medical negligence (MN), Medicolegal (ML), Neonatal/premature intensive care units (NICU), Pediatric intensive care units (PICU)

Aim: Defenses available to doctor after a difficult situation created by sudden and unexpected death.

Objective: A doctor may defend against a medical malpractice claim by arguing that emergency is well documented and same was diagnosed and treated diligently prudently yet patient's died natural death as per the IPD papers writing.

INTRODUCTION

It is rather impossible to find a medical professional who would say that they never faced a medicolegal (ML) situation called "Difficult situation of unexpected death" and world at large gazing in their face as if they were responsible for death. This type of scenario where treating team of doctor is made to feel guilty about difficult situation of unexpected death by relatives is not uncommon. A spectrum of ML reactions from patient party affecting medical professional may be: (1) sometimes in the event of unexpected death occurring in front of lot of accompanying relatives then at slightest provocation they may take law in their own hands and bash pediatricians and other staff members along with destroying medical equipment and hospital property. (2) Some other times, no sooner than expected instead relatives asking you explanations about unexpected death, you have a policemen coming to make ML questioning to you and your staff as to what happened to deceased child as they have received an ML complaint from relatives. (3) So often in the event of difficult situation of unexpected death, you may receive a politicians telephone to resolve the issue amicably or some social worker actually walking in your office to pay for unexpected death or a local goon threatening you to cough up money immediately for unexpected death without asking your explanation. (4) So often in the event of difficult situation of unexpected death, you may find media and press people gathering around you and your staff members to speak details of difficult situation of unexpected death, which are flashed in defamatory way on TV or newspapers leaving you disgusted. (5) In the event of unexpected death, you should feel lucky and blessed if police does not walk to make inquiry about difficult situation created by unexpected death but so often your comfort is disturbed weeks later or sometimes months later by a lawyers notice probing in situation of unexpected death and asking for case papers related to medical treatment of deceased along with compensation. (6) As per the media projection[1] one out of ten pediatricians are receiving dragged in unnecessary prosecutions for medical negligence (MN). Court summons for situation of unexpected death and complains narrating absurd allegations and asking astronomical sum of money as compensation is going to be on rise coming days.

It is surprisingly true that in spite of wearing good, empathetic, sympathetic attitude and observing courteousness in communications allegations of MN in difficult situation of unexpected death may put medical professional in an ML maze of alleged MN and leave them disgusted. Medical professionals feel they are framed in alleged MN even though there is no ML issue in unexpected death. A new breed of legal advisors in ML issues of MN on internet are on rise who lure relatives confronting unexpected death and show them big money in prosecuting doctor which cannot be traded off by medical professional wearing good, empathetic, sympathetic attitude, and observing courteousness in communications in event of difficult situation of unexpected death. Ultimate answer lies in insuring oneself for professional work with insurance companies. This article is designed to reduce the trauma accompanied with alleged MN in difficult situation of unexpected death, where there is no MN of doctor. Some knowledge of ML aspects of difficult situation of unexpected death may sharpen your record-keeping skills and also communication skills while dealing with relatives, police, and politician or for that matter a goon walking in your office.

WHY ML PROBLEMS ARE ON RISE IN DIFFICULT SITUATION OF UNEXPECTED DEATH IN PEDIATRICS?

As such two decades ago a difficult situation of unexpected death in a nursing home or hospital would not invite much hue and cry. Ever since branch of pediatrics has matured and ushered in new era of critical care (CC) and emergency treatment (ET) with advent of better patient monitoring facilities and advancement in knowledge and skills CC and ET. A number of small to big tertiary care centers in the form of neonatal/premature intensive care units (NICU) and pediatric intensive care units (PICU) with huge investment in infrastructure have come up, even in small towns and talukas apart from big cities in India. State of art infrastructure costs a fortune and escalates cost of quality care in pediatric treatment.

Understanding ML Mindset of Courts in Case of Unexpected Death in Alleged MN

In today's scenario,[2] medical professional(s) are assuming role of health risk managers of ill child patients. So often, children are prone to get into acute crisis for various reasons. Law differentiates between what was the original disease, which pushed the child in to acute crisis. Law also probes in, why original disease pushed child in to acuter crisis. Law finds out whether it was lack of treatment or delay in treatment, which pushed the child into acute crisis or as such nature of disease was such that it galloped its way to acute crisis leaving no time for medical professional to treat it. Law also finds out who was responsible for delay in treatment or for lack of treatment pushing child in acute crisis. Sometimes under treatment and apparently well child is pushed in acute crisis due to anaphylaxis caused by a drug. Sometimes postsurgical complication of internal bleeding or severe sepsis puts the child into crisis. In the event of unexpected death, such situations if there is alleged MN and it comes up for hearing in the law courts then courts find out after developing of complication what remedial measures were taken in the interest of patient. Was patient referred to proper specialist and proper medical care was made available to child in acute crisis as soon as possible. Medical professional should keep this in mindset of courts and accordingly pediatricians should be careful enough to reflect this mind set in case paper writings. Case paper writings showing above-mentioned details as required by courts are helpful in pleading and proving no MN of pediatricians in courts. Any action or inaction (act of omission or commission) of medical professional that accelerates or increases the health risks of a critically ill patient may result in an allegation of breach of duty of medical professional.[3] Amount of money asked is mind-boggling.[4] Patients may sue a medical professional for compensation by asking usually lakhs of rupees and many times in crores.[5]

Making Relatives of Patient Party Understand Difficult Situation during Unexpected Death

The ML problems related to difficult situation of unexpected death in children have become commonplace with the advent of better patient monitoring facilities and advancement in knowledge in maintaining vital parameters till basic pathology causing havoc in critically ill child is managed of by appropriate specific treatment. Pediatrician's perspective in treating fervently acute conditions causing destabilization of vitals and not so vigorously addressing basic pathology in tandem creates confusion in the minds of relatives of patient. So often just monitoring and maintaining vitals cost a fortune, whereas relatives perceive as if specific treatment for basic disease was going on, e.g., septicemia due to a large abscess destabilizing vitals, hence abscess is not drained, because of unstable vitals since it cannot withstand anesthesia. Sometimes vitals remain unstable and original disease pathology dominates so much that it reaches to point of no return and child develops unexpected death. This misunderstanding of relatives is not able to differentiate between maintaining vitals by monitoring costs in money, inflating bills, which are different from medical treatment cost for treating basic pathology. So often difficult situation of unexpected death occurs causing confusion of relatives as to what needed to be done by doctor was not done and doctor wasted time in monitoring vitals and did nothing for basic disease. This mix up of laymen thinking and loose talk by hospital staff gets jumbled up with misunderstanding and misinterpretation of unpalatable scientific explanations given by treating doctor regarding treatment of basic disease and CC and ET for maintaining vitals pave its way to ML cases. Even though CC and ET have significantly advanced in field of pediatrics, which has saved unsalvageable, lives but ushered every one of us in high cost treatment arena. High cost of CC most often results in cure but when it leads to difficult situation of unexpected death, as outcome then it becomes source of ML problems. It is not uncommon to see or hear or read in newspapers that relatives took law in their own hand, e.g., Sinhania Hospital

Thane was turned to ashes due to difficult situation of unexpected death of local Shiv Sena politician Shri Anant Dighe. It is not true for high-profile unexpected death, but also true for common people facing difficult situation of unexpected death culminating in abuse of medical person and their property. We see alleged ML cases being registered as first information report (FIR) under S. 154 of Criminal procedure code (Cr.PC) for difficult situation of unexpected death at local police stations all over the India and police arresting pediatricians under Section 304 A of Indian Penal Code (IPC). This tendency of arresting pediatricians in difficult situation of unexpected death is brought under control by the Supreme Court decision of Jacob Mathews versus State of Punjab.[6] Even the fourth estate is not much behind in reporting unexpected death in TV, press every day in defamatory way against pediatricians. Each such news articles shakes medical professional to core, who wishfully thinks, god, let this not happen to me. Let me practice defensively. This has eroded confidence of innovative and motivated dedicated pediatricians. It is not a good signal.

Already existing S. 304 A of IPC has got a boost in prosecution of pediatricians by enactment of Consumer Protection Act-2019 (CPA) and it has accelerated prosecutions related to alleged ML. Both criminal and civil remedies are on fast tract of judicial remedy in alleged ML cases. Already existing criminal courts along with establishment of consumer courts[7] have put the cases of alleged MN[8] on fast tract remedy. There is no limit set by legislature and judiciary for asking of compensation by prosecution for alleged MN cases. Patient party approaching police stations and law courts is better than they taking law in their own hands.

What is the Definition of MN in Difficult Situation of Unexpected Death?

Heavy cost of CC and ET has made this emerging pediatric subspecialty, a hotspot of prosecution in alleged MN cases. In today's scenario, medical professional(s) are health risk managers of the critically sick children, who need vigilant monitoring with various gadgets and timely treatment to maintain vital parameters to avert any further crisis due to common and foreseeable complications, So corollary is that medical professional(s) are expected to chart the course of the health of their critically ill patients with minimal health hazards by use of state of art and costly monitoring equipment. Any action or inaction of medical professional in emergency room that accelerates or increases the health risks may result in allegation of breach of duty of medical professional.

Document Clinical Findings and Obtain Written Consents and Dissents

Very often when treatment charts and case papers are reviewed by court, when a case of MN related to unexpected death is heard it finds that so often medical professional(s) were busy treating acute cardiac failure, acute respiratory distress, acute renal failure, acute liver failure, acute severe brain edema, and acute shock to maintain life. Court finds and points out that causative disease took a back seat while vigorous treatment for acute crisis was going on. So along with treatment of acute crisis, clinical notes also write notes related to basic pathology being treated on day-to-day basis and it should be reflected in clinical notes and it should appear as if both acute crisis and basic pathology were being treated with same vigor. Similarly, relatives need to be explained about need to monitor and maintain vitals and it does not constitute the treatment of basic pathology. Medical professional should make it abundantly clear to relatives that monitoring vitals is different from treating the original basic disease. High-risk consents, informed consents, and dissents need to be recorded in writing on case papers and signed by relatives and a witness to allow court to evaluate whether relatives were informed time to time without confusion.

Legal Proof of Documenting Continuous Monitoring

Very often when treatment charts and case papers are reviewed by court, when a case of MN related to unexpected death is heard, it finds that so often medical professional(s) claim that they did continuous monitoring of patient related to heart rate/pulse, blood pressure, respiratory rate, temperature, oxygen saturation, and electrocardiograph but clinical notes of case papers do not reflect any mention of these readings. Case papers do not showing any entry of vital parameters make court to conclude that monitoring was not done.

Legal View Regarding Diagnosis

We as pediatricians view diagnosis with great respect. Making an accurate diagnosis makes a doctor feel as if he has reached to zenith of his mental abilities. Courts are not very serious about accuracy of diagnosis but at the same time are not ready to condone palpably wrong diagnosis. Very often when case papers are reviewed by court, when a case of MN related to unexpected death is heard and so often medical professional(s) vehemently claim that they made accurate diagnosis so there is no MN on the part of doctor. Even if diagnosis is not accurate but usual conduct of care of patient by doctor is correct then courts take lenient view regarding making errors in diagnosis of main disease. This is because so many diseases present to medical professional with common signs and symptom complexes and medical professional(s) may make an error of judgment, if the disease presents with rare, atypical signs and symptoms. Medical professional has liberty to choose treatment after arriving at tentative diagnosis. This liberty is related to causative disease and not to acute emergency syndrome management.

Deficiency in Attending the Patient and Conducting a Procedure

Very often when treatment charts and case papers are reviewed by court, when a case of MN related to unexpected death is being heard it finds that so often medical professional(s) did not attend the patient[9] then courts take very strict view. Courts take very strict view if there is deficiency in procedure of putting intravenous lines, intragastric tubes, urine catheters, and tracheal intubation. Courts take very strict view if there is deficiency in continuous monitoring system readings related to pulse/heart rate, blood pressure, respiratory rate, temperature, oxygen saturation, and electrocardiograph finding no entry in clinical notes on case papers. Deficiency in procedures or conducts of treatment of acute cardiac failure, acute respiratory distress, acute renal failure, acute liver failure, acute severe brain edema and acute shock or anaphylaxis to maintain life is also taken as gross negligence. If difficult situation of unexpected death occurs due to such breach of duty of medical professional in emergency room then he may have to defend himself from the charges of MN in courts. Since treatment costs are high and results of critically ill sometimes may result in difficult situation of unexpected death so compensations asked by patient litigant are astronomical.

Difficult Situation of Unexpected Death and Insurance

Medical indemnity insurance policy[10] is the only way out to practice pediatrics and only safe way to practice emergency and CC pediatrics peacefully even when unexpected death occurs. Looking into such an unequal and odious ML scenario where risks of litigations shall continue to increase in days to come. Then where lies the answer? Highest level of record keeping and best communication skills may not be too effective to trade off the compensation benefits patient party gets by dragging you in court of law. This is not a corollary or license for improper record keeping or arrogant communication with patient party. These risks could possibly be managed and if any claim arises, it could be paid by buying indemnity cum hospital error and omission policy issued by private and public insurance companies in India.

LIKELY SITUATIONS OF ML IMPORTANCE IN DIFFICULT SITUATION OF UNEXPECTED DEATH REQUIRING INFORMATION TO POLICE

Difficult Situation of Unexpected Death in ML Cases

The ML situation where one may get patients who mysteriously develop difficult situation causing unexpected death either after entry to emergency unit/room/ward or sometimes afterward. Medical professional should continue to treat patient with meticulous history recording, examination, investigations needed, and treatment as per reasonable norms of medical practice. As per ML norms, it is mandatory to inform law enforcers and/or legal authorities (usually it is local police station[11]). Why? Because medical professional(s) duty is to receive and treat the ill/critical patient and duty of police[12] is to find out whether any crime was been committed on child victim/patient for making him/her suffer from problems listed below:

- Difficult situation of unexpected death happens in Tetanus, gas gangrene, significant burns, head injuries, significant violence[13] needing indoor admission, motor vehicular[14] and other accidental fractures, accidental falls needing indoor admission, attempted suicides,[15] attempted poisoning, attempted homicide,[16] human or animal or snakebite, rape,[17] minor's pregnancy and MTP,[18] battered baby. Insist for postmortem in difficult situation of unexpected death.

Difficult Situation of Unexpected Death in Poisoning

Difficult situation of unexpected death in case of attempted/alleged/suicidal/homicidal or accidental poisoning[19] medical professional is duty bound to preserve specimen stomach wash as per protocol (usually 100 mL or more in a clean glass bottle), blood samples in EDTA and plain bulbs (usually 2 mL each), as applicable and feasible and hand it over to police with proper labeling of name, sex, age, time of collection, brief or detailed history as per the direction of police and full treatment record be given. In case of difficult situation of unexpected death due to poisoning, insist for postmortem. Law demands consent for postmortem to be obtained from relatives by postmortem performing doctor and not by treating medical professional.

Following are other difficult situations of unexpected deaths which need to be informed to police:

- Difficult situation of unexpected death happening in indoor admitted child falling from cot or in hospital bathroom.
- Difficult situation of unexpected death happening on operation table or difficult situation of unexpected death in postoperative patients.
- Difficult situation of unexpected death resulting from anaphylaxis due to a drug.
- Difficult situation of unexpected death due to Steven–Johnson syndrome.
- Difficult situation of unexpected death as a postprocedure event, for example, after lumber puncture, liver biopsy and other biopsies.
- Difficult situation of unexpected death happening due to internal or incessant external bleeding and disseminated intravascular coagulation.
- Difficult situation of unexpected death during or postanesthesia.

How to tackle situation of difficult situation of unexpected death when it occurs in presence of many relatives: If there are many relatives when difficult situation of unexpected death then immediately divide medical professional's working team into two parts. One team shall continue "So-called" sham treatment in difficult situation of unexpected death till relatives are explained about difficult situation of unexpected death and are satisfied and then only death is declared. Second team tackles the leader among relatives about difficult situation of unexpected death by telling that our team of other medical professional(s) is trying hard. Try and make relatives understand and differentiate between the basic disease leading to acute crisis and explain that monitoring vitals is not treatment but guiding pediatricians in treating illness and maintaining vital parameters. Medical professional should wear empathetic, sympathetic attitude, and observing courteousness in communications while explaining difficult situation of unexpected death to relatives.

What to do before declaring death in difficult situation of unexpected death?
"So-called" sham treatment should continue in difficult situation of unexpected death till relatives are completely satisfied and disperse. At the same time, see that all documentation of clinical notes is complete. Preserve all empty vials of injection and injection syringes. Collect 10 mL of blood in plain bulb, EDTA bulb, and Sugar bulb and label them. This is to meet the allegation of relatives that either a poison or overdose of medicine was given.

When to declare death in difficult situation of unexpected death: Where numbers of relatives slowly increase as the time passes in hospital premises when "so-called" treatment in difficult situation of unexpected death is going on. If number increases then one should surely inform police for self-protection as well as safety of property. Declare finally death in front of police and hand over body of patient with collected blood samples and empty injection vials and ampoules and syringes. Do not move the body of unexpected death from OT to ICU if patient dies in OT.

No loose talk in difficult situation of unexpected death: Warn pediatricians and staff members to be careful of loose talk about unexpected death as it may spark physical abuse of medical team or destruction of hospital property.

Reason for "so-called sham treatment": Declaration of death in difficult situation of unexpected death should be essentially preceded by "so-called sham treatment", even putting in intravenous line or starting nasal oxygen or even putting on respirator is a good trick. This will buy time and wisdom for medical team to declare death in difficult situation of unexpected death at the terms and conditions desired by medical team rather than getting swept away by unruly behavior of relatives by untimely declaration of death in absence of police. Kindly do not charge for treatment as it may spark another fury of relatives.

How to transport sick and serious dying patient:
- Medical professional and nurse team should accompany the dying patient[20]
- Ambulance should have enough variety and stock of emergency medicines, injections, intravenous fluids, and oxygen[21]
- Monitoring equipment like stethoscope, blood pressure instrument, cardiac monitor machine with preferably a defibrillator and a ventilator[22]
- In case difficult situation of unexpected death occurs, bring back the child to your hospital and declare death after proper explanations satisfying the relatives.

Legal standards of reasonable medical care in emergency rooms in case of difficult situation of unexpected death: Standards of medical care in emergency room are higher because emergency rooms[23] care claims giving state of art services being given to patient admitted as below:
- Duty of care in emergency room (which means actively avoiding all kinds of dangers, i.e., health risks from all sources, i.e., from disease, drugs, and surgery, all the time) to your patients by continuous monitoring of all relevant vital parameters and investigations to avoid any further acceleration in disease process.[24]
- Law requires higher proportionate degree of medical care in emergency room. Higher the risks undertaken then higher are the standard of monitoring and medical procedural skill demanded by law in caring for critically ill.
- Any lack or shortcoming or deficiency of medical care on the part of medical practitioner in monitoring or treatment of critically ill, medical professional's actions, which causes acceleration of disease process leading to unexpected death, is actionable under law. Under law for actionable negligence, such breach of duty should cause acceleration of unexpected death.
- There should be close nexus between negligence leading to acceleration of unexpected death.

ABOUT CONSENT, DISSENT, ASSENT, COUNSELING, FOREWARNING IN DIFFICULT SITUATION OF UNEXPECTED DEATH

- In emergency rooms, standards for consent, informed are much lower than usual cold situations. In dire emergency courts waive of consent in favor of giving lifesaving treatment, even though nature of treatment may amount to adventure.[25] In a case of a road side accident, victim's (in case of accident victim court takes very strict view if no attempt is made to save life)[26,27] vitals were stabilized by giving ET before shifting to higher center, where one limb had to be amputated because of delay in referral, court did not hold medical professional negligent in causing delay in referring because stabilization of vitals was crucial before transfer of patient otherwise patient would have suffered unexpected death during transit. Defendant would be liable for such unexpected death occurs if vitals were not stabilized before transferring. In another case of vehicular accident, a reasonable delay in preparing for operation and arranging for 19 bottles of blood was permitted by court even though patient postoperatively was in difficult situation later died.[28]

- Some times in emergency omission to perform operation for want of consent may amount to negligence.[29] Here, emergency appendectomy not done, for want of consent nor dissent from patient taken in writing, doctor was held liable. In this case, appendix later burst and unexpected death occurred. Remember written dissent is more important than consent for invasive procedure, surgery, investigation, transfer, and referral in emergency situations.[30]

ABOUT MONITORING AND RECORD KEEPING PRIOR TO DIFFICULT SITUATION OF UNEXPECTED DEATH OCCURRENCE

- Monitoring[31] serious patients by keeping record[32] and using available gadgets and investigations or refer by providing ambulance to transfer. Bottom line for monitoring is recording pulse, respiration temperature, blood pressure, and intake and output chart.
- Remember proper record is valid defense in MN case as the law asks for show of care rather than cure[33]

ABOUT CRITICALLY ILL PATIENTS WHERE "KNOWN COMPLICATION" WHICH CANNOT BE PREVENTED PRIOR TO DIFFICULT SITUATION OF UNEXPECTED DEATH OCCURRENCE

Son bitten by cat. ARV given. He developed neuroparalytic reaction.[34] Hospitalized unexpected death occurred in ICU. No negligence, as standard textbooks and WHO report of 1984 which mentions neuroparalytic reactions well-known complication of ARV. Hence, proper ICU treatment given with care.

ABOUT CASES RELATED TO ANAPHYLAXIS[35] CAUSING DIFFICULT SITUATION OF UNEXPECTED DEATH

Medical professional did not do penicillin test dose also did not keep emergency medicines ready for treating anaphylaxis of penicillin and failed to treat complication, patient developed unexpected death, medical professional held negligent for not treating complication.

EMERGENCY BLOOD TRANSFUSION PRIOR TO DIFFICULT SITUATION OF UNEXPECTED DEATH OCCURRENCE

Sometimes emergency blood transfusion may belong to wrong blood group causing mismatch[36] transfusion reaction leading to unexpected death. It is better to be safe than sorry by following proper blood checking norms.

SUMMARY

This write up is intended to provide ML information as to what a medical professional should do in the event of unexpected death. How a medical professional and CC and ET provider should deal with relative, police, press, politicians, social workers, lawyers and what kind of mindset the law courts pursue. The knowledge of mindset of nonmedical people should allow you to refocus on your clinical notes documentation. This ML knowledge and wisdom to bridge the gap of ignorance of relevant laws as applicable to practicing medical professional and CC and ET provider to prevent solve and understand the ML problems related to difficult situation of unexpected death. All of us know and have experienced in our life that ignorance breeds and feeds uncertainty. Uncertainty breeds and feeds unfounded fears. We also know unfounded fears usually never become true or actually happen in one's life but makes life stressful and unlivable. In the light of basis legal knowledge, let us dispel these unfounded legal fears and do right things in right direction. Let us not give up and practice defensive medicine for fear of legal wrangles.

LEARNING KEY POINTS

These are practical points to remember.
- Keep crisis trolley along with designated team member to communicate to relatives.
- Keeping all resuscitative measures ready all 24 hours. They include emergency drug tray with drugs within expiry date. Resuscitation equipment, oxygen cylinder if there is no central oxygen, tubes, etc.
- One person specially trained in communication skills be designated team member to talk to relatives during crisis in separate room.
- Moment sudden unexpected cardiac arrest or respiratory difficulty arises then immediately tell politely all the relatives and bystanders to leave the ward or resuscitation room or else wheel the patient to resuscitation room.
- Keep one of designated team member during "sudden death crisis" for informing the seriousness of the health and assurance that all measures are being taken to revive the patient.
- Designated team member should also take additional high-risk consents, informed consents, and dissents which should be in writing and need to record in writing on case papers and signed by relatives and a witness. This exercise is presumably for police and law courts to evaluate whether relatives were informed time to time without confusion.

TAKE-HOME MESSAGES

Do not be in hurry to declare death, assess patient party mood, situation, counsel, and slowly first say patient is serious, all necessary treatment is going on, you can call any other pediatrician for second opinion, transfer of patient is not possible. The chief must speak to decision makers of patient party.

MUST AVOID THINGS

Getting in heated arguments with patient party.

DO NOT DO

Never ever threaten postmortem in retaliation.

WARNINGS

The entire thing is recorded in CCTV camera, which patient party should be humbly made aware.

MESSAGES WHICH THE READER MUST BE AWARE

Keep discharge cum death summary ready in duplicate, get its receiving signed and acknowledged by legal guardian with two witnesses.

MUST DO THING

Inform police by dialing number 100 in case you anticipate violence.

MEDICAL NEGLIGENCE PEARLS

It is surprisingly true that in spite of wearing good, empathetic, sympathetic attitude and observing courteousness in communications allegations of MN in SUD may put medical professional in a ML maze of alleged MN and leave them disgusted.

ONLY ONE FACT TO REMEMBER

Amount of money asked is mind-boggling. Patients may sue a medical professional for compensation by asking usually lakhs of rupees and sometimes in crores under new CPA 2019.

MCQs

Choose one correct answer
1. What to do before declaring death in SUD?
   a. Treatment continue in SUD till relatives are completely satisfied
   b. Documentation is complete.
   c. Preserve all empty vials of injection and injection syringes.
   d. Collect 10 mL of blood in plain bulb, EDTA bulb, and sugar bulb and label them.
   e. All of the above
2. Enumerate few causes of sudden and unexpected death in clinical practice.
   a. Anaphylactic shock
   b. Shock due to embolism
   c. Endotoxic shock
   d. Hemorrhagic shock
   e. All of above
3. Deaths which needs to be informed to police:
   a. Falls in hospital
   b. Operation table death
   c. Death due to drug anaphylaxis
   d. Death due to accident of any type
   e. All of the above

Answers
1. e   2. e   3. e

FAQs
1. What is sequel of sudden unexpected death?
   a. Mob violence
   b. Breakage of ICU property
   c. Brought dead
   d. Nonsettlement of bills and dues

REFERENCES
1. Outlook magazine April 2002 issue.
2. The Consumer Protection Act 2019 as amended up to date.
3. Indian Medical Association & Ors. v. V.P. Shantha & Ors. JT 1995(8) SC 119: AIR 1996 SC 550: 1995 (6) SCC 651: 1995 (3) CPJ 1 (SC): 1995 (3) CPR 412(SC).
4. Spring Meadows Hospital & Anr. v. Harjot Ahluwalia (through K.S. Ahluwalia) & Anr.,1998(3)CPR1(SC):1998(I)CPJI:JTI998(2) SC620.
5. Charan Singh v. Healing Touch Hospital & Ors., 2003 (2) CPR 95: 2003 (3) CPJ 62: 2003(6) CLD46(NCDRC).
6. Jacob Methews versus State of Punjab.
7. The Consumer Protection Act 2019 as amended up to date.
8. The Law of Tort.
9. Maruti Eknath Masane versus shushusha hospital and others.
10. The Indian Insurance Act, 1937 governs general insurance group of companies viz; New India, United India, National & Oriental insurance companies offer at nominal premium.
11. S. 154 of The Criminal Procedure Code, 1973.
12. S. 173 of Code of criminal procedure, 1973 empowers police to investigate a case.
13. S. 319 to 338 of Indian Penal code, 1860.
14. Motor Vehicle Act.
15. S. 309 of Indian Penal code, 1860.
16. S. 299 of Indian Penal code, 1860.
17. S. 375,376 of Indian Penal code, 1860.
18. Medical termination of pregnancy Act, 1971.
19. The Poisons Act, 1919.
20. Mr. Shakil v. Dr P. Irani and ors 1999(2) CPR 515.
21. P.S. Govindarajan v. General Manager, Integral Coach Factory & Ors., 1993 (2) CP J 1211(TNSCDRC).

22. D.C. Bhawani Prasad v. Krishna Nursing Home, 1997 (I) CPJ 483 (Karn. SCDRC)s.
23. Laxman Balkrishna Joshi (Dr.) v. Dr. Trimbak Bapu Godbole, 1968 ACJ 183 (SC): AIR 1969 SC 128: 1969 (1) SCR 206.
24. Guru Teg Bahadur Sahib (Charitable) Hospital v. D.K. Nayyar, 2002 (I) CPR 442 Punj. SCDRC).
25. Lekhraj v. Bharaj Nursing Home & Anr., 1998 (2) CPJ 335 (Punj. SCDRC).
26. Paschim Banga Khet Mazdoor Samity & Ors. v. State of West Bengal & Anr., 1996 (4) Supreme 260: AIR 1996 SC 2426: 1996 (4) SCC 37: IT 1996 (6) 43 (SC).
27. Parmanand Katara v. Union of India, 1989 (4) SCC 286: AIR 1989 SC 2039: 1989 ACl 1000: 1989 (4) SCC 286.
28. Amir Ali Shakir v. St. John's Medical College Hospital, Bangalore, 1996 (1) CPJ 169: 1995(3) CPR 174 (Karn. SCDRC).
29. T.T. Thomas (Dr.) v. Smt. Elisa, AIR 1987 Ker.-HC 52: 1986 Ker. LT 1026.
30. P.N. Sudhakar Gupta v. Anugraha Vittala Nursing Home, 1997 (1) CPJ 266.
31. Guru Teg Bahadur Sahib (Charitable) Hospital v. D.K. Nayyar, 2002 (I) CPR 442 Punj. SCDRC).
32. Saraswati Parakhoi v. Grid Corporation of Orissa, 2001 ACJ 874 (Ori.) (DB).
33. V Chandra Sekar v. Malar Hospitals Ltd., 2001 (I) CPJ 137: 2001 (I),CPR 628 (TN SCDRC).
34. Dipti De Sarkar v. Steel Authority of India & ors, 1993 (1) CPR 640:1993(2) CPJ 1289 Orissa SCDRC.
35. Chin Keo v. Govt of Malaysia, 1967 ACJ 379 P.C.
36. Calcutta Medical Research Institute v. Bimalesh Chatterjee & Ors., 1999 (1) CPR 3 (NCDRC).

CHAPTER 16

Prevention of Violence Against Doctors

Hemant R Gangolia, Bela Amichandra Verma, Samik Basu, Rajakumar Marol

"An eye for an eye only ends up making the whole world blind".
—Mahatma Gandhi

Keywords: Doctor Violence Protection Act, Mob violence, Violence

Aim: To examine cues for predictable mob violence or violence in field of medicine.

Objective: The healthcare provided from physical and mental abuse from patient party while in workplace.

INTRODUCTION

Malcom X said "Sometimes you have to pick the gun up to put the gun down. If someone puts their hands on you make sure they never put their hands on anybody else again". The irony was that both Mahatma Gandhi and Malcom X were shot dead. In today's era of consumerism, violence seems inevitable.

The Indian Medical Association (IMA) survey states:[1,2]
- 82.7% of doctors in India feel stressed out in their profession.
- 46.3% fear violence is the main cause of stress in many doctors.
- 24.2% doctors fear being sued.
- 62.8% of the doctors surveyed are unable to see their patients without any fear of violence.
- 57.7% have thought of hiring security in their premises.
- 2014 survey states 75% of surveyed doctors in India have suffered some form of physical violence while on duty.

As the society evolves and the population becomes more and more literate it is expected that vandalism against doctors would decline but it is not so. Recently, we have noticed not only a rise in the incident but there is major change in the trend. It was believed that mob violence is commonly seen in clinics and establishments in communally sensitive or politically sensitive area or in slums and industrial belts. However, recent incidents show us that the culprits involved in such incident are surprisingly well educated and well placed economically.

Who are at risk?
- Doctors
- Nurses
- Ward boys and ayahs
- Reception and office staff
- Security guards and watchmen
- Any healthcare provider.

The causes of violence are multifactorial and following are those:[3-5]
- *Sudden death:* Mob involvement
- Lack of proper communication and poor communication
- High volume of patient load

- Cost of healthcare
- Billing
- Mob mentality
- Emergency department manned by doctors lacking EM training
- Understaffed emergency department
- Inadequate care by hospital staff
- Lack of understanding of patient's illness
- Low health literacy
- Meagre health budget and poor-quality healthcare
- Vulnerability of small and medium healthcare establishments
- Poor image of doctors and the role of the media
- Lack of faith in the judicial process
- Nonavailability of medicine and equipment
- Lack of security
- Patient transportation
- Hospital rules.

Following are the aggravating factors:
- Criticism by own colleagues (doctor jousting)—43%
- Death of the patient—22%
- Deformity or disability—18%
- Complications of treatment
- "Ambulance Chaser Advocates"
- "So-called Social Workers".

Following are the types of violence which one comes across:
- Offensive language and abuses
- Threats of assaults
- Physical assaults
- Destruction of building, property, and medical equipment
- Disrupting the hospital routine and treatment of other patients
- Homicidal attacks.

PREVENTION IS BETTER THAN CURE

As each one knows that the prevention is better than cure, therefore the prime objectives are the prevention of assaults on doctors and the prevention of damage to hospital property. The law will decide the prima facie of the medical negligence.

NO UNIVERSAL, BLANKET SOLUTION

There is no universal, blanket solution to prevent the violence but one to devise one's own methods to be tailor-made as per the individual's needs.

CHANGE IN LAW: CPA

Over last three decades, many case laws and consumer protection act have changed the medical practice and at present, the faith has been replaced by contract. Therefore, one has to change with time and one has to accept and face the mishaps which are now the part and parcel of the medical practice.

POSSIBLE SOLUTIONS

We can find the solution to any issue in our practice if we apply following six words while approaching any issue:
1. *Anticipation* during our OPD, indoor formats of the practice.
2. *Documentation* which should be justified informed one.
3. *Communication* which should be an informed documented one.
4. *Limitations* should be always kept in the mind, qualifications, infrastructure wise. One should not mind in having second opinion if one is not sure of the diagnosis keeping the ego apart.

5. *Ethics* described by four principles of respect, do good, do no harm and the equality should be tried to be achieved as near as to the perfection.
6. *Introspection* to be done by auditing ourselves by thought of putting near and dear ones in the shoes of the patient at the end of the day. Does one is accumulating the heap of nonsatisfiers, critics, etc. by one's practice format, staff behavior, huge billing, etc.

LEARN TO ANTICIPATE

It is high time that one should learn to anticipate the ringing bell of the probable violence in following scenarios:

- *Occurrence of the anaphylaxis at the clinic after giving injectables:* The mainstay of the management of the anaphylaxis is adrenaline but it should be easily accessible and one should be aware of its short expiry. The important steps are the resuscitative measures and its documentation as in the event of death which is a known complication of anaphylactic reaction, the attempt of the resuscitative measures and panchnama in case of complaint saves from the gross medical negligence. Hence, the clinic and office practice should be well equipped with oxygen cylinder, Ambu bag, resuscitative equipment, emergency medicines, etc. The communication skill is very important in handling such situation.
- *When the gasping patient is brought as an emergency and dies:* At the outset, the emergency patient cannot be refused as per the Parmanand Katra versus Union of India[5] case law; therefore, it has to be managed by the one's capacity, ability, and infrastructure available. In case of death, one has to document the chronology of the given treatment and inform the police. The communication and documentation is very important and one should not give the death certificate but one can declare the death and as soon as police comes, police takes over the charge of dead body and decides the further action of line. Ideally, the police ask for postmortem.
- *Occurrence of sudden death in hospitalized patient or while treating the patient at the hospital set up:* The sudden death is shocking to both relatives of the patient and treating doctors. The body language is very important as hurry and worry may create the doubts. One has to remain calm, maintain confidence, to behave in a polite and dignified manner and the most important to share the sorrow professionally without being overemotional but be empathetic. One should keep all resuscitative measures ready and to avoid chaos, shouting, and loud orders. One should not retaliate as offence cannot be always the best defense.

While treating the patient, the communication, counseling, and documentation of the communication/counseling is very important on day-to-day basis. One can maintain the transparency by giving xerox papers of day-to-day treatment but one has to be sure of proper documentation.

One has to complete all the documents, check for the various instruments/drugs before informing the relatives. The team leader has to inform the responsible relatives present, especially the decision makers, after briefing to the junior doctors and the staff as all should be on same page. There should be no loose talk. One has to inform police on

letterhead with the following details and get acknowledgement:
- Patient's name and age
- Time of arrival/admission
- Date and time of death.

One should not mention the cause of the death, and once the police take over the charge of the body, decide about the further line of action such as postmortem.
- *Occurrence of the table deaths:* Whenever table deaths occur, one should complete the papers with the appropriate documentation and inform the police. The best option is to declare the death after the arrival of the police and never to give the death certificate, insisting on postmortem.
- *When brought dead at the clinic/hospital:* The dead patient cannot be referred hence one has to inform the police and not to give the death certificate. If it is a known person or seen within last 14 days and there is no suspected foul play then one may give the death certificate but the bottom line is one should be able to justify the cause of death if summoned by the court of law.
- The syndrome of VIP effect has to be kept in the mind and one has to take care of 6 Ps namely police, press, politicians, prosecutors (lawyers), professors (teachers), and peers.
- The huge billing issue and nonpayment of the bill has to be handled delicately.

ANTICIPATION OF VIOLENCE AND PREPARATIONS

As anticipation makes one mentally prepared, let us see the practical tips as how to go about in above stated scenarios:
- *Emergency exit:* There should be always an emergency exit/escape exit/lifesaving exit while designing the workplace which many knows but reluctant to make the change.
- *The emergency room* should always be well equipped with all lifesaving medicines and equipment. It is very important to avoid the chaos and panicky situation in the emergency states.
- *The Doctor Protection Act* board should be displayed in each clinical establishment at the prominent places and with due permission of the local police station, one can put the name of the police station on the board. The soft copy of the act should always be available in one's smart phone so as to show or forward to the police station as sometimes police not aware of it in view of other priorities. The display board should have the below mentioned points:

DOCTOR VIOLENCE PROTECTION ACT AND MEDICAL ASSOCIATION MANAGING POLICE

The (State name) Medicare Service Persons and Medicare Service Institutions (Prevention of Violence and Damage or loss to Property).[6-8]

Important Sections

Section 3: Any act causing damage or loss to the property of the hospital or any act of violence against any of the employee of hospital or abusing such an act is prohibited.

Section 4: The offender could be punished with imprisonment which may extend to 3 years and fine of ₹50,000/-.

Section 5: The offence would be cognizable and nonbailable and tried by the court of JM of 1st Class.

Section 6: In addition to above punishment, the offender would be liable to pay compensation of twice the amount of damage or loss caused to the property of hospital.

It is important to know because when one files FIR after the mishap and later on the charge sheet, the filing is under the above said act and the IPC sections as applicable.

Whenever the office bearers of the local association change, one can pay a courtesy visit to the local police station so as to establish the rapport with the police authorities.

DOES AND DON'TS IN HOSPITAL

- Each clinical establishment should be equipped with CCTV with the display of "One is under CCTV (video/audio) surveillance". The CCTV recording is taken as an evidence in court of law subject to the certification of the recording by the CCTV service provider or if needed by forensic laboratory.

  The smart phones can be used for the audio/video recording with the consent to explain the seriousness, prognosis, treatment of the diseases with the patient/relatives/decision makers. The smart phone can be used for the SMS rush team group messaging in case of the mishap.

- The assistant or the responsible staff should have the list of emergency phone numbers of the responsible colleagues, benevolent persons of the society, benevolent local politicians, police station to call them immediately in case of the mishap. One can have the rush team concept whereby the team arrives immediately in case of mishap call. The presence of colleagues and benevolent persons besides giving the moral support definitely dilutes the situation and helps out to ease the situation.

- One has to have the competent, umbrella insurance cover besides the professional indemnity of at least 1 crore or the amount as per the infrastructure. There are many private, association medicolegal insurance agencies which besides the insurance cover provide the medicolegal support. One has to choose the firm wisely and judiciously.

- One should be a member of the local medical association as well one should develop the local rush team concept. The local rush team should reach the mishap site immediately on the call of the concerned person. As a medical association one should develop the rapport with the local police station time to time, may be at the time of the change of the office bearers as well during the visit to exchange the information of the local medical issues as well the related laws to the medical practice.

- The clinical establishment should outsource the security measures which may be individual or association wise. One should learn the self-defense measures as well the staff of the clinical establishment should be well trained in self-defense measures and as a group to decide the role of each one in case of the mishap. One can wisely and judiciously decide to get the licensed arms.

- There should be restricted entry to emergency, intensive care rooms such as NICU, PICU, MICU, and SICU may be based on identity cards such as Aadhar card, the time of the visiting hours should be designed effectively in order to prevent the overcrowding and the respective guidelines to be displayed in the clinical establishment.[8]

- The names of the miscreants should be uploaded in the electronic medical record system if available.

- The staff, paramedics of the clinical establishment should be trained by means of the mock drill[8] time to time so that each one gets acquainted and get to know the exact role one has to play in case of mishap more so at the reception/emergency areas of the clinical establishment. They should be trained in the elements of documentation and communication which are the important pillars of the defense.

ACTUAL SCENE OF MOB VIOLENCE RECREATED

In spite of the anticipation and above-mentioned practical tips being observed, one gets victimized of assault, mob violence, etc. Let us see the genesis of such incidences. As the news of the mishap spreads in the area where the patient stays, the local population gets instigated to visit the site. These may include local goons, local politicians, local social workers, local dissatisfied old patients, and also some who come just to watch the fun. The mob mentality lacks intelligent reasoning and wishes to have fun and a call by even one person "Maro" "Todo" can instigate the crowd to barge in and start the vandalism.

PRACTICAL PREVENTIVE ACTIONS

The situation in such can go out of hand in no time, therefore one has to act swiftly and following are the measures to be taken:
- The responsible staff has to trigger the alarm system for the rush team.
- One has to call the colleagues immediately.
- One should inform and call the police immediately and once they arrive, they take over the situation.
- Involving the politicians is double-edged sword, hence one has to be wise in calling them and more often if not called happen to be there from side of the patient. If one is in good rapport with the politician, they do help in diffusing the situation but they do take the advantage later on.
- One should take the photographs of the damages immediately which will be helpful in the court of law and the insurance process. It is better to take these photographs or videos before the police and politicians arrive at the site.
- To send all the injured staff and doctors for medical check-up and first aid preferably to nearby Government hospital and to make the medicolegal case that hospital and preserve all the injury reports.
- One should register the FIR at the police station and to mention the names of the miscreants if known otherwise in the name of unknown persons. One should hand over the copy of the CCTV footage. The police themselves come to the site for CCTV footage and take the same.
- To inform the insurance company immediately and to submit the photographs/FIR copy to the company.
- One should never compromise and one should not succumb to the requests/pressures by politicians/social workers to compromise.
- Sometimes one has to handle the delayed reaction of police. The police may want to delay immediate arrest of culprits because it can worsen the law-and-order situation. However, if police are delaying arrest even after the cremation, make a complaint to senior police officers or one can make use of RTI or we may have to go ahead with writ petition.

Crisis management committee: If possible and feasible, to form Crisis Management Committee at taluka level or district level consisting of Doctors, Social Workers, Politicians, Legal Personalities, Press reporters, etc.

SOME IMPORTANT ASPECTS FOR DAY-TO-DAY PRACTICE

- When police arrive and take over the situation, they ask and collect the original papers of the case and dose the panchnama. One should complete all the papers, number them, sign on each page with the counter signature of the police officials, take the xerox of the pages, and take the acknowledgment of receiving the originals with the number of pages received.
- The communication skill is an art and to be practiced which is very important while declaring/sharing the bad news, explaining the seriousness/prognosis of the disease, explaining the day-to-day status of serious patient, and informing the treatment options available and the pros/cons of the treatment options. The seniors have the important role to play and to take the lead in such situations.
- The documentation in the aggravating scenarios of anaphylaxis, sudden death, and table death is very important and one should learn to write the notes in order, the most important being the resuscitative notes.
- One has to learn the art of facing media, press, social media, newspapers, television news more often it gets flashed as the breaking news. One should relax, people have short memory, and many do not read the newspapers. One should not ignore the press/reporters but to answer their questions in a scientific manner and one can resort to your colleague for help. One has to face the problem, accept the challenge, time is the best healer but one should take appropriate medicolegal guidance.
- One finds difficult to face the colleagues after any such incidences but each one of us are liable to come across such a problem at any moment, hence each one of us requires moral support of others and hence the importance of an association. Each one of us is in same boat; hence, we have to learn from the mistakes of others rather than deriving pleasure from it or criticizing it.
- In view of freedom of speech and expression, it is common to find the scenarios of defamation posts, remarks, pictures, videos, etc. on social media. One can file the defamation case but in view of long-time frame, it is really difficult preposition.
- One should introspect by auditing oneself treatment wise at the end of the day by putting our near, dear ones in the shoes of the patients and whether one is accumulating the heap of nonsatisfiers, critics by one's practice format, staff behavior, huge billing, etc.
- One should know one's limitation and practice accordingly specialty wise, ability wise, capacity wise, and infrastructure wise. If one is not sure of diagnosis, one should mind in having second opinion and to avoid egoism.
- One should follow the four basics principles of the medical ethics namely, autonomy (respect the patient's ability to take decisions on behalf of themselves), beneficence (do good), nonmaleficence (do no harm), and justice (treat equitably and distribute benefits fairly).

How to address the press?
- Establish the site/venue
- Appoint a Media Liaison
- Communicate through press briefings
- Establish the facts
- 5 Ws (Who, What, When, Where, Why)
- 1H (How)
- Express emotions.

The most common FAQs by media or relatives are:
1. What went wrong?
2. What caused this?
3. Did you have any prior indication that there was a problem?
4. Who made the critical decision?
5. Who was in charge at the time?
6. How will the case be investigated?
7. How was the negligence discovered, by whom and when?
8. What action will be taken against those responsible?
9. When was the family notified?
10. What was said to them?
11. What state and local authorities have been notified and when?
12. What is being done to avoid a repeat scenario?
13. Has anything like this happened before?

SUGGESTIONS TO AVOID VIOLENCE

- All hospitals should develop a comprehensive violence prevention program.
- No universal strategy exists to prevent violence.
- The risk factors vary from hospital to hospital and from unit to unit.
- Hospitals should form multidisciplinary committees that include direct-care staff as well as union representatives (if available) to identify risk factors in specific work scenarios and to develop strategies for reducing them.
- All hospital workers should be alert and cautious when interacting with patients and visitors.
- They should actively participate in safety training programs and be familiar with their employers' policies, procedures, and materials on violence prevention.

SUMMARY

Under the shadows of violence fright and laws still, the bottom line is if we have honesty, transparency, punctuality, in our profession and practice, we can overcome the stress of our practice.

LEARNING KEY POINTS AND TAKE-HOME MESSAGES

- DPR is deteriorating globally and situation is appalling
- But the situation is not totally hopeless
- Be a patient listener
- Show genuine concern
- Maintain proper records
- Refer the patient whenever necessary
- Update your knowledge
- Establish a good rapport with patient
- Do not overreach
- Consent
- Documentation
- Proper communication
- Be alert
- Restrict entry
- Standard operating procedure (SOP)
- Insurance
- No universal solution
- To be tailor made as per individual's needs.

MUST AVOID THINGS

Do not overreach.

DO NOT DO

Poor or no communication with patient party.

WARNINGS
You are under CCTV surveillance 24 × 7.

MESSAGES WHICH THE READER MUST BE AWARE
For everything and anything, take fresh consent again and again.

MUST DO THING
Maintain proper records and keep ready for police.

MEDICAL NEGLIGENCE PEARLS
Dial 100 and call police.

ONLY ONE FACT TO REMEMBER
Restrict entry of too many relatives at one time; make passes for two at a time.

REFERENCES
1. The Hindu. (2017). Most doctors concerned about violence at work, Survey conducted by IMA shows that 80 per cent of doctors report having faced some degree of aggression from patients. [online] Available from: https://www.thehindu.com/news/cities/Delhi/Most-doctors-concerned-about-violence-at-work/article17043948.ece. [Last accessed December, 2023].
2. The Hindu. (2017). Majority of doctors in India fear violence, says IMA survey. [online] Available from: https://www.thehindu.com/sci-tech/health/majority-of-doctors-in-india-fear-violence-says-ima-survey/article19198919.ece. [Last accessed December, 2023].
3. Baldwa M, Baldwa V, Padvi N, Baldwa S. Legal issues in Medical Practice, 1st edition. New Delhi: CBS Publishers & Distributors; 2019.
4. Tiwari S. Textbook on Medicolegal Issues, 2nd edition. New Delhi: Jaypee Brothers Medical Publisher; 2018.
5. Pt. Parmanand Katara vs Union Of India & Ors on 28 August, 1989. https://www.bing.com/ck/a?!&&p=f61be3d02b8b42ecJmltdHM9MTY3NjMzMjgwMCZpZ3VpZD0yZjI4YjY4MC00YTFkLTY3YmItMjU3Ny1hNzhmNGI4NjY2ODcmaW5zaWQ9NTMwMw&ptn=3&hsh=3&fclid=2f28b680-4a1d-67bb-2577-a78f4b866687&psq=parmanand+katara+vs+union+of+india+summary&u=a1aHR0cHM6Ly9pbmRpYW5rYW5vb24ub3JnL2RvYy80OTgxMjYv&ntb=1.
6. The Prevention of Violence Against Doctors, Medical Professionals And Medical Institutions Bill, 2018 By Dr. Shrikant Eknath Shinde, M.P., A Bill https://www.bing.com/ck/a?!&&p=75cd97cb73427613JmltdHM9MTY3NjMzMjgwMCZpZ3VpZD0yZjI4YjY4MC00YTFkLTY3YmItMjU3Ny1hNzhmNGI4NjY2ODcmaW5zaWQ9NTE4OA&ptn=3&hsh=3&fclid=2f28b680-4a1d-67bb-2577-a78f4b866687&psq=doctor+protection+act+2010&u=a1aHR0cDovLzE2NC4xMDAuNDcuNC9iaWxsc3RleHRzL2xzYmlsaHRleHRzL2FzaW50cm9kdWNlZC8yMjY5YXNMucGRm&ntb=1.
7. Maharashtra Act No. XI Of 2010. https://www.bing.com/ck/a?!&&p=ed929fce6fe897d1JmltdHM9MTY3NjMzMjgwMCZpZ3VpZD0yZjI4YjY4MC00YTFkLTY3YmItMjU3Ny1hNzhmNGI4NjY2ODcmaW5zaWQ9NTE4Mw&ptn=3&hsh=3&fclid=2f28b680-4a1d-67bb-2577-a78f4b866687&psq=+maharashtra+doctor+protection+act+2010&u=a1aHR0cHM6Ly9sai5tYWhhcmFzaHRyYS5nb3YuaW4vc2l0ZXMvZGVmYXVsdC9maWxlcy9UaGUtUERGLnBkZg&ntb=1.
8. Pandey SK, Sharma V. Aggression and violence against doctors. How to address this frightening new epidemic? Indian J Ophthalmol. 2019;67(11):1903-5.

SUGGESTED READING
1. Baldwa M, Baldwa V, Padvi N, Baldwa S. Legal Issues in Critical Care. New Delhi: CBS Publishers & Distributors; 2022.
2. Baldwa M, Baldwa V, Padvi N, Baldwa S. Legal Issues in Medical Practice, 2nd edition. New Delhi: CBS Publishers & Distributors; 2023.

CHAPTER 17

Medicolegal Issues in Pediatric Critical Care

Dnyanesh DK, Suma Dnyanesh

Keywords: Emergency treatment, Indian Penal Code, Medical negligence, Medicolegal case (MLC), Pediatric intensive care units

Aim: Pediatric critical care must adhere to a complex body of laws, regulations, and ethical standards. This includes complying with requirements for informed consent, surrogate decision-making, end-of-life care, medical record documentation, and reporting of adverse events.

Objective: Medicolegal issues are prevalent in pediatric critical care, as healthcare providers navigate complex ethical dilemmas, manage critically ill children, and interact with families facing difficult decisions. These issues stem from the delicate balance between providing life-saving treatment, respecting patient autonomy, and adhering to ethical and legal principles.

INTRODUCTION

No greater opportunity, no greater responsibility, and no greater obligation can fall to any other human being than to become a medical professional.[1] In the care of suffering, the medical professionals need scientific knowledge, technical skill, moral understanding of profession, and awareness about the relevant laws of the land. Primarily doctors, especially physicians, dealing with emergency and critical care have several ethical and legal obligations in performance of their duties. The doctors who are involved in critical care should know their legal obligations to avoid allegations and safeguard themselves against medical negligence. This chapter discusses important medicolegal issues in emergency room and critical care.

MEDICOLEGAL ISSUES RELATED TO REFUSAL OF EMERGENCY PATIENT CARE

Case scenario: A 4-year-old child with history of continuous convulsions was brought to appropriate nursing home. But the doctor refused to treat the child because child was requiring mechanical ventilatory care but the patient was poor. So without giving any treatment sent the child to a government hospital. The child died on the way to the hospital. Now can the doctor of the private nursing home be booked under medical negligence?

Explanation: First of all, we should know what medical emergency is. Medical emergency means sudden, unforeseen condition of the patient and/or where the question of life and death is there.[2]

In the case of "Paramanand Katara versus Union of India", the honorable Supreme Court has observed that: "There can be no second opinion that preservation of human life is of paramount importance. That is so on account of the fact that once life is lost, status quo ante cannot be restored as resurrection is beyond the capacity of man. Every doctor whether at a government hospital or otherwise has professional obligation to extend his services with due expertise for protecting life. No law or state action can interfere to avoid or delay the discharge of the paramount obligation cast upon members of the medical profession".[3]

So in conclusion, "Doctors cannot refuse emergency treatment to a patient irrespective of his caste, creed, ability to pay, etc. because saving human life is of paramount importance. It is a legal obligation on each doctor".[4]

In the above case scenario, doctor knows that it was a medical emergency. He could have intubated the child and given oxygen, anticonvulsants, and IV fluids. Since patient was not affordable, then he could have transported the child to a government hospital where ventilator facility is available. This is the legal and professional obligation.

A doctor is free to choose his patients, say according to their capacity to pay his fees or according to his level of competence. But this liberty does not extend to medical emergency cases, accidents, and injury cases.

Hospitals, nursing homes, clinics of doctors who declare that they provide emergency services are legally bound to attend all medical emergency cases, accidents, and injury cases. They cannot refuse the treatment to such cases.

MEDICOLEGAL ISSUES RELATED TO EMERGENCY MLC CASES

Case scenario: Mr "X" met with an accident. He had head injury and fracture of right femur. He was bleeding heavily and was taken to nearby hospital. But the doctor did not attend the case saying that it is a medicolegal case (MLC) and advised the attendants to take him to a government hospital. But on the way, the patient died. Can the doctor be held responsible for this?

Explanation: In the case of "Paramanand Katara versus Union of India", the honorable Supreme Court has observed that: "There are no provisions in the Indian penal code, criminal procedure code, motor vehicle act, etc., which prevent the doctor from attending the seriously injured persons before the arrival of police. The treatment of the patient would not wait for the arrival of police or for completing the hospital formalities".[5] Hence for the doctors, the cases should not matter from the treatment point of view whether MLC or non-MLC. First priority is to save the life of the patient, next comes the legal formalities. In MLC cases, the only thing the doctor has to do is informing police after stabilizing the patient or after the death of the patient.

Remember, no doctor should refuse to attend the emergency cases, accidents, and injury cases. Try to stabilize the patient as per your skills and competence and refer to higher centers in case if it is required, with suitable mode of transport.

In the above case, the doctor is found to be negligent.

Can government hospitals refuse emergency cases saying "no vacant bed" or specialist doctor is not available?

Case scenario: Mr "M" fell from a height and sustained serious head injury and brain hemorrhage. He was taken to a primary healthcare center (PHC). But since necessary facilities for the treatment were not available, he was referred to a district government hospital. There his admission was refused saying *"no vacant bed"*. Then he was taken to a state government hospital. There also, he did not get admission saying *"no vacant bed"* and no neurosurgeon is available. Then he was treated in a private hospital with heavy expenditure. Can the state government be held responsible for this?

Explanation: Honorable Supreme Court, in the case of "Paschim Bengal Khet Mazdoor Samity and others versus West Bengal", has stated that Article 21 of Indian constitution imposes an obligation on the state to safeguard the right to life of every person. Preservation of human life is thus of paramount importance. The government hospitals run by state and doctors employed there are duty bound to provide medical assistance for preserving human life. Failure to provide timely medical treatment to a person in need results in violation of his right to life guaranteed under Article 21.[6] So, it is the responsibility of state government to upgrade the hospitals at district and sub-divisional level, so that serious cases can be treated there and government should make sure the all government hospitals are well equipped and adequate staff and specialist are there. Otherwise, government has to pay the compensation.

MEDICOLEGAL ISSUES RELATED TO CONSENT IN CRITICAL CARE

Case scenario:
1. An 18-year-old boy was brought to emergency room with history of severe abdominal pain with distension. Patient was in altered sensorium and was diagnosed to have ruptured appendix with peritonitis and requiring immediate laparotomy surgery to save the patient. The patient attender after leaving him to the hospital was not available for giving consent. Can surgeon take the patient for laparotomy without consent?
2. A 16-year-old boy was admitted in pediatric intensive care unit (PICU) for the treatment of severe broncho-pneumonia. He was in PICU for 10 days. But there was no much improvement in his condition, was on verge of requiring mechanical ventilation. Since the parents were very poor, they were asking for leaving against medical advice (LAMA). But the boy was requesting to continue the treatment including ventilation. Can 16-year-old boy give consent for major treatment?

Explanation: When a patient >12 years approaches a physician, the consent for physical examination is implied. Sections 88 and 90 of IPC 1860 say that any person who is conscious, mentally sound, and >12 years old can give consent for physical examination, diagnosis, and treatment.[7] But when the patient is requiring hospitalization and invasive procedures, written informed consent of the patient is a must. In case if the patient is <18 years, mentally not sound, or is in unconscious state, written informed consent from the parents or relatives or guardian is a must. Otherwise, it amounts to an offence. The doctrine of written informed consent is premised on the notion that "every human being of adult years and sound mind has a right to determine what shall be done with his body".[8]

The informed written consent should include the following things:
- Diagnosis
- Nature and purpose of proposed procedure or treatment

- Risks, side effects, and consequences of proposed procedure
- Reasonably available alternatives and their risks
- Expected outcome without the procedure.

Informed consent should be in the language that patient/relatives can understand and it should not contain any medical or technical language which an ordinary person cannot understand. It should be signed by doctor, patient/guardian, and witnesses. Remember blanket consent is not considered as consent legally.

There are some legally recognized exceptions to the doctrine of informed consent in the context of emergency care.
- Medical emergency where patient cannot give consent, nobody is there with patient and delay in treatment can lead to death of the patient, then the life-saving procedures can be done even without the consent (Section 92 IPC)[9]
- *Section 92 IPC*: The well-being of the patient is of paramount and medical rather than legal considerations come first. No delay in medical intervention is expectable for want of consent.

In the case of Barnett versus Bacharach, the court held that in a medical emergency, in which patient lies unconscious on the operating table, the surgeon may lawfully carry out the duties of a physician in the best interest of the patient, even if these duties entail the performance of a procedure that was not originally contemplated. In Barnett versus Bacharach, a patient who complained of abdominal pains was diagnosed with ectopic pregnancy. The patient was consented only for the removal of ectopic pregnancy. On incision, the surgeon found that the patient did not have ectopic pregnancy but had acute appendicitis. The surgeon in the best interest of the patient, appendectomy was performed. The patient recovered well, but refused to pay the hospital bills, saying she had not given consent for the removal of appendix. The trial court found that the surgeon acted properly because of the seriousness of the patient's condition.[10]

It is essential to note that for the unconscious patient exception to apply, the relevant emergency situation must require immediate medical attention with insufficient time to fully inform the patient or seek consent from another authorized person.

In the case of Tabor versus Scobee, the court found that, a violation of informed consent had occurred. During the surgery of appendectomy, the surgeon found infected fallopian tubes and decided to remove the tubes at that point in the best interest of patient. The court held that removal of tubes in this case did not fall within the exception to informed consent in an emergency situation.[11]

Note that, conscious refusal of the patient in case of emergency will not come under the exceptions to doctrine of informed consent. Physician must respect the refusal of treatment by the patient even during medical emergency.

Physicians are generally not held liable for treating a minor without a parental consent, when an emergency exists. As immediate injury or death could result from the delay, associated with attempting to obtain parental consent. In case of Jackovach versus Yocom, court held that when a minor patient's condition is life-threatening and requiring immediate medical attention, does not require parental informed consent. But in the case of Rogers versus Sells, court held that when a minor patient's condition is life threatening, yet not requiring immediate medical attention, the emergency exception does not apply. Therefore, parental concern or consent from another legally authorized individual must be obtained.[12]

Younts versus St Francis Hospital is an example of the mature minor exception. In this case, court held that if the minor patient has the ability to understand and comprehend the nature of the proposed treatment as well as associates the risks and potential results in view of surrounding circumstances then law allows the minor to give informed consent.

Emergency blood transfusion in a minor patient: If a minor is in need of life-saving blood transfusion and parents of the minor are refusing because of religious beliefs, the majority of courts may order to transfuse the blood to preserve the life of the child.

MEDICOLEGAL ISSUES RELATED TO NEGLIGENCE OF JUNIOR DOCTORS/POSTGRADUATE STUDENTS

Case scenario: A 10-year-old boy was admitted with severe shock, no IV access for fluids. Since the consultant was out of station, he asked the postgraduate to put central line in the neck. The postgraduate put the line and went for food. After 3 hours when he came back, the child was found to be gasping. Immediately it went into cardiac arrest and died. Whether the consultant is vicariously liable?

Explanation: Improper delegation of responsibility would itself qualify as negligence. Doctors have a duty to satisfy themselves that the persons to whom the work is delegated are qualified and have the appropriate experience to discharge the delegate task.

In "Spring Meadow hospital versus Harjot Ahluwalia", it was held that a consultant could be vicariously liable where he delegates the responsibility to his juniors with knowledge that the junior was incapable of performing his duties properly. Similarly, hospital is liable for the negligence of its staff.[13] In the case of "Cassidy versus Ministry of health", it is stated that the hospital authorities are responsible for the negligence of their staff including nurses, physicians, surgeons, anesthetists, etc. It does not matter whether they are permanent or temporary, full time or part time. Similar observations were made in the case of KK Radha versus GU Shekhar.[14]

In the above case, the consultant is vicariously liable.

MEDICOLEGAL ISSUES RELATED TO TRANSPORT OF EMERGENCY PATIENTS

Most of the doctors will be worried about the transport of accident and critically ill patients to higher centers because of fear of legal process. But in the strict sense, the law requires the victims to be transported even by the nonmedical public and if not, it amounts to negligence. The transport could be accomplished with medicos as even with paramedical people.[15] Even if the patient dies during the transport, the law just requires the matter to be informed to the police personnel, if the death is under suspicious circumstances or if it is an MLC. Naturally as a responsible law abiding citizen, we have to oblige the summons from the court as and when necessary.

MEDICOLEGAL ISSUES RELATED TO TELEPHONIC ADVICE GIVEN BY A CONSULTANT TO A RESIDENT DOCTOR IN ICU, CAUSING HARM TO THE PATIENT: CAN IT AMOUNT TO NEGLIGENCE?

Explanation: It is better to avoid giving medical advices on phone. In case you know about the patient, you may give some instructions and advice on phone to the resident doctors. But ask the resident doctor to write down the instructions and to read it out what he has written, to confirm. Otherwise, any harm caused by telephonic advice amounts to negligence.[5] Best way is to follow Telemedicine Practice Guidelines issued by National Medical Commission.

MEDICOLEGAL ISSUES RELATED TO ISSUING DEATH CERTIFICATE IN "BROUGHT DEAD" CASES

Explanation: This is not an uncommon scenario in emergency rooms. Patient will be brought dead and the attenders will be forcing the doctor to give death certificate. Routinely death certificate is issued by Registered Medical Practitioner who has attended the last stages of life of the patient. So if the patient is brought dead to the hospital or dies unattended, the death certificate cannot be issued. In this situation, it is given after postmortem.[16]

Case of unnatural (MLC) deaths, on table anesthetic and operative deaths, should always be reported to the police for conducting inquest and postmortem. No consent is required for medicolegal PM as it is done as per the requirements of law.

MEDICOLEGAL ISSUES RELATED TO LEAVING AGAINST MEDICAL ADVICE

Explanation: All patients/patient attenders have right to refuse further medical care. They can leave against medical advice to the extent that it does not contravene any law. They have a right to obtain details of investigations and treatment undergone. But the doctor, before sending the patient LAMA, should talk to the patient/patient attenders, regarding the patient conditions and treatment given. Document the discussion in the case sheet properly and take the consent signature of patient/patient attenders.[5]

MEDICOLEGAL ISSUES RELATED TO POST DEATH DIAGNOSTIC PROCEDURE

Case scenario: A 6-month-old child was admitted in PICU with a history of jaundice and hepatosplenomegaly noticed since 1 month of age. Probable diagnosis was storage disorder. The child died after 2 days of admission. Post death, the doctor did liver biopsy without the consent of parents. Is the doctor right?

Explanation: No—Even after death of the patient, if you want to do any procedure, you have to take the consent of parents/relatives. You have to explain them how does this postdeath diagnostic test helps them. The senior doctors often encourage their junior colleagues to "practice procedure" in dead or on dying patients like endotracheal intubation. But before doing such procedures, the sensitivities of the family should be taken into consideration.[4]

MEDICOLEGAL ISSUES RELATED TO "NOT PAYING HOSPITAL BILLS": CAN THE HOSPITAL KEEP THE DEAD BODY TILL THE CLEARANCE OF PAYMENT?

Explanation: Keeping a dead body is not an offence under any sections of IPC. But in some states like Karnataka under KPME Act 2017, it is an offence. So the doctor should not do this. Hand over the body immediately to the relatives and file a civil suit in the court against the relatives who had admitted the patient after signing informed written consent.[15]

MEDICOLEGAL ISSUES RELATED TO A MOB ATTACKING THE HOSPITAL AND DAMAGING THE PROPERTY

Explanation: This is a very common scenario nowadays. If there is any death of a close relative/friend, due to a serious medical problem, some people come in group and attack the doctors, equipment of the hospital and cause heavy damage. To prevent such violence against doctors and hospitals, some of the states like Karnataka, Maharashtra, Tamil Nadu, etc. are having laws, Karnataka Prohibition of Violence against Medicare Personnel and Damage to Medicare Service Institutions Act 2009. According to this Act, any violence against doctor and hospital is a nonbailable cognizable offence and punishment includes imprisonment of up to 3 years with fine. The fine is estimated based on damage, usually double charge of damaged things.[17] This law has really helped the doctors and the states where still this law has not been implemented, it is the responsibility of doctors of that state to put pressure on that government to bring this law. Whenever there is mob attack on the hospital first thing you should do is inform the police and all hospitals should have CCTVs at different places of hospitals so that you will be saving evidences.

MEDICOLEGAL ISSUES RELATED TO WITHHOLDING OR WITHDRAWAL OF LIFE SUPPORT

Case scenario: A 17-year-old patient was admitted in ICU for the treatment of pneumonia and meningitis. Patient was on ventilation for 14 days but there was no improvement. Later his relatives wanted to take him home and requested the doctor to withdraw the life support measures as it was not helping the patient. Legally can the doctor withdraw the life support or does it amount to euthanasia?

Explanation: Legally there is no difference between withholding or withdrawal of life support. Both have same intention to stop futile interventions. Withholding treatment means not starting treatment, withdrawal of treatment means stopping the treatment.

In a recent SC case, Aruna Ramachandran Shanbag versus Union of India, SC has legalized withdrawal of life support measures in patients with persistent vegetative state.[18] It is acceptable for terminally ill cases where further intervention, treatment is futile. But before withdrawing the life support measures, you should discuss with patient relatives, document the whole discussion in the case sheet and take signature on written informed consent form. Rarely in some cases for withdrawal of the life support measures, we need to take permission from high court. Remember that doctor alone cannot take unilateral decision in withdrawal of the life support measures. It amounts to "helping to commit suicide" (IPC sections 306 and 309).

Doctors are expected to give life, not to take it away. Law does not give this power to doctor to act independently. Only after patient relatives consent, you should withdraw the life support. In spite of this, some patient relatives approach the court claiming negligence. Then the IPC sections 76, 81, and 88 protect the doctors (nothing is offence which is done in good faith without criminal intention).

Withdrawal of the life support measures or withholding of the life support measures in terminally ill patients does not amount to euthanasia. Because in euthanasia, the intention is to cause death by some means but in withdrawing or withholding of the life support allows the disease to take its natural course, it may result in death later.

Still, there are no clear guidelines regarding withdrawing or withholding of the life support in terminally ill patients. Hence, it is better to adopt ISCCM (Indian Society of Critical Care Medicine) guidelines.

When you find that further treatment is going to be futile explain the prognosis to patient relatives, if the relatives are ready for the withdrawal of therapy, then record the discussion in the case sheet, take consent signature of the relatives and follow the ISCCM guidelines, i.e.:

- DNR (do not resuscitate)
- De-escalation of therapy
- Do not start any new medication.

With these measures, patient will die in few hours and you can declare the death. Here, the legal problems of withdrawing or withholding of the life support will not arise.

Do not Attempt Resuscitation ICMR Consensus Guidelines

These guidelines help treating physician on their decision concerning do not attempt resuscitation (DNAR). These guidelines preserve dignity in death and avoid prolonged suffering through nonbeneficial CPR (cardiopulmonary resuscitation). Treating physician should initiate discussion with the parent of critically sick child or patient/surrogate and explain in detail about the patients disease, prognosis and benefits, harms of CPR in case patient develops cardiac or respiratory arrest. All discussion must be noted in patient's case records and DNAR form. Good communication and documentation are very crucial. DNAR is distinct from withdrawal or withholding of other life supporting treatment. It guides to continue other curative and supportive care.

Preventive Measures Against Complaint of Medical Negligence in Critical Care

Lord Denning: The doctor's professional reputation is as dear to him as his body, perhaps more so and an action for negligence could wound his reputation as severely as a dagger could injure his body.

A doctor should always keep in mind, the following "3D" principles during practice to avoid a complaint of medical negligence.

- *Duty:* The doctor should do his duty sincerely. Always attend to an emergency and to your patient regularly. Manage the case properly as per the treatment given in standard textbooks. Law is just expecting reasonable care and skills as per your qualification. There may be errors in the diagnosis but it should not be gross. It is the duty of a medical practitioner to keep his professional knowledge up to date as medical science changes day by day.
- *Dialog:* Communication with patient/patient's family is an important part of medical management. Most of the

legal problems arise when there is a communication gap between patient and the doctor. Communication with the patient should be regular and in the language the patient understands. Always communicate the diagnosis, details of treatment, surgery required, likely complications, prognosis, and probable expenditure.

- *Documentation:* A good medical record is the physician's best defense. The case sheet is the important medical record for the treatment of patient in the emergency department as well as in the court of law. The case sheet should have name, father's name, address, and hospital number on each page. All entries should be dated and timed. The physician's notes should not be at variance with that of the nurse. All major events during the patient's stay should be recorded with date and time. A complete well-documented record that convincingly gives the diagnosis and records actions which are appropriate for the diagnosis and the clinical conditions of the patients suggests to the lawyer not to proceed any further. No attempts should be made to change in the record at a later stage.

SUMMARY

To effectively address medicolegal issues in pediatric critical care, healthcare providers should cultivate a comprehensive understanding of ethical and legal principles, establish clear guidelines for navigating ethical dilemmas, promote open communication and collaboration among healthcare professionals and families, seek guidance from legal counsel and ethics experts when faced with complex situations, and continuously evaluate and refine practices to align with evolving ethical and legal standards.

LEARNING KEY POINTS

- *Comprehensive understanding:* Healthcare providers in pediatric critical care must acquire a thorough comprehension of both ethical and legal principles relevant to their field.
- *Guidelines establishment:* It is essential to establish clear and well-defined guidelines for effectively navigating ethical dilemmas that may arise in the course of pediatric critical care.
- *Open communication:* Promoting open and transparent communication among healthcare professionals and involving families in the decision-making process is crucial for ethical and legal practice.
- *Collaboration:* Collaborative decision-making involving multidisciplinary healthcare teams can lead to better ethical outcomes and legal compliance in pediatric critical care.

TAKE-HOME MESSAGES

To always prioritize the best interests and well-being of the child when making medical decisions, and ensure thorough documentation of these decisions.

MUST AVOID THINGS

Do not appoint unqualified and unregistered subordinates.

DO NOT DO

Do not hesitate to take second opinion from qualified specialist when available.

WARNINGS

Restrict to your specialization.

MESSAGES WHICH THE READER MUST BE AWARE

Written informed consent from parents/guardian is a must before each invasive procedure.

MUST DO THINGS

Medical documentation. It is only available defense for doctors in medical negligence.

MEDICAL NEGLIGENCE PEARLS

Always follow standard treatment protocols from standard textbooks and standard guidelines.

ONLY ONE FACT TO REMEMBER

Do not refuse medical emergency cases, accidents, and injury cases.

REFERENCES

1. Singh AK, Singh K. Study of Medico-legal case management in tertiary care hospital. J Ind Acad Forensic Med. 2011;33(4):337-41.
2. Black HC. (1990). Black's Law Dictionary, 6th edition. [online] Available from: https://karnatakajudiciary.kar.nic.in/hcklibrary/PDF/Blacks%20Law%206th%20Edition%20-%20SecA.pdf. [Last accessed December, 2023].
3. Paramand Katara V union of India, 1989 ACJ1000 (SC).
4. Chugh K. Ethical and Legal Issues in Emergency Care. Textbook on Principles Paediatrics and Neonatal Emergencies, 3rd edition. New Delhi: Jaypee Brothers Medical Publisher; 2011.
5. Singh J. Text book on Medical Negligence and Compensation, 4th edition. Jaipur: Bharat Law Publications; 2014.
6. Paschim Bengal Khetmazdoorsamity and others V West Bengal. 1996 (4) Supreme 260: AIR 1996. SC 2426.
7. Sections 88 and 90 IPC 1860.
8. Kurt M. Exceptions to inform consent in emergency medicine, Hospital physician, 1999.
9. Section 92 IPC 1860.
10. Barnett V Bacharach. 34 A: 2d 626 (1943).
11. Tabor V Scobee 254 S.W. 2d 474 (1951).
12. Roger V Sells 178 okla 103 (1936).
13. Spring Meadow Hospital V Harjot Ahluwalia CPRI (SC) 1998: 1998 (I) CPJI.
14. KK Radha V Dr. GU Sekher 1994 (3) CPJ 376 (Kerala SCDRC).
15. Meenakshi S. Medico-legal aspects of critical care medicine. Ind J of Anae. 2007;51:344-46.
16. Singhal SK. The doctor and law, 1st edition. New Delhi: The National Books; 1999.
17. Karnataka prohibition of violence against medicare personnel and damage to medicare service institutions act 2009.
18. Aruna R Shanbagh V union of India.

SUGGESTED READING

1. Baldwa M, Baldwa V, Padvi N, Baldwa S. Legal Issues in Critical Care. New Delhi: CBS Publishers & Distributors Pvt Ltd; 2022.
2. Baldwa M, Baldwa V, Padvi N, Baldwa S. Legal Issues in Medical Practice, 2nd edition. New Delhi: CBS Publishers & Distributors Pvt Ltd; 2023.

CHAPTER 18

Medicolegal Aspects of Vaccinations

Jyoti Kumar Gupta, Vivek Saxena, Raj Tilak, Sanjay Niranjan

You can have the best vaccines for children, but if you cannot reach them then they will not work.

Keywords: Adverse event following immunization (AEFI), Consumer Protection Act (CPA), Indian Penal Code (IPC), Vaccine-associated paralytic poliomyelitis (VAPP), Vaccine Injury Compensation Program (VICP)

Aim: To protect doctors from medicolegal issues in vaccination like catastrophic anaphylaxis to mild and major reactions while giving vaccines.

Objective: Doctor is ready to help for immunizing. No vaccine is 100% safe or 100% effective. Thus leaving place for litigation. Immunization helps protect future generations by eradicating diseases. Many infectious diseases are rare or eradicated now as a result of immunization programs, but new infectious diseases are appearing around the world. The National Immunization Program is one of the biggest public health programs in India.

■ INTRODUCTION

Vaccines are one of the most successful health interventions that bring about significant reductions in infectious diseases and adverse health consequences and improve quality of life. Vaccines have provided cost-effective improvements to human health by reducing avoidable human suffering, costs of care and treatment, and loss of work. More and more diseases are becoming vaccine preventable and with the advent of coronavirus disease (COVID) era awareness about vaccinations have reached to new dimensions. Since vaccines are administered to healthy people, especially children, it is pivotal to ascertain they are safe and cost-effective. Although most of the time vaccination is safe but at times adverse reaction and vaccination error do occur which poses medicolegal issues to the vaccinator.

■ NEED OF IMMUNIZATION

There has been a "cleavage of opinion" and different schools of thoughts regarding need of immunization. Many of us also believe that the population in developing nations is being used as "guinea pigs" for these "under trial vaccines". But COVID vaccination has changed the global perception and at present time even a common man is aware about the need and importance of vaccination. But since there is long list of vaccines to be given to our children, a sense of complacency still prevails in society. Issue arises whether all the vaccines those are available in market shall be administered to each and every child or there shall be selection bias.[1] Aim of the immunization is to protect the children against various communicable diseases and every child has right to be protected from vaccine preventable disease. So it is duty of doctor to inform parent about the vaccines recommended by National Immunization Schedule and Indian Academy of Pediatric Schedule and should pass the relevant information about vaccines available which would help parents in taking decision whether to immunize child or not depending upon their own understanding, willingness, and affordability. Decision of not immunizing child with particular vaccine despite of getting knowledge from doctor has to be honored.

MANDATORY VERSUS OPTIONAL VACCINATION

Few years ago there were two categories of vaccines—compulsory and optional. But now all vaccines are mandatory and should be administered to all children. There is a separate category of vaccines which may be given in special situation after discussion with parents.[2] So as of now there is no optional vaccine category. Actually every child has right to be immunized against vaccine preventable diseases. Parents who are unable to afford private vaccine should be counseled for vaccination from government center. Doctor should vaccinate himself and should motivate hospital or clinic staff for getting themselves vaccinated as they may get infection from some vaccine preventable disease such as hepatitis B and rabies. Pediatrician show advice vaccination in discharge card of neonate and should administer it in initial clinic visits. Adolescent patients should be motivated for catch up vaccinations. Patients with asthma, recurrent respiratory infections, and immunocompromised states should be counseled for pneumococcal and influenza vaccination.

DUTIES DURING VACCINATION

- Taking general history and complete routine examination of babies.
- Taking history of allergies and any previous adverse event during vaccination.
- As vaccination is a traditionally a part of Well Baby Clinic, so developmental and growth assessment, high-risk newborn screening referral, and explanation of prognosis and risk of neurodevelopmental sequelae should also be done.
- For performing earlier mentioned duties and documenting it, routine outpatient department (OPD) prescription should be made and prescription fee should be charged as a proof of performing these duties.
- If attendants not brought Old Treatment Record and Vaccination Record, better to defer vaccination or document the fact of not carrying these records.
- Preparedness for dealing any adverse event following immunization (AEFI) and vaccination errors.
- Informed consent about vaccination.
- Visible as well as oral instruction to stay for half an hour after vaccination.
- Reporting of AEFI within 24 hours.

HISTORY TAKING

The past history of any adverse reactions to any vaccine is very important, as it may decide whether to inject a particular vaccine or not. History of any severe reaction to vaccine or floppiness must be taken and vaccination must not be done in such cases. History of egg allergy may give warning signal at times to some vaccination like influenza. Proper history of any previous complications must be recorded in writing, e.g., before giving triple vaccine take history of any neurological complications, existing neurological deficits, and excessive irritability with previous dose. A visible notice should be displayed in consultation chamber and visiting area to inform about any previous reaction to any vaccine before going for vaccination. In *Tapan Kumar Nayak versus State of Orissa II (1997) CPJ 14 NC,* a child developed severe reaction and brain damage after a triple vaccine. No other child suffered such complications. The National Commission while confirming the order passed by the Orissa State Commission, that there was no scope for awarding relief to the complainant under Consumer Protection Act, strongly recommended to the State Government to render all possible assistance in proper rehabilitation of the child.

History of immunocompromised disorder, history of taking any drug causing immunocompromised state, history of blood transfusion in near past should also be taken, and documented and immunization to be deferred accordingly. History of febrile seizure and breath holding spell should also be taken prior to vaccination to avoid such events following vaccinations.

CONSENT

In the present era of internet with ease of information, it is important that basic information related to immunization should be given to the parents or guardians. Judiciary and various courts are also of the opinion that health is the fundamental right of an individual including the right of refusal for trial or treatment. Hence, an informed consent may be considered as one of the prerequisites before vaccinating any child. An informed consent in relation to immunization may include information regarding need of the vaccine, its cost, what are the consequences of not taking a particular vaccine, and also the known adverse effects (a model consent form is attached in the form of appendix). It is also important to inform that in some cases disease can result even after successful vaccination. The Centre for Disease Control and Prevention (CDC) requires that even the vaccination information statements (VIS) be given to parents in advance.[3] In United States of America, parental consent for immunization is standard practice in 43 states. At present there is no such law in India, but remember that most of us including judiciary/government are following Western countries.

Medicolegal issues following vaccination may arise at the time of vaccination for adverse reaction also. Consent becomes relevant at the time of AEFI as issues of nonpassage of information about vaccines may arise. Similar issues may arise at the time of ineffectiveness also. One time consent should be taken for passing general information and overall risk of vaccination and it may be printed on vaccination card itself alongside of vaccination chart and consent may be obtained there from the parents. Although consent for vaccination deemed to be implied as patient has vaccinated himself after knowing all about vaccine. Still detailed inform consent is the need of hour. Documentation of routine each time consent may be done on OPD prescription in following way *"Given_____Vaccine today I/M or S/C or I/D at _____(Vaccination Site) after getting informed consent with aseptic precautions".*

DOCUMENTATION

Not only informed consent should be taken but also it should be documented on

Vaccination Card and Prescription paper. Unwillingness to opt recommended vaccine should also be documented. Documentation of vaccination should be done at proper column of vaccination Chart and next vaccination date should also be mentioned. Placing labels of vaccination over vaccination card or mentioning batch number of vaccine is a good practice. Apart from documentation over vaccination card, vaccination should also be documented over the prescription paper. The documentation is also important because the parents or individual may need a certificate at the time of travel or school admissions in the future life.

If attendants are not carrying Vaccination Record, then it is better to defer vaccination or document the fact of not carrying these records. Vaccination should not be done in absence of vaccination card solely on memory of attendant due to chances of unwarranted repeat vaccination. If new vaccination card need to be prepared for compiling multiple ones or issuing on attendant's memory basis, then date of reissuing should be documented on vaccination card. Entry in vaccination card should be made at appropriate column and in legible writing. False certificate of vaccination should never be issued. As vaccination is a traditionally a part of Well Baby Clinic so developmental and growth assessment, anthropometry, high-risk screening, and referrals should be done and documented on prescription paper.

RECORD KEEPING

The vaccine administrator must record the type of vaccine, brand name, and date of administration of the vaccine in the patient's file/immunization record. In addition, recording of the batch number of the vaccine is also recommended. Record keeping is very important as guidelines issued for reporting of AEFI are also applicable to the private practitioners. Traditionally vaccination is an OPD practice and physicians are not obliged to maintain OPD record as per Medical Council of India (MCI) Regulation 1.3.2 as of now still vaccination record may be cross checked with OPD or Indoor Case register. So these registers and infantry are to be maintained till 6 year as per section 44AA and Rule 6F of Income Tax Act 1961.

ADVERSE EVENTS FOLLOWING IMMUNIZATION

The only safe vaccine is one that is never used.
Dr James R. Shannon (Former Director, National Institute of Health).[4]

Vaccines are among the safest medicines to use and these are considered very effective tool for preventing infectious diseases. Like any other drug, no vaccine is 100% effective or 100% safe. As with other drugs, adverse events can occur with vaccines too. In addition to the vaccines themselves, the process of administration of vaccines is a potential source of an AEFI.

An AEFI is any untoward medical occurrence which follows immunization and which does not necessarily have a causal relationship with the usage of the vaccine, i.e., might have not been caused by vaccine ingredients or the process of vaccination or immunization but have a temporal relationship with administration of vaccine. It can be any unfavorable or unintended sign, abnormal laboratory finding, symptom, or disease. Sometimes, mass use of vaccines can cause anxiety in community and even such responses can be considered as AEFI. AEFI surveillance system is usually a passive system to enable spontaneous reporting of all adverse events. It is a part of the National

Regulatory Authority (NRA) for vaccines. The primary purpose of spontaneous AEFI reporting is to monitor the known adverse events associated with vaccine use, and to identify the new adverse events, i.e., safety signals after a product is marketed.

CAUSE-SPECIFIC TYPES OF ADVERSE EVENT FOLLOWING IMMUNIZATION

Vaccine Product-related Reaction

An AEFI that is caused or precipitated by a vaccine due to one or more of the inherent properties of the vaccine product (or ingredients), e.g., extensive limb swelling following diphtheria, tetanus, and pertussis (DTP) vaccination. In this scenario, vaccine might have been used correctly without compromising with manufacturing process, transport, or storage. Thus, absolutely correct use of vaccine may also cause this type of AEFI.

Vaccine Quality Defect-related Reaction

An AEFI that is caused or precipitated by a vaccine is due to one or more quality defects of the vaccine product including its administration device as provided by the manufacturer, e.g., failure by the manufacturer to completely inactivate a lot of inactivated polio vaccine (IPV) leads to cases of paralytic polio.

Immunization Error-related Reaction

An AEFI that is caused by inappropriate vaccine handling, prescribing, or administration and thus by its nature is preventable, e.g., transmission of infection by contaminated multidose vial.

Immunization Anxiety-related Reaction

An AEFI arising from anxiety about the immunization, e.g., vasovagal syncope in an adolescent following vaccination. The anxiety may spread to community too, at times.

Coincidental Event

An AEFI that is caused by something other than the vaccine product, immunization error, or immunization anxiety, e.g., fever after vaccination (temporal association) and malarial parasite isolated from blood.

EMERGENCY MANAGEMENT OF ANAPHYLACTIC REACTIONS

If symptoms are generalized, activate the emergency medical system. Assessment of airway, breathing, circulation, and level of consciousness of the patient should be made. Vital signs should be monitored continuously. The first-line and most important therapy in anaphylaxis is epinephrine. There are no absolute contraindications to epinephrine in the setting of anaphylaxis. Recommended dose is 0.01 mg/kg body weight up to 0.5 mg maximum dose. It may be repeated every 5–15 minutes up to three times while waiting for emergency medical services (EMS) to arrive. Antihistamines may be given for relief of itching or hives. The patient should be monitored closely and should be shifted to hospital as soon as possible. Cardiopulmonary resuscitation (CPR) may be needed to perform if necessary, and airway should be maintained and oxygen should be given if available. Patient's reaction (e.g., hives and anaphylaxis) to the vaccine, all vital signs, and medications administered to the patient, including the time, dosage, response, and the name of the medical personnel who administered the medication should be documented. Incident should be reported to authorities within 24 hours or a soon as possible.

PREPAREDNESS TO DEAL WITH AEFI

The various side effects shall be informed before vaccinating the child. It is advisable to inform common as well as remote adverse reactions. Various adverse reactions must be diagnosed and treated within proper and adequate time to avoid allegations of deficiency or negligence. Oxygen, adrenaline, intravenous (IV) fluids, and steroids shall be available in case reaction occurs. Various facilities needed to tackle or manage such adverse reactions shall be available in the hospital in case need arises. Visible instructions should be placed in form of notice in consultation chamber and in waiting area for passing information to doctor or vaccinator about any previous reaction to any vaccine in past and patient to stay for half an hour for observation after vaccination.

COMMON VACCINATION ERRORS

- Not using a screening checklist to identify patient's contraindications and precautions to vaccination
- Administering the wrong vaccine due to similarities in vaccine names and packing
- Using the wrong diluent or administering the diluent only
- Administering a vaccine after the expiration date
- Administering vaccine in the wrong site or by the wrong route
- Giving a vaccine dose earlier than the recommended age or interval
- Giving two doses of live injectable or nasally administered vaccines too close together (leading to potential interference between these vaccines)
- Giving the wrong dosage amount for the patient's age.

DUTY IN PREVENTING AND MANAGING VACCINATION ERRORS: SOME PRACTICAL TIPS[5]

Vaccination in Contraindicated Patients

To avoid this history of previous vaccination reaction, immunocompromised disorder, drug causing immune compromised state, history of recent blood transfusion, and history of previous infection for which vaccine is intended should be noted and for this questionnaire may be used.

Administering the Wrong Vaccine due to Similarities in Vaccine Names

To avoid this vaccine vial label should be checked three times! Store such vaccines separately and mark them clearly on the patient's vaccine tray. Prepare vaccines needed for one family member at a time, and always verify names and birth dates for the patient receiving the vaccines. The parent/patient should be told the wrong vaccine was given. Provide the correct vaccine, if necessary, with correct spacing.

Using the Wrong Diluents or Administering the Diluents Only

To avoid this use careful labeling. Keep vaccines and their diluents together if storage requirements are the same. If the wrong diluents is used, the vaccine needs to be repeated [except in the case of mixing up the diluents between measles, mumps, and rubella (MMR), measles, mumps, rubella, and varicella (MMRV), varicella, and zoster vaccines use the same sterile water diluents]. If an inactivated vaccine is reconstituted with the wrong diluents and is administered, the dose is invalid and should be repeated ASAP. If a live vaccine is reconstituted with the wrong diluents and is administered, the dose is invalid and if it cannot be repeated on the same clinic day, it needs to be repeated no earlier than 4 weeks after the invalid dose.

Administering a Vaccine after the Expiration Date

If a dose of expired vaccine is inadvertently given, it should be repeated. If the expired dose is a live virus vaccine, you must wait at least 4 weeks after the expired dose was given before repeating it. The repeat dose of an expired inactivated vaccine can be given on the same day or any other time.

Administering Vaccine in Wrong Site or by Wrong Route

The deltoid muscle and anterolateral thigh are preferred site for vaccination. If a vaccine is given by the wrong route (subcutaneously instead of intramuscular, or intramuscular instead of subcutaneously), it does not need to be repeated with four exceptions: hepatitis B, rabies, human papillomavirus (HPV), and inactivated influenza vaccine.

Giving a Vaccine Dose Earlier than the Recommended Age or Interval

A dose administered 5 or more days earlier than the recommended *minimum interval* between doses is not valid and should be repeated.

WHAT AMOUNT TO NEGLIGENCE?

Medical negligence in vaccination can be alleged if there is deficiency or damage because an act of commission or omission associated with the process of immunization. Vaccination errors as enumerated earlier and AEFI and side effects may be alleged as negligence. Vaccination errors can be avoided by measures suggested earlier and by taking all the precautions in vaccination. Corrective measures should be adopted in case of vaccination error and if such error does not cause any damage allegation of negligence may not have leg to stand. AEFI prevention is usually beyond the scope of clinician but proper management of emergency and timely referral and reporting can save doctors from allegation of negligence. Vaccination done by clinic or hospital staff or in vaccination camp may attract vicarious responsibility on part of consultant in charge.

RESPONSIBILITY FOR INADEQUATE PROTECTION

It is established fact that no vaccine can be 100% efficacious. Doctor has to choose the vaccine as per scientific studies passed to him and printed on packing insert of vaccines, the WHO prequalification and endorsement from government authorities and academic associations. Efficacy data and side effect profile are available to both doctor and patient party. So if clinician has properly maintained cold chain and has passed documented information about efficacy of vaccines available in packing insert or available online or in other printed material to patient or parents and inform consent has been received in consequence, there should be no issue of inadequate protection. If a serological correlates of protection are not known for a vaccine, one should avoid recommending vaccines till authentic seroprotection data and recommendation is available.

MEDICOLEGAL ISSUES IN VACCINATION ERRORS OR ADVERSE REACTION

If vaccination error or adverse reaction following immunization has occurred and corrective measures have been taken and no damage have occurred then there should be no criminal liability as per defense available in Section 95 of Indian Penal Code which says that act causing slight harm can be used as defense against criminal prosecution. But definition of harm is broad in Section 2(22) in Consumer Protection Act 2019 and "harm" includes mental agony or emotional distress attendant to personal injury or illness or damage to property and may attract litigation. But if duty to manage vaccination error and AEFI has been performed with due diligence and seniority there is very little scope of award, for this duty performed in pursuance must be documented.

INADVERTENTLY ADMINISTRATION OF EXPIRED VACCINE

If any expired vaccine has been administered inadvertently, then vaccine dose should not be counted as valid and vaccine has to be repeated as per CDC guidelines.[6] Certain ingredients can stop working after expiry, which could render a vaccine less effective. There are not many documented cases that using an expired vaccine could cause harmful reactions.[7] There is no existing data that taking an expired COVID-19 vaccine is dangerous.

IMPORTANT JUDGMENTS IN MEDICAL NEGLIGENCE DURING VACCINATION

Dr Durga Nursing Home versus K. Dhanasekharan before the State Consumer Disputes Redressal Commission, Chennai, F.A. Nos. 1070/2011 and 683/2012.

Petitioner approached the district consumer court, alleging negligence and the use of expired vaccines. District Forum concluded that the nursing home did not have an effective storage system and its ambulance facility was inadequate, and thus services were deficient. It awarded a compensation of INR 100,000 for mental agony and hardship and INR 5,000 toward costs. Both parties then appealed in the state consumer court. The court awarded compensation of INR 300,000 for mental agony + 5,000 toward costs.

State of Gujarat and Others versus Shahenazbanu Ashrafali on July 13, 1995 Gujarat High Court. 1997 ACJ 176, AIR 1996 Guj 136.

State of Gujarat appealed against a compensation of INR 100,000 awarded on the ground that the petitioner had suffered permanent deformity and disability following negligent administration of a DPT. After 15 years the High Court reversed the decree of the trial court and stayed the execution of the money decree. While dismissing the claim, it maintained that the claimant had been unable to establish a causal linkage or the fact that there had been negligence.

District court in New Delhi directed the Delhi government to pay INR 2 lakh as compensation to the parents of an infant who died after being administered with Pulse Polio drops in 1999.[8] Court held that:

"The constitutional obligation of the Government to improve public health is not confined to introducing programs and administering medicines but extends to protecting a child under such a program from all the consequential effects".

"In any program of immunization involving administration of drops, the possibility of side-effects cannot be ruled out and it is necessary for the government to gear up its machinery to meet such an eventuality".

Sama: Resource Group for Women and Health and others versus Union of India and others (Writ Petition (Civil) No. 921 of 2013)

In 2013, a civil writ petition was filed in the Supreme Court by Sama: Resource Group for Women and Health and Others against the Union of India and Others, demanding compensation for the deaths of seven girls during the "observational study" of HPV vaccines by the Program for Appropriate Technology in Health (PATH). The case is still pending in the Supreme Court and no decision had been taken on compensation.

Deaths due to vaccine-associated paralytic poliomyelitis (VAPP) and the triple vaccine DTP occur on a regular basis, but no remedial action has been undertaken by the government till date.[9-11]

NO FAULT INSURANCE FOR VACCINE INJURY

Since AEFI are accidental injuries in true sense, many countries are having No Fault Insurance for Vaccine injury. In United States of America such type of insurance has been in practice since a quite long time. US Congress passed National Childhood Vaccine Injury Act of 1986. The Act established the National Vaccine Injury Compensation Program (VICP) in 1988 to compensate victims. VICP, funded by a 75 cent tax on each vaccination given, is a "no fault" system designed to compensate the injured while protecting healthcare providers and vaccine manufacturers from lawsuits.[12] Claims must be made to the VICP within 3 years of the onset of symptoms for an injury victim. Awards for a vaccine-related death are limited to $250,000, plus attorney's fees and costs. The Vaccine Damage Payments Act 1979 (the "VDP Act") in the United Kingdom established a national fund administered through the Department for Works and Pensions to compensate people injured by vaccines. To qualify for a vaccine damages payment, a person must have been injured by a vaccine for a disease on the statutory list; the vaccination must have been received in the United Kingdom before the age of 18 years; and the injury must have resulted in that person becoming 60% disabled.[13] Similarly 19 other countries are providing such compensation on vaccination injuries.[14] Swedish government started an insurance program for patients in 1975 which was followed by pharmaceutical insurance, launched by pharmaceutical companies in 1978. Finland, Norway, and Sweden use the manufacturers' levy to finance compensation. Taiwan (China) like USA has centralized government program funded from a vaccine tax. New Zealand and Japan have scheme financed from several sources.

NEED OF COMPENSATION POLICY FOR VACCINE RELATED INJURIES AND DEATH IN INDIA

India necessitates the recognition of an injury following vaccination and the formulation of an appropriate compensation policy. In the absence of such a policy, the affected parties will be left with no option other than to approach the legal system under tort law which would not be justice to affected party as well as vaccinator and will shake the confidence in vaccination process and it would not be good for national health. No-fault insurance policy may be formulated for vaccination separately on joint contribution from vaccine industry and government or may be designed separately to cover all sort of medical treatment accidents.

SUMMARY AND CONCLUSION

Vaccines are among the most cost-effective interventions in healthcare, and the public health benefits of vaccination are clear. Some years ago, the WHO estimated that >2.5 million deaths have been prevented through the use of vaccine immunization programs.[15] And a key to increased use of preventative care and early vaccination is increased trust in and understanding of vaccinations.[16] This trust in vaccination can only be maintained by avoiding vaccination errors, managing, and avoiding AEFI judicially with utmost sincerity. Deaths and adverse events following compulsory immunization must be adequately compensated on the basis of "no-fault". Till the time Vaccination Injury Compensation Program is not there, we have no option other than having handsome professional indemnity insurance and practice with maximum care and diligence.

LEARNING KEY POINTS

- Inform consent for vaccination may save from medicolegal issues in case of AEFI.
- Never vaccinate solely based on memory without documentary proof of previous vaccination.
- Always make prescription and do health checkup and developmental assessment at the time of vaccination. Charging the fee for prescription at the time of vaccination is indirect proof of examination done.
- Always purchase vaccine from authorized dealer with tax invoice.
- Display a notice in waiting area 'Give prior history of reaction to any vaccine or drug and stay for half hour after vaccination or injection'.

TAKE-HOME MESSAGES

- Vaccination errors are those avoidable errors which can put vaccinator in trouble and may create medicolegal issues. These errors must be avoided by showing diligence and utmost sincerity during vaccination.
- Corrective steps to vaccination error, truthfulness, and fair communication are tools to avoid litigation.
- AEFI are usually unavoidable events during vaccination. Preparedness to tackle AEFI is warranted from vaccinator and quick judicious management of AEFI along with communication and documentation may avoid medicolegal issues in AEFI.

MUST AVOID THINGS—DO NOT DO

- Never vaccinate solely based on memory without documentary proof of previous vaccination.
- Never vaccinate multiple patients at same time to avoid mixing of vaccination.
- Never issue false vaccination certificate.

MUST DO THINGS

- Always make entry of vaccination legibly in vaccination card in appropriate column.
- Always make prescription and do health checkup and developmental assessment at the time of vaccination. Charging the fee for prescription at the time of vaccination is indirect proof of examination done.
- Give vaccine on anterolateral aspect of thigh and deltoid muscle only.
- Always keep drugs like epinephrine handy while doing vaccination.

MESSAGES WHICH THE READER MUST BE AWARE

Vaccination is not just giving immunization but is traditionally a part of Well Baby Clinic, so examination of baby, growth assessment, neurodevelopmental assessment, high-risk newborn screening, physiotherapy referral, prognosis explanation, etc. should also be done.

WARNINGS

- Check expiry date of vaccine twice before immunization.
- Do vaccinate yourself.
- Keep injection adrenaline at vaccination place along with oxygen.

MEDICAL NEGLIGENCE PEARLS

AEFI prevention is usually beyond the scope of clinician but proper management of emergency and timely referral and reporting can save doctors from allegation of negligence.

ONLY ONE FACT TO REMEMBER

Taking history of allergies and any previous adverse event during vaccination is as vital as having injection adrenaline at vaccination center.

MCQs

Choose one correct answer
1. Which of the following is not true?
    a. Vaccine gives 100% protection
    b. Missed vaccines can be given
    c. Inform consent for vaccination should be taken
    d. A/L thigh or deltoid is ideal site for vaccination
2. Adverse effect following immunization should be reported to authorities within:
    a. 24 hours
    b. 1 week
    c. 5 days
    d. Need not to be reported
3. The first-line and most important therapy in anaphylaxis during vaccination is:
    a. Pain killer
    b. Steroid
    c. Antihistaminic
    d. Epinephrine

Answers

1. a   2. a   3. d

REFERENCES

1. Tiwari S. Medical ethics: are we going in right direction? Mathur GP, Mathur S (Eds). Current Trends in Pediatrics, 1st edition. New Delhi. Academic Publishers; 2006. pp. 67-71.
2. Indian Academy of Pediatrics. IAP Guidebook on Immunization 2018–2019, 3rd edition. New Delhi: Jaypee Brothers Medical Publishers (P) Ltd.; 2020.
3. Centers for Disease Control and Prevention. Vaccine Information Statements (VISs). [online] Available from: http://www.cdc.gov/vaccines/pubs/vis/default.htm. [Last accessed December, 2023].
4. Shannon JR. (2008). Vaccine Quotes Worth Repeating. [online] Available from: http://drrimatruthreports.com/resources/dr-laibows-codex-newsletter-archives-4/vaccine-quotes-worth-repeating/. [Last accessed December, 2023].
5. Immunization Action Coalition. Don't Be Guilty of These Preventable Errors in Vaccine Administration. [online] Available from: https://oeps.wv.gov/immunizations/documents/vfc/manual/7/vaccine_storage_errors.pdf. [Last accessed December, 2023].
6. Centers for Disease Control and Prevention. (2023). Storage and Handling of Immuno-biologics. [online] Available from: https://www.cdc.gov/vaccines/hcp/acip-recs/

general-recs/storage.html. [Last accessed December, 2023].
7. Sherman J. (2021). What happens if you get an expired vaccine. [online] Available from: https://health-desk.org/articles/what-happens-if-you-get-an-expired-vaccine. [Last accessed December, 2023].
8. Anand U. (2009). 10 yrs after side effects of polio drop kills infant, court orders govt to pay Rs 2 lakh to family. [online] Available from: https://indianexpress.com/article/cities/delhi/10-yrs-after-side-effects-of-polio-drop-kills-infant-court-orders-govt-to-pay-rs-2-lakh-to-family/. [Last accessed December, 2023].
9. Suryanarayan D. (2013). 2-month-old dies after vaccination in Mumbai. [online] Available from: http://www.dnaindia.com/mumbai/report_2-month-old-dies-after-vaccination-in-mumbai_1320922. [Last accessed December, 2023].
10. Rajadhyaksha M. (2009). New panel will study reaction to vaccines. [online] Available from: https://timesofindia.indiatimes.com/city/mumbai/new-panel-will-study-recation-to-vaccines/articleshow/4536828.cms. [Last accessed December, 2023].
11. Kanhema T. (2009). DTP "poisoning" blamed for infant deaths. [online] Available from: http://www.informante.web.na/index.php?option=com_content&task=view&id=3458&Itemid=100. [Last accessed December, 2023].
12. Health Resources & Services Administration (HRSA). (2023). National Vaccine Injury Compensation Program. [online] Available from: https://www.hrsa.gov/vaccine-compensation. [Last accessed December, 2023].
13. Vaccine Damage Payments Act 1979 (c.17), United Kingdom.
14. ResearchGate. Countries and provinces that have introduced vaccine injury compensation schemes. [online] Available from: https://www.researchgate.net/figure/Countries-and-provinces-that-have-introduced-vaccine-injury-compensation-schemes_fig1_51111456/download. [Last accessed December, 2023].
15. Kesselheim A. Safety, Supply, and Suits—Litigation and the Vaccine Industry. N Engl J Med. 2011;364:1485-7.
16. Quinn SC, Parmer J, Freimuth VS, Hilyard KM, Musa D, Kim KH. Exploring Communication, Trust in Government, and Vaccination Intention Later in the 2009 H1N1 Pandemic: Results of a National Survey. Biosecur Bioterror. 2013;11(2):96-106.

SUGGESTED READING

1. Baldwa M, Baldwa V, Padvi N, Baldwa S. Legal Issues in Critical Care, 1st edition. New Delhi: CBS Publishers and Distributors Pvt. Ltd.; 2022.
2. Baldwa M, Baldwa V, Padvi N, Baldwa S. Legal Issues in Medical Practice, 2nd edition. New Delhi: CBS Publishers and Distributors Pvt. Ltd.; 2023.

APPENDIX: CONSENT FOR VACCINATION

(These forms should be printed or filled in local vernacular language)

I/we have been informed about various vaccines available for the immunization for my/our child. We have also been explained about advantages and side effects or complications occurring after the vaccination. I/we have been explained that in rare cases there can be a risk of life also following vaccination.

We are informed in details about all mandatory and optional vaccines as per national immunization schedule and schedule recommended by Indian Academy of Pediatrics. We are willing to immunize our child as per our affordability and own understanding about the need of vaccination.

I/we have been informed that the most of the vaccines may not give 100% and there may be possibility of disease even after vaccination.

I/we have been explained all these in language known to me/us and we consenting for vaccination after satisfying all the queries/doubt.

Name of vaccine recipient: Age/sex:
Signature of parents/guardian: Relationship:
Date & Time: Place:

Medicolegal Aspects of Transferring the Acute Ill Patients, Transit Death, Inadvertent use of Expiry Drug

CHAPTER 19

Jyoti Kumar Gupta, Anurag Mehrotra, Satish Sharma, Ambrish Gupta

"The adversarial dynamics of medical lawsuits often left doctors emotionally wounded."

Keywords: Interhospital transfer (IHT), Off-label drug use (OLDU), Placebo drugs, Shelf Life Extension Program (SLEP), Stabilization

Aim: Healthcare providers must comply with all applicable laws and regulations related to patient transfer, including those governing informed consent, patient safety, and documentation. The inadvertent use of expired drugs raises potential legal concerns for healthcare providers due to the possibility of compromising patient safety and violating applicable regulations.

Objective: The medicolegal aspects of patient transfer should facilitate coordination of care between different healthcare providers, ensuring that patients receive the best possible care throughout their transfer. Train staff on proper medication administration protocols, including the importance of checking expiration dates and following established procedures.

TRANSFER OF THE PATIENT

Introduction

Transfer of patient may be primary or secondary. Primary transfers to hospital from a prehospital site of illness or injury are commonly the responsibility of attendants and the ambulance service. These systems may be supported or supplemented by doctors. Secondary transfers include both intrahospital and interhospital transport, and are inevitable for all critically ill patients in the emergency department. An interhospital transfer (IHT) is needed when the diagnostic and therapeutic facilities required for a patient are not available at the given hospital. IHT may take place from emergency department, ward, or intensive care unit (ICU) of one hospital to that of another. Regionalization of specialized care and increased requirement of superspecialty treatment have contributed to an increase in IHT. IHT may sometimes also be needed for nonclinical reasons such as nonavailability of bed or issues of funding of medical treatment. Thus, IHT of patients is now an integral process and essential component of healthcare system.

Objective of Transfer

Optimal health and well-being of the patient is the underlying goal of IHT. Therefore, the decision to transfer is patient centered and is undertaken when the benefits of transfer outweigh the risks.[1] Choice of the destination hospital should be based primarily on infrastructure, availability of specialized care, and proximity to the referring hospital, the aim being to seek transfer to a hospital nearby providing the highest quality care. Once the decision is made, the transfer process must be initiated and completed as soon as possible. Both the referring and receiving hospitals should thereafter focus on the continuity of medical care and not just on administrative procedures of discharge and readmission. IHT carries its own risk and a poorly and hastily conducted transfer increases morbidity and mortality risk for patients.[2] Therefore, a well-organized system with appropriate equipment and personnel is crucial for a safe IHT.

Key Elements of Safe Transfer

The Pediatric Intensive Care Society has also laid the guidelines for the transport of the critically ill children.[3] Majority of these guidelines have stressed pretransport coordination and communication, qualified and trained accompanying personnel, appropriate transport equipment, standard monitoring, and documentation as key elements of a safe transfer. These are briefly described here.

Pretransport Coordination and Communication

Patients or their guardians should be involved in the decision for IHT and their consent should also be taken after thorough discussion of its risks and benefits. The destination hospital should be identified and its agreement to accept patients should be obtained in advance. The responsibility for the transfer primarily lies on the physician at the referring hospital until the patient is taken over by the medical personnel at the receiving hospital. However, when a patient is transferred by a specialized retrieval team sent by the receiving hospital, the responsibility of care is taken over by the retrieval team.

There should be direct communication between the referring and receiving physicians. Important patient information that should be shared includes clinical condition of patient, treatment given, reasons for transfer risks of deterioration during the transfer, any treatment or investigations required before initiating transfer, mode of transport, and approximate time-line of the transfer.

Accompanying Personnel

All doctors and other personnel undertaking the transfer should be appropriately trained, qualified and certified. In addition to the vehicle operator, trained medical personnel should accompany critically ill-patients during IHT.

Transport Equipment

For transport of critically ill patients, the transport ambulance should have all equipment needed for airway management, oxygenation, hemodynamic monitoring, and all drugs for resuscitation.

Monitoring during Transport

Critically ill patient should be transferred in ambulance equipped with monitoring facility. Pulse oximeter, blood pressure monitoring instruments, electrocardiogram (ECG), etc. should be there. Critical care ambulance may be equipped with additional monitoring facility. Accompanying staff should be trained for proper monitoring and managing emergencies.

Documentation

Documentation of the decision to transfer should include the following details:

Referring physician's name, designation, contact details, date and time at which decision to transfer was taken, and reasons for transfer. Patient's clinical status and vital parameters before, during, and after transfer should be documented, so also the medical management during the transport. Copy of patient's medical records and results of investigations should be given to the receiving hospital.

Pretransfer Preparation of the Patient

Before undertaking IHT, patient should be resuscitated and stabilized to the maximum extent possible without wasting undue time, keeping in mind that in some cases complete stabilization may not be feasible until definitive treatment at the receiving hospital.[4] During the pretransfer preparation, "ABC" or "airway, breathing, and circulation" check should be performed to identify and correct any preventable problems.

Pretransfer Checklist

- *Airway:* Is the airway patent and protected against aspiration?
- *Breathing:* Is the breathing adequate? Are the blood gases levels satisfactory?
- *Circulation:* Does the patient have adequate intravenous (IV) access? Has hypotension been treated?
- *Disability or neurological status:* Is the evaluation for disability and neurological status done?
- *Environmental condition:* Have appropriate precautions been taken to protect the patient against possible adverse environmental conditions during transport?
- *Investigation, monitoring, and Infusions:* Are the baseline investigations done? Are appropriate monitoring and necessary infusions in place before transfer?

Adverse Events during Transfer

Understanding various types of possible adverse events and risk factors predisposing patients to these is important for improving the safety of IHT.[5] Transport impacts the patient via two main mechanisms, movement and its physiology and change from the environment and equipment of the initial care unit to that of the medical ambulance. These may lead to adverse events that can be either minor (i.e., >20% change in physiological parameters from baseline) or critical (i.e., a life-threatening incident requiring urgent therapeutic intervention). The adverse events that may occur during transfer include:[6]

- Medical:
  - *Cardiovascular:* Severe hypotension or hypertension, arrhythmia, and cardiac arrest
  - *Respiratory:* Hypoxia, aspiration, accidental extubation, selective intubation, bronchospasm, pneumothorax, and patient-ventilator dyssynchrony
  - *Neurological:* Agitation and intracranial hypertension
  - Hypothermia
- *Equipment malfunction or technical:* Electrical failure, uncharged batteries, gas failure, oxygen or IV-line disconnection, monitoring equipment malfunction, and vehicle breakdown
- *Human error:* Drug error and patient mix-up.

Risk Factors for Adverse Events

The risk factors can be categorized as follows:[7]
- *Equipment related (technical factors):* The common equipment problems are related to mechanical ventilation, infusion pumps, and drainage or monitoring lines. A technical understanding of functioning

of medical equipment and familiarity with the equipment used during transport is therefore important for identifying and resolving these problems.
- *Transport team related (human factors):* Lack of training and lack of supervision. This can be minimized by transport team training programs and physician education.
- *Transport organization related (collective factors):* Inadequacies in communication and coordination between the referring and receiving teams can delay transfer process, increase total transport time and incidence of adverse events. Ideally, the IHT should be organized such that the patient bypasses the emergency department admission and directly reaches the intended destination like the operating room or ICU.
- *Patient-related (including clinical instability):* Increased severity of illness, hemodynamic instability, and oxygenation failure are all risk factors. The risk can be reduced by patient stabilization before and during transfer.

A retrospective study of IHT of critically ill patients transferred using standard ground ambulance in the Netherlands reported a 34% incidence of adverse events. The researchers estimated that 70% of these events were due to poor patient preparation by referring hospital while the remaining 30% events were due to equipment or technical problems, many of which were avoidable.[8] There have been a few studies carried out to evaluate the outcome for patients admitted after IHT. Durairaj et al. reported significantly higher ICU mortality rates (25% vs. 21%) for post-IHT admissions as opposed to direct admissions.[9] Another study showed that Acute Physiology and Chronic Health Evaluation III (APACHE III) scores, hospital and ICU mortality rates, and duration of hospital or ICU stay were significantly greater for transferred patients as opposed to those directly admitted.[10]

Standards of Medical Care in Emergency Room are Higher

Standards of medical care in emergency room are higher because emergency room care claims giving state of art services to patient admitted as follows:
- Duty of care in emergency room (which means actively avoiding all kinds of dangers, i.e., health risks from all sources, i.e., from disease, drugs, and surgery, all the time) to your patients by continuous monitoring of all relevant vital parameters and investigations.
- Law requires proportionate degree of care in emergency room. Higher the risk undertaken higher is the standard demanded by law in caring for critically ill.
- Any lack of care on the part of medical practitioner in monitoring or treatment of a critically ill and doctor's actions which causes acceleration of disease process leading to death or disability are punishable/actionable under law.
- Under law for actionable negligence, such an acceleration should be caused by breach of duty of a doctor (lack of due care of critically ill and lack of caution in monitoring critically or delaying or omitting to give treatment to critically ill) which should results in actual (proved) physical or mental damage to patient.
- There should be close nexus between such acceleration of disease process caused by negligence of doctor and not because of inherent nature of disease. Such acceleration should cause disability

or death due to breach of duty (lack of due care and caution) resulting in damage.

Legally if there is no resultant damage due to lack of care, then no compensation can be given to patient.

Transfer of Patients Who Leave Against Medical Advice

Transfers of patients who leave against medical advice (LAMA) are both a concern and a challenge for individuals in the healthcare field. Skilful communication, flexible routines, policies and procedures, negotiable management options, good clinical care, and thorough documentation constitute the cornerstones of dealing with this problem. The need for a clearly documented system or guidelines for assessing and managing such patients is highlighted. Clinical Establishment Act Standards for Hospital (Level 1A 1B) Standard No. CEA/Hospital–001 mention in point number 10.25 that "Discharge/Death summary shall also be given to patient and/or attendant in case of transfer LAMA/discharge against medical advice (DAMA) or death".

Medicolegal Aspect of Safe Transfer: Global Scenario

In the United States, there is a statute called Emergency Medical Treatment and Labor Act (EMTALA) which was enacted by introducing it in 1986 into the Consolidated Omnibus Budget Reconciliation Act, 1985 (COBRA). This Act is also known as the Patient Anti-Dumping Act. It imposed a mandatory duty on hospitals to give medical treatment to patients in emergency medical condition and women under labor. Hospital must screen and stabilize such persons with emergency medical treatment. After screening, if the hospital has no facilities, it must transfer the person to another hospital having necessary facilities.

The EMTALA governs how patients may be transferred from one hospital to another. Under the law, a patient is considered stable for transfer if the treating physician determines that no material deterioration will occur during the movement between facilities and that the receiving facility has the capability to manage the patients' medical condition. Patients with incompletely stabilized emergency medical condition may still be transferred under if one of the two following conditions exists:

1. The patient (or someone on the patient's behalf) provides a written request for transfer despite being informed of the hospital's EMTALA obligations to provide treatment; or
2. A physician certifies that medical benefits reasonably expected from transfer outweigh the risk to the individual.

Once a doctor has decided to transfer the individual, (points out the guide), the following steps must be taken:
- The transferring hospital must provide all medical treatment within its capacity, which minimizes the risk to the individual's health.
- The receiving facility must accept the transfer and must have space available and qualified personnel to treat the individual.
- The transferring hospital must send copies of all medical records related to the emergency medical condition. If the physician on call refuses or fails to assist in the patient's case, the physician's name and address must be documented on the medical records provided to the receiving facility.

- Qualified personnel, with the appropriate medical equipment, must accompany the patient during transfer.

Under EMTALA, the patient care during transport is the responsibility of the transferring physician/hospital until the patient arrives at the receiving facility. The transferring physician is also responsible for the orders as to transfer and for the treatment orders to be followed during the transport. Certificate of necessity for transfer is a requirement for reimbursement by the Centers for Medicare and Medicaid Services (CMS).

Safe Transfer After Stabilization as per Indian Law

Section 12-2 of Clinical Establishment Act 2010 imposes condition for registration of clinical establishment as "The clinical establishment shall undertake to provide within the staff and facilities available, such medical examination and treatment as may be required to stabilize the emergency medical condition of any individual who comes or is brought to such clinical establishment" Section 2 (d) defines "emergency medical condition" as a medical condition manifesting itself by acute symptoms of sufficient severity (including severe pain) of such a nature that the absence of immediate medical attention could reasonably be expected to result in— (1) placing the health of the individual or, with respect to a pregnant women, the health of the woman or her unborn child, in serious jeopardy; or (2) serious impairment to bodily functions; or (3) serious dysfunction of any organ or part of a body.

Clinical Establishment Act Standards for Hospital (Level 1A 1B) Standard No. CEA/Hospital–001 mentions in point number 10.10 "In case of nonavailability of beds or where clinical need warrants, the patient shall be referred to another facility along with the required clinical information or notes". Point number 10.15 mentions that "The Clinical Establishment shall undertake to provide within the staff and facilities available, such medical examination and treatment as may be required to stabilize the emergency medical condition of any individual who comes or is brought to such clinical establishment".

Guidelines to Medical Officers (MOs)[11] also pose obligation on Government MOs for taking precautions for sick transfer. It says that "It is incumbent upon all MOs/Specialist Officers ordering sick transfer to properly assess the condition of the patient and fitness to undertake the journey by the selected mode of transfer. The sick attendant will be properly briefed and provided necessary wherewithal to manage the patient en route. Patients traveling without a sick attendant should carry a card giving the identification, diagnosis, treatment, and important contact telephone numbers in case of any emergency".

National Medical Commission Ethics and Medical Registration Board Notification issued on 2nd August 2023 in regulation no 27 says that "Only such follow-up consultation should be planned as required by the patient. An update/summary of the clinical condition and reasons for referral must be documented and provided at the referral".

Indian Judiciary on Safe Transfer of Patients

Supreme Court regarding need of transfer or referral of patient has said in *Parmanand Katara versus Union of India and Ors. 1989 SCC (4) 286: AIR 1989 SC 2039*

"We would also like to mention that whenever on such occasions a man of the medical profession is approached and if he finds that whatever assistance he could give is not sufficient really to save the life of the person but some better assistance is necessary-it is also the duty of the man in the medical profession so approached to render all the help which he could and also see that the person reaches the proper expert as early as possible".

In *Paschim Banga Khet Mazdoor Samity versus State of West Bengal, 1996 (4) SCC 37*, the Supreme Court took cognizance of US Congress enacted COBRA of 1986 which mandates emergency treatment of patient and need to stabilize before transfer to higher center in case of necessity. Apex Court held that we are of the view that in order that proper medical facilities are available for dealing with emergency cases it must be that: "facilities are available at the Primary Health Centers where the patient can be given immediate primary treatment so as to stabilize his condition ... Proper arrangement of ambulance is made for transport of a patient ... The ambulance is adequately provided with necessary equipment and medical personnel".

The NCDRC has expressed need of transfer in prescribed form with consent in *Pravat Kumar Mukherjee versus Ruby General Hospital and Ors.*[12]

"In our view, therefore, the contention of the Hospital that the passer-by who brought the patient to the Hospital wanted to take him to Government Hospital is baseless. In any case, the transfer from one Hospital to the other Hospital was required to be done in the form prescribed and after taking a written undertaking. Nothing was done".

In *D.C. Bhawani Prasad versus Krishna Nursing Home, 1997 (1) CPJ 483* Karnataka State Consumer Disputes Redressal Commission (SCDRC) has said that "Complainant's son suffered from continuous vomiting and so he was admitted to Nursing home. At the time of admission he developed fits. Treatment was started, and a pediatrician's and neurologist's opinion was sought and since the condition continued to deteriorate he was shifted to St. John's Medical College Hospital but the patient died on the way. The State Commission held that all that possible was done, and dismissed the case".

201st Law Commission Report on Emergency Medical Care 2006[13]

The 201st Law Commission Report under the chairmanship of Mr Justice M Jagannadha Rao has discussed the emergency medical care and need of proper transfer. Law Commission has made the draft bill based on the principles of the COBRA of 1985. This report emphasized that the emergency medical service (EMS) has to be legislated so that the patients can enforce their rights. This report recommended that the Parliament should legislate this issue and make it an absolute duty of the healthcare institution, whether it is public or private to provide emergency medical care. Report mentions in paragraph 5 of "Proposed Model Law bill" that patient in emergency needs to be stabilized first then if such facilities are not available with the hospital or the medical practitioner, or the person requests for a transfer, the transfer of the person should be arranged. Paragraph 7 of Model Bill restricts transfer till patient is stabilized. Paragraph 8 describes appropriate transfer and paragraph 9 emphasizes on maintenance of record.

Summary

The IHT is undertaken to obtain additional care for the patient after carefully weighing the risk benefit ratio. Rather than haphazardly following a "scoop and run" approach, IHT should be guided by a policy of "stabilize and shift", keeping in mind that complete stabilization of the patient may be achieved only at the receiving end and until then, it is important to maintain continuity of care. The transport crew should be trained and skilled to anticipate and manage any technical and medical contingencies that may arise during the transfer. As IHT is often critical for making best possible medical care available to patients, there is a need to maximize its safety and efficiency. Hence, while several countries such as USA, UK, and Australia have formulated guidelines to regulate and improve the standards of IHTs, most other countries particularly the developing nations including India are yet to do so.

TRANSIT DEATHS

Many a time death of serious patient happens in shifting during transit despite of all precautions. In such situation not only medicolegal issues arises but also question arises about issuing of death certificate and postmortem.

When patient is referred by a hospital to other hospital, responsibility of shifting safely lies on referring hospital. If expiry occurs, then death certificate should be issued by referring hospital. If responsibility of shifting has been shouldered by hospital referred, then death certificate has to be issued by hospital referred.

For Government MOs, guidelines are available at National Health Systems Resource Centre website for transit death of patient.[11]

Death of Patient not Accompanied by Sick Attendant

Transfer by Rail

In case of death of sick patient not accompanied by attendant, inquest and postmortem is arranged by Railway police. The train guard usually contacts the Station Master of the next station having Government Railway Police (GRP) for necessary formalities. The death certificate and autopsy report in such cases is obtained from the civil hospital where the body was taken for autopsy and necessary documentation completed accordingly.

Transfers by Road

In case the patient is traveling by ambulance, the driver of the ambulance will inform the nearest civil police, or/and nearest Station headquarters, the unit of the deceased, the referring hospital, and the hospital to which he is being transferred/referred to for necessary action.

Guidelines in Case of Death of Patient Accompanied by Sick Attendant

As per AHQ Policy Letter No. 11952/DGMS-5A (31305/Pol/DGMS-5A) Dated 28 Jan/19 Feb 88, in case of death of patient during sick transfer the receiving hospital is to admit the case as "found dead". Where there is no possibility/suspicion of foul play, the cause of death will be recorded as the disease from which the patient was suffering and a clinical postmortem is to be carried out. In case death occurs at a place which is far away from the destination, the sick attendant should immediately contact the nearest Station headquarters and the civil police (railway police in case of transfer by rail) for further action.

MEDICOLEGAL ASPECTS OF EXPIRY DATE DRUGS

Drug Expiry Date

Drug expiration is the date after which a drug might not be suitable for use as manufactured.

It is the date appearing on a pharmaceutical product beyond which the manufacturer will not guarantee the potency, purity, uniformity, or bioavailability of the product. It printed on the label or stamped onto the bottle or carton. It is usually 2-5 years from production date. It should be standard practice that for proper disposal, expired drug should be kept in a separate shelf with proper record maintenance.

What do the Expiry Date/Use by Date Mean?

The expiry date usually means that you should not take the medicine after the end of the month given. For example, if the expiry date is July 2023, you should not take the medicine after 31 July 2023. If your medicine has a "use by" or "use before" date instead of an expiry date, this usually means that you should not take the medicine after the end of the previous month. For example, if the use by date is July 2023, you should not take the medicine after 30 June 2023.

Issues with Expiry Drug

Losing potency and efficacy is not a one-time process just after expiry date. It is true that the effectiveness of a drug may decrease over time, but much of the original potency still remains even a decade after the expiration date. There are little scientific evidences that expired drugs are toxic. Renal tubular damage is reported due to degraded tetracycline. Excluding nitroglycerin, insulin, and liquid antibiotics, most medications are as long-lasting as the ones tested by the military. It has been shown that placing a medicine in a cool place, such as a refrigerator, will help a drug remain potent for many years. Solid dosage forms, such as tablets and capsules, appear to be most stable past their expiration date. Drugs that exist in solution or as a reconstituted suspension, and that require refrigeration (such as amoxicillin suspension), may not have the required potency if used when out dated. Loss of potency can be a major health concern, especially when treating an infection with an antibiotic. In addition, antibiotic resistance may occur with subpotent medications. Drugs that exist in solution, especially injectable drugs, should be discarded if the product forms a precipitant or looks cloudy or discolored.

Accidental Use of Drug After Expiry Date: What do Evidences Say?

Expired drugs have not necessarily lost their potency and efficacy. The expiration date is only an assurance that the labeled potency will last at least until that date. Expiry date is not just a point at which the medication is no longer effective or has become unsafe to use. Most medicines stored under reasonable conditions retain at least 70-80% of their original potency for at least 1-2 years after the expiration date, even after the container has been opened. Placing medication in a cool dry place, such as a refrigerator, will help it remain potent for many years.

Ongoing research shows that stored under optimal conditions, many drugs retain 90% of their potency for at least 5 years after the labeled expiration date, and sometimes longer. Even 10 years after the expiration date many pharmaceuticals retain a significant amount of their original potency.[14]

A study by Khanchandani on efficacy, safety concern and disposal practices followed for expired drug preparations among medical personnel, found that about 90% were safe and effective as long as 15 years past their original expiration date. Loel Dawis, expiration date chief said that with a handful of exception notably nitroglycerin, insulin, and liquid antibiotic most drugs are probably as durable as the agency tested.[15]

A study done by Simons on outdated EpiPen and EpiPen Jr autoinjectors: Past their prime, noted that, drugs differ in terms of their forms, dosage, and stability. Usually, drugs in liquid forms (e.g., solutions and suspensions) are not as stable as those in the solid forms (e.g., tablets and capsules). It has been reported that bioavailability of EpiPen˚ (epinephrine autoinjectors) were reduced when administered between 1 and 90 months after the labeled expiration date compared with those that were not yet expired.[16]

Shelf Life Extension Program/ Expiration Date Extension—USA

The best evidence of acceptable potency of the medications beyond their expiration date is provided by the Shelf Life Extension Program (SLEP) undertaken by the Food and Drug Administration (FDA) for the Department of Defense. The aim of the SLEP program was to reduce medication costs for the military. SLEP has found that 88% of 122 different drugs stored under ideal conditions should have their expiration dates extended >1 year, with an average extension of 66 months, and a maximum extension of 278 months.[17] Primarily the FDA approved prescription nominated as SLEP candidates are military significant contingency use products such as anti-tetanus serum (ATS), antibiotics, nonsteroidal anti-inflammatory drug (NSAID), and drugs with limited commercial use—nerve agent antidotes, antisnake venom (ASV), and drugs purchased in large quantities.

The 2015 commentary in Mayo Clinic Proceedings, "Extending Shelf Life Just Makes Sense", suggested that drug makers could be required to set a preliminary expiration date and then update it after long-term testing. An independent organization could also do testing similar to that done by the FDA extension program or data from the extension program could be applied to properly stored medications.[18]

Drugs that should Never be Used Post Expiration Date

- *Narrow therapeutic index drugs:* Anticonvulsants, digoxin, and warfarin
- Drugs losing potency very quickly such as phenytoin, phenobarbital, nitroglycerin, theophylline, epinephrine, and insulin.
- *Eye drops*: Eyes are particularly sensitive to any bacteria that might grow in a solution once a preservative degrades.
- Tetracyclines
- Other drugs such as Procan SR—sustained release procainamide, thyroid preparations, paraldehyde, and oral contraceptives.

Health Hazard of Expired Drugs

- The presence of unused and expired medications in cabinets and cupboards is a potential danger and can be harmful to humans, environment, and wildlife.
- Diclofenac has appeared to incite renal failure in vultures following the ingestion of remains from cows treated with this drug.
- In USA, many drugs such as acetaminophen, verapamil, and estradiol are found in waterways.
- The presence of antibiotics in water may prompt antibiotic resistance.

How to Safely Dispose of Unused or Expired Medicine[19]

The best way to dispose of most types of unused or expired medicines (both prescription and over the counter) is to drop off the medicine at a drug take back site, location, or program immediately. If you cannot get to a drug take back location promptly, or there is none near you, and your medicine is on the FDA flush list, your next best option is to immediately flush these potentially dangerous medicine down the toilet, not on the flush list, you should follow these instructions to discard the medicine in your trash at home.

Medicolegal Implication of Inadvertent Use of Expiry Drug

If inadvertently expiry drug has been administered to a patient and no damage have occurred, then there should be no criminal liability as per defense available in Section 95 of Indian Penal Code which says that Act causing slight harm can be used as defense against criminal prosecution. But definition of harm is broad in Section 2(22) in Consumer Protection Act 2019 and "harm" includes mental agony or emotional distress attendant to personal injury or illness or damage to property and may attract litigation. In light of scientific evidences available which mentions that most drugs do not have any significant side effect if given inadvertently after expiry date, rather there are chances of potential decrease in efficacy; there are less chances of penalization of doctors by courts.

Summary

Expired medical products can be less effective or risky due to a change in chemical composition or a decrease in strength. Certain expired medications are at risk of bacterial growth and subpotent antibiotics can fail to treat infections, leading to more serious illnesses and antibiotic resistance. So, one should be vigilant and avoid accidental use of any drug after expiry date. Now time has come to formulate a SLEP list of drugs in India with laboratory backup to save economy and also lawsuits against medicos.

MEDICOLEGAL ASPECTS OF OFF-LABEL USE OF DRUGS

Off-label Use of Drugs

Off-label use is the use of pharmaceutical drugs for an unapproved indication or in an unapproved age group, dosage, or route of administration. Off-label drug use (OLDU) is prescribing for an indication, or employing a dosage or dosage form, that has not been approved through the FDA process.

Both prescription drugs and over-the-counter (OTC) drugs can be used in off-label ways. Off-label use is very common and generally legal unless it violates ethical guidelines or safety regulations. The ability to prescribe drugs for uses beyond the officially approved indications is commonly used to good effect by healthcare providers. For example, methotrexate is commonly used off-label because its immunomodulatory effects relieve various disorders. However, off-label use can entail health risks and differences in legal liability. Marketing of pharmaceuticals for off-label use is usually prohibited.

Is Off-label Drug Use Common?

Off-label use is very common. Generic drugs generally have no sponsor as their indications and use expands, and incentives are limited to initiate new clinical trials to generate additional data for approval agencies to expand indications of proprietary drugs.

Up to one-fifth of all drugs are prescribed off-label and among psychiatric drugs, off-label use rises to 31%.[20] Radley et al. reported in 2006 that in a group of commonly used medications, 21% of prescriptions were for an off-label use. In certain subpopulations of patients, this rate may be even higher. For example, a study by Shah et al.[21] found that 78.9% of children discharged from pediatric hospitals were taking at least one off-label medication. In addition, in a pediatric emergency department, the rate of OLDU was estimated to be 26.2%.[22] The off-label use of antidepressant, anticonvulsant, and antipsychotic medications is high and is more prevalent with increasing patient age. In an ICU, Lat et al.[23] reported that 36.2% of medication orders were for an off-label use.

Use of Off-label Drug in Pediatrics

Since the patient population in pediatrics is often excluded from clinical drug studies, examples of OLDU are especially abundant. For example, morphine has never received an FDA indication for pain treatment in children, but it is extensively used for this indication in hospitalized pediatric patients.[21] In another example, researchers discovered in the 1970s that the nonsteroidal anti-inflammatory agent indomethacin was efficacious as a medical therapy for closing a persistent, symptomatic patent ductus arteriosus in newborns.[24] Thus, a trial of indomethacin became the treatment of choice for many affected newborns in an attempt to avoid curative surgery. Indomethacin has never been approved for this indication and, as such, this use remains an OLDU. In addition, many inhaled bronchodilators, antimicrobials, anticonvulsants, and proton pump inhibitors are often used in the pediatric population without formal FDA approval.

Factors for Use of Off-label Drug

Off-label drug use can be motivated by several factors. First, a medication may not have been studied and approved for a specific population (e.g., pediatric, geriatric, or pregnant patients). Second, a life-threatening or terminal medical condition may motivate a healthcare professional to give any treatment that is logical and available, whether approved by the FDA or not. Third, if one medication from a class of drugs has FDA approval, physicians commonly use other medications in the same class without specific FDA approval for that use for the same indication.

Can an OLDU for a Given Drug become a Widely Accepted Practice or Even a Standard of Care?

Off-label drug uses can become widely entrenched in clinical practice and become predominant treatments for a given clinical condition. For example, tricyclic antidepressants do not have FDA approval as a treatment for neuropathic pain, yet this class of drugs is considered a first-line treatment option OLDU. Aspirin was widely used before the introduction of the Food, Drug, and Cosmetic Act of 1938. Therefore, aspirin was grandfathered and approved as an existing drug without the rigorous testing that modern medications undergo.

If Efficacious, Why is Government Approval not Obtained to Convert Off-label uses of Drugs to On-label Uses?

Obtaining a new FDA approval for a medication can be costly and time-consuming. To add additional indications for an already approved medication requires the proprietor to file a supplemental drug application, and, even if eventually approved, revenues for the new indication may not offset the expense and effort of obtaining approval.[25] Finally, generic medications may not have the requisite funding foundations needed to pursue FDA-approval studies. For these financial reasons, drug proprietors may never seek FDA approval for a new drug indication.

Medicolegal Implications of Use of Off-label Drug Usage

Physicians have been involved in legal claims due to an adverse reaction related to a medication prescribed for an off-label use. The FDA makes it clear that it does not regulate the practice of medicine and that the federal Food, Drug, and Cosmetic Act of 1938 will not play a role in creating physician liability for OLDU.[26]

No court decision to date has mandated that a physician must disclose, through an informed consent process, the off-label use of a drug.[27] Two arguments are often voiced by those who oppose any routine requirement for disclosure: (1) disclosure may unduly frighten patients and (2) the extensive burden placed on physicians to constantly review and communicate medication risk and benefit information may divert attention away from other more important patient care issues.

Off-label use cannot be considered illegal as long as ethical and safety concerns are not violated.[28]

In *Canterbury versus Spence* case, the Canterbury court held that "The test for determining whether a particular peril must be divulged is its *materiality* to the patient's decision.[29]" A material risk is one in which "a reasonable person, in what the physician knows or should know to be the patient's position, would be likely to attach significance to the risk or cluster of risks in deciding whether or not to forego the proposed therapy."

Klein versus Biscup case, Ohio court held that off-label use of medical devices was a "matter of medical judgment. "According to the court, physicians may be subject to professional liability for medical negligence involving OLDU but will not be held liable for nondisclosure.[30]

A physician's duty of care is defined as the same degree of care provided by other physicians practicing under similar circumstances. Use of off-label medication alone does not result in liability under negligence standards.[31] When a patient believes that he or she was harmed by an off-label use of a medication, it must be established that the prescribing physician deviated from the standard of practice.

Off-label Drug Usage Regulation in India

In India, the Drug Controller General of India (DCGI) is the regulatory authority for granting approval for new drugs but, unfortunately, there are no clear-cut guidelines on the off-label use of drugs. Indian law does not currently allow drugs to be prescribed for indications for which they have not been approved. Off-label marketing by pharmaceutical companies are regarded as a violation of law in India, and it is an offence under the drug and magic remedies (objectionable advertisements) Act, 1954. Despite the Indian Medical Association's (IMA's) positive opinion about off-label prescribing, any rule about the off-label prescribing is yet to come in India. Many are of the opinion that authorizing off-label prescribing will set a bad example because of ignorance of patients and domination of pharmaceutical companies on prescribing patterns in India. In a policy statement submitted to the health ministry, the association said doctors in India should be allowed to prescribe drugs for unapproved indications when there is scientific evidence and medical opinion to justify such "off-label" treatment.

Document the Reasoning for Off-label Use

Clear documentation of failed medication trials and course of treatment leading to OLDU can help reinforce the fact that standards of practice are being met. Part of supportive documentation involves maintaining updated knowledge of the medication and having scientific literature (peer-reviewed, if possible) that supports the reasonable application of a medication and its nonexperimental status. This documentation can be useful to physicians defending themselves in malpractice cases involving alleged wrongful prescriptions for off-label indications.

Obtain Appropriate Informed Consent

Given the lack of precedent establishing a legal requirement for what constitutes informed consent in off-label treatment, there is no official best practice to guide clinicians. Thus, it may be prudent to clearly communicate benefits and risks associated with off-label medications, including the lack of strong clinical evidence supporting its use for off-label purpose. Inclusion of this information in informed consent discussions may also serve to reduce the risk of a negligent practice claim. These practices should also be considered and discussed when promoting off-label prescription to other physicians.

Summary

The term "off-label" refers to circumstances in which a physician prescribes a drug to a patient in a manner that varies in some way from the drug's (or device's) FDA-approved labeling. Off-label prescription occurs when a physician prescribes a drug in any manner that varies from labeling specifications. The term "off-label" represents no more than a regulatory description of the administratively approved use or uses of a medical drug or device. Thus, off-label only references a drug's legal status and does not refer to scientific facts or accepted medical practices. Off-label use of drugs (and medical devices) is recognized to be a legitimate part of the practice of medicine and, as a practice, is legal. Off-label uses also are considered to be ethical and are thought to represent neither experimentation nor research. Furthermore, the courts have found that a treatment found to be "in accordance with generally accepted standards of medical practice" would hardly be "experimental" and similarly, a procedure found to be of "scientifically proven value" would similarly not be "experimental".[32]

MEDICOLEGAL ASPECTS OF PLACEBO DRUGS

A placebo is any medication or procedure with no known therapeutic effect. Placebos are often given for the psychological, rather than physiological, benefit of the patient and are also used as a control measure in the testing of new drugs. Common placebos include sugar pills, saline injections, or drugs given in such miniscule doses that there is no beneficial effect. A placebo can be roughly defined as a sham medical treatment. Placebos are also popular because they can sometimes produce relief through psychological mechanisms (phenomenon known as "placebo effect"). The placebo effect is defined as the positive response experienced by some patients after receiving a placebo, which is thought to be brought about by a combination of patient expectations and beliefs, genetic factors, and the context in which the placebo is given.

Mechanism of Action of the Placebo

Generally, a placebo is seen as an inert substance or procedure and the placebo effect (or response) is something that follows the administration of a placebo. There are basically two main mechanisms by which placebos are claimed to exert effect on patient.

1. *Psychological mechanisms*: From the psychological viewpoint, a multitude of mechanisms contribute to placebo effects. These include expectations, conditioning, learning, memory, motivation, somatic focus, reward, and reduction of anxiety
2. *Neurobiological mechanisms*: The neurobiology of placebo effects is commonly considered in terms of opioid and nonopioid mechanisms. Several studies have demonstrated that placebo effects can be completely or partially reversed by the opioid antagonist naloxone, supporting the involvement of endogenous opioids in some analgesic effects of placebo. Studies have demonstrated that some mechanisms of placebo operate by altering the activity of both cholecystokinin (CCK) and endogenous opioids.

Factors Influencing the Power of the Placebo Effect

Children seem to have a greater response than adults to placebos.[33] If the person dispensing the placebo shows their care toward the patient, is friendly and sympathetic, or has a high expectation of a treatment's success, then the placebo would be more effectual.

Placebo in Clinical Trials

The placebo, a pharmaceutically inert substance (typically sugar pill), is the clinical researcher's analog to the scientist's control experiment. To prove a new treatment effective above and beyond the psychological results of a simple belief in the ability of the drug to cure, a researcher compares the results of the experimental treatment for an illness with those obtained from the placebo. The placebo controlled trial "is widely regarded as the gold standard for testing the efficacy of new treatments".

Ethics of Placebo Controlled Trials

The use of a placebo in clinical research continues to be a topic of debate in the medical community in recent times. Some argue that the use of placebos is often unethical because alternative study designs would produce similar results with less risk to individual research participants. Others argue that the use of placebos is essential to protect the society from the harm that could result from the widespread use of ineffective medical treatments. Another argument proposed against placebo controlled trials is that they potentially violate the concept of clinical equipoise when proven effective therapy is available. Clinical equipoise refers to the state where clinicians are unsure whether the new treatment or intervention is as good as the standard treatment. Those who reject the use of placebo controlled trials argue that they violate the therapeutic obligation of physicians to offer optimal medical care. In other words, they compromise the right of the patient to receive the best care possible and violate the ethical principle of therapeutic beneficence. Critics of placebo controlled trial or trials that include an untreated control group cite Article 11.3 of the Declaration of Helsinki: "In any medical study, every patient including those of control group, if any should be assured of the best proven diagnostic and therapeutic methods and no patient should suffer from unnecessary pain".

Guidelines of the Office for Human Research Protection on Placebo

The Office for Human Research Protection (OHRP) published guidelines in 2008 for the use of placebo and methods to minimize the risk associated with it.[34] The guidelines state, "placebos may be used in clinical trials where there is no known or available (i.e., FDA approved) alternative therapy that can be tolerated by subjects." The use of placebos in controlled clinical trials must be justified by a positive risk benefit analysis, and the subjects must be fully informed of the risks involved in the assignment to the placebo group.

If a placebo is used in a study, the informed consent form must include all of the following information:

- The subjects must be informed that they may be given a placebo.
- A clear lay definition of the term "placebo" must be given to the subjects.
- The rationale for using a placebo must be explained to the subjects.
- If applicable, the subjects must be informed of any viable medical alternatives to being placed on placebo.
- The duration of time that a subject will be on a placebo, degree of discomfort, and potential effects of not receiving medication must all be explained.
- Any consequences of delayed active treatment must be explained to the subjects.
- A statement in the risk section of the consent that the condition of the subject may worsen while on placebo should be included.
- Clinical drug trials or other research involving patients or volunteers must comply with the Indian Council of Medical Research (ICMR) guidelines and the New Drugs and Clinical Trials Rules, 2018.
- Consent taken from any patient or participant for the trial of drug or therapy which is not as per the guidelines shall be construed as misconduct. National Medical Commission Ethics and Medical Registration Board Notification issued on 2nd August, 2023.

Ethics of Placebo in Children

The use of placebo in children is more restricted than in adults, because children cannot consent. Placebo should not be used when it means withholding effective treatment, particularly for serious and life threatening conditions. The use of placebo is often needed for scientific reasons, including pediatric trials. The use of placebo may be warranted in children as in adults when evidence for any particular treatment is lacking or when the placebo effect is known to be very variable (e.g., pain and hay fever). As the level of evidence in favor of an effective treatment increases, the ethical justification for the use of placebo decreases.[35]

Medicolegal Implications of Use of Placebo

The practice of doctors prescribing placebos that are disguised as real medication is controversial. A chief concern is that it is deceptive and could harm the doctor–patient relationship in the long run. While some say that blanket consent, or the general consent to unspecified treatment given by patients beforehand, is ethical, others argue that patients should always obtain specific information about the name of the drug they are receiving, its side effects, and other treatment options. This view is shared by some on the grounds of patient autonomy. There are also concerns that legitimate doctors and pharmacists could open themselves up to charges of fraud or malpractice by using a placebo. For clinical trials one should strictly follow OHRP guidelines.

Summary

Placebo controlled trials are justifiable when they are supported by sound methodologic consideration and when their use does not expose research participants to excessive risk of harm. Consideration should be given to the "best available therapy" control groups in the evaluation of a new therapy or intervention over an existing therapy.

MEDICOLEGAL ASPECTS OF DRUGS USED IN PEDIATRICS WHERE MANUFACTURER SAYS DO NOT

There have been many instances when doctors are tempted to use the medicines in good faith for the treatment of their patients on the basis of experience. Many a times there are no issue in using drugs where there is no recommendation from manufacturer or guidelines from government or academic bodies but in era of medicolegal awareness some times medicolegal issues do arise. Judiciary has shown varied responses to such litigations but for safe practice it is highly recommended that physician should be aware of the recommendations and avoid temptation to use them even if their past experience permits such usage. Some judgments are being presented here for awareness.

Judicious Use of Floxacins

Uttar Pradesh SCDRC in Dr Rakesh Nath Mehrotra versus Atul Pradhan and others[36] has to deal the administration of ciprofloxacin in child of 1 year 6 months treated with the drug for enteric fever in 1994. Baby cured within 7 days and no side effects shown. Same illness was treated with same medicine in 1996 when it was 3 years of age. Court held doctor was not negligent in prescribing the drug. It cannot be said that Dr R.N. Mehrotra was in any way negligent in treating the child patient and has caused any sort of permanent damage to the child by prescribing ciprofloxacin which, according to some medical opinion, should not be given to children below 12 years of age. Some of the medical literature advocates the use of this medicine in children also. It is for the doctor, who is treating the patient, to see as to which drug will be very effective and will cure the patient at a particular time. According to Dr R.N. Mehrotra, when the child has been treated and responded well to the administration of ciprofloxacin in the year 1994 when he was only 1.5 years of age and was completely cured so the same medicine was safely repeated for treatment of same type of disease again in the year 1996 when the child was about 3 years of age, the doctor had taken reasonable care and caution and his previous experience in prescribing this medicine for the benefit of the child patient. In the present case, the doctor was not negligent in prescribing ciprofloxacin to the child patient and there is no evidence on record to prove or suggest that any permanent damage of any kind to any organ or the body of the child has been caused or the growth of the child in any way been affected by this treatment.

Nimesulide Prescribed by Opponent No. 1 Hospital was at That Time a Banned Drug as per Government of India Notification Dated 10/02/2011—No Negligence

In Kum Sakshi Satyajeet S versus Ashwini Prasad Hospital case[37] tablet Nise (nimesulide) was prescribed by opponent No.1 Hospital which was at that time a banned drug as per Government of India Notification dated 10/02/2011. It was held that for proving negligence on the part of prescribing doctor, complainant is under obligation to establish at the first instance that it is a banned drug and said ban was within conscientious knowledge of the doctor—complainant must establish a nexus between act of complained and the injury alleged to have sustained—no adverse effects shown to have been taken place on patient/complainant after taking this particular drug—complainant failed to substantiate her such case—arguments of the opponents that had there being any adverse effect of the drug, complainant-Sakshi's father would not have purchased drug again and, certainly, would have complained about it to the chemist—no interference warranted—appeal disposed of.

Vijaya Laxmi versus Krishna Kumar (Dr) Supreme Court of India 2006

Syrup nimesulide prescribed by opponent claimed to be banned in India. Syrup nimesulide 30 mL one bottle in 40 kg child was not cause of fulminant hepatic failure and death of 12-year old boy. The child died due to typhoid and malaria along with possibility of hepatitis A. No negligence. Upheld, National commission judgment.

Wrong Administration of Grilinctus Syrup to 5-Month Old Child—Negligence

Sri Rabindra Nath Poddar versus Colombia Asia Hospital, (WBSCDRC), Complaint Case No. CC/203 of 2016.D/d. 10.06.2022.

Wrong administration of Grilinctus syrup to 5-month old child—no damage to child. Negligence—human error—pay one lakh.

Aminoglycosides May Cause Deafness but in this Case it Appears to be Congenital

In Sidharth Batta versus Dr Maj. Gen. M. L. Magotra, 2003 (2) CLD 266: AIR 2003 NOC 477 (Jammu and Kashmir-HC), administration of drugs—child having medical problems since its birth, suffered from jaundice and acute diarrhea—he was given the drug gentamicin by the doctor—complainant alleges that because of excess injection of said drug the child became deaf and thus the doctor was negligent in treating the child that resulted in deafness—medical opinion reveals that the drug administered under permissible limits—doctor not be held negligent or deficient in service—a doctor would not be guilty of negligence if he has acted in accordance with the practice accepted as proper by a responsible body of medical men skilled in that particular art and if he has acted in accordance with such practice then merely because there is a body of opinion that takes a contrary view will not make him liable for negligence. Dr M, who is an Assistant Surgeon, stated that the deafness from which the appellant is suffering is a congenital defect. Dr A, another Assistant Surgeon stated that whatever he had mentioned in the certificate was not on the basis of personal observations. The question arises as to whether the deafness from which the appellant came to suffer was congenital or this occurred on account of excess injunction of gentamicin. Dr M has stated in categorical terms that the appellant is suffering from deafness which is congenital in nature. Dr J has given an opinion that gentamicin can be given to a child suffering from diarrhea and has further opined that the dose which was prescribed was within permissible limit. In the present case, the medical opinion which has come on the record is that gentamicin could be given to a child and it has been further stated that the same has been given under permissible limits. If above be the situation, then, it is difficult to record a finding that the respondent doctor was negligent.

MEDICOLEGAL ASPECTS OF USE OF SECRET DRUG FORMULATIONS

Indian Medical Council (Professional Conduct, Etiquette and Ethics) Regulations, 2002 puts obligation on every physician under regulation 1.5 for using drugs with Generic names only. Regulation says that "Every physician should, as far as possible, prescribe drugs with generic names and he/she shall ensure that there is a rational prescription and use of drugs".

Regulation 3.2 says that consultation should be for patient's benefit. So physician is obligated to ensure rational prescription and should use known drugs with their generic names. Regulation 6.5 specifically prohibits use of any sort of secret remedies. Regulation 6.5 says that "The prescribing or dispensing by a physician of secret remedial agents of which he does not know the composition, or the manufacture or promotion of their use is unethical and as such prohibited. All the drugs prescribed by a physician should always carry a proprietary formula and clear name". So it is clear that using secret drug formulation is not only unethical but also prohibited.

National Medical Commission Ethics and Medical Registration Board Notification issued on 2nd August, 2023 also says in regulation no 3 (D) that every Registered Medical Practitioner (RMP) shall practice the system of medicine in which he/she has trained and certified (for this purpose referred to as modern medicine or allopathic medicine). "Modern medicine" or "allopathy" is defined as a healthcare discipline that involves a scientific understanding of disease processes and uses rational and evidence-based treatment methods. This notification in regulation 8 also puts an obligation on physician for prescribing generic medicines. Regulation says that "Every RMP should prescribe drugs using generic names written legibly and prescribe drugs rationally, avoiding unnecessary medications, and irrational fixed-dose combination tablets".

The Drugs and Cosmetics Act (1940) demands the fact that every patented or proprietary medicinal preparation under this act must display a label on the container mentioning the exact formula or list of ingredients in it. This act empowers the Central Government to form a drug technical advisory board and to establish a central drug laboratory to help and advice both the central and states government. It controls the quality, purity, and strength of drugs for safety.

It regulates the import, manufacture, distribution, and sale of these drugs. The amended act has enhanced the scale of punishment for various offences, including sale of spurious drugs, adulteration of drugs and cosmetics, toxic contamination, etc. In order to facilitate the analysis or testing of drug samples to assess their quality, the central drugs laboratory was established in 1962 under the Drugs and Cosmetics Rules. Stringent punishments have laid down for manufacture, stocking, or sale of substandard or spurious drugs

The Drugs and Magic Remedies (Objectionable Advertisement) Act, 1954 ensures that ethical standards are maintained when drugs are advertised by manufacturers. This act bans the objectionable advertisements of magical remedial drugs for curing conditions such as venereal diseases, impotency, menstrual disorders, infertility, abortion, misconception, and insanity. Advertisements offending decency or morality can be banned under this Act.

SUMMARY

As per the Indian Law prescribing secret drug formulation is strictly prohibited. Manufacturing and advertising of any spurious drug or secret formulation is prohibited. Manufacturer are bound to display drug formulation and doctors are obligated to prescribe only those drug who are generic and licensed by DCGI as per scientific understanding of disease processes and rational and evidence-based treatment methods.

LEARNING KEY POINTS AND TAKE-HOME MESSAGES

- Inter Hospital Transfer (IHT) carries its own risk and a poorly and hastily conducted transfer increases morbidity and mortality risk for patients. Therefore, a well-organized system with appropriate equipment and personnel is crucial for a safe IHT.
- Inter Hospital Transfer should be guided by a policy of "stabilize and shift", keeping in mind that complete stabilization of the patient may be achieved only at the receiving end and until then, it is important to maintain continuity of care.
- One should be vigilant and avoid accidental use of any drug after expiry date.
- The prescribing or dispensing by a physician of secret remedial agents of which he does not know the composition, or the manufacture or promotion of their use is unethical and as such prohibited.
- One should avoid using those drugs where there is no recommendation from manufacturer or guidelines from government or academic bodies.

MUST AVOID THINGS— DO NOT DO

- Never prescribe secret formulation drug.
- Never transfer a patient without referral letter and documents with a proper receipt.
- Never be tempted to use expired drug even of few weeks or months.

MUST DO THINGS

- Always stabilize patient before making transfer to other hospital.
- Keep checking expiry dates of drugs. Be vigilant of expiry dates.
- Always keep expired drug in separate shelf and return or destroy them as soon as possible.

MESSAGES WHICH THE READER MUST BE AWARE

The transport crew should be trained and skilled to anticipate and manage any technical and medical contingencies that may arise during the transfer.

WARNINGS

- Check expiry date of drug twice before using them.
- Use of expired drugs or secret formulation drug may give rise to medicolegal issues.
- Placebo drugs must be used in trials after taking inform consent.

MEDICAL NEGLIGENCE PEARLS

Discharge/death summary shall also be given to patient and/or attendant in case of transfer LAMA/DAMA or death.

ONLY ONE FACT TO REMEMBER

Pretransport coordination and communication, qualified and trained accompanying personnel, appropriate transport equipment, standard monitoring, and documentation are key elements of a safe transfer.

MCQs

Choose one correct answer

1. Which Law Commission Report has discussed "emergency medical care and need of proper transfer"?
    a. 201st
    b. 145th
    c. 154th
    d. None of the above
2. Which statement is true regarding off-label use of drug?
    a. Off-label use is the use of pharmaceutical drugs for an unapproved indication or in an unapproved age group, dosage, or route of administration
    b. It is common seen in intensive acre, pediatric, and psychiatry practice.
    c. There are no clear-cut guidelines on the off-label use of drugs
    d. All of the above
3. In which case Supreme Court took cognizance of US Congress enacted Consolidated Omnibus Budget Reconciliation Act of 1986 which mandates emergency treatment of patient and need to stabilize before transfer to higher center?
    a. Parmanand Katara versus Union of India
    b. IMA versus VP Shantha
    c. Jacob Mathews versus State of Punjab
    d. Paschim Banga Khet Mazdoor Samity versus State of West Bengal
4. Which statement is true?
    a. Losing potency and efficacy is not a one-time process just after expiry date.
    b. Effectiveness of a drug may decrease over time, but much of the original potency still remains even a decade after the expiration date.
    c. Solid dosage forms, such as tablets and capsules, appear to be most stable past their expiration date.
    d. All of the above

Answers

1. a   2. d   3. d   4. d

REFERENCES

1. Singh JM, MacDonald RD. Pro/con debate: Do the benefits of regionalized critical care delivery outweigh the risks of interfacility patient transport? Crit Care. 2009;13:219.
2. Barry PW, Ralston C. Adverse events occurring during interhospital transfer of the critically ill. Arch Dis Child. 1994;71:8-11.

3. Paediatric Intensive Care Society. Retrieval and transfer of the most critically ill children. In: Standards for the Care of Critically Ill Children, 4th edition. London: Paediatric Intensive Care Society; 2010.
4. Harrahill M, Bartkus E. Preparing the trauma patient for transfer. J Emerg Nurs. 1990;16:25-8.
5. Haji-Michael P. Critical care transfers: a danger foreseen is half avoided. Crit Care. 2005;9:343-4.
6. Lim MT, Ratnavel N. A prospective review of adverse events during interhospital transfers of neonates by a dedicated neonatal transfer service. PediatrCrit Care Med. 2008; 9:289-93.
7. Rokos IC, Sanddal ND, Pancioli AM, Wolff C, Gaieski DF; 2010 Academic emergency medicine consensus conference Beyond regionalization: Intergrated networks of emergency care. Inter-hospital Communi-cations and Transport: Turning One-way Funnels Into Two-way Networks. Acad Emerg Med. 2010;17:1279-85.
8. Ligtenberg JJ, Arnold LG, Stienstra Y, van der Werf TS, Meertens JH, Tulleken JE, et al. Quality of interhospital transport of critically ill patients: A prospective audit. Crit Care 2005;9:R446-51.
9. Durairaj L, Will JG, Torner JC, Doebbeling BN. Prognostic factors for mortality following interhospital transfers to the medical intensive care unit of a tertiary referral center. Crit Care Med. 2003;31:1981-6.
10. Golestanian E, Scruggs JE, Gangnon RE, Mak RP, Wood KE. Effect of interhospital transfer on resource utilization and outcomes at a tertiary care referral center. Crit Care Med. 2007;35:1470-6.
11. National Health Systems Resource Centre. Medicolegal Issues: Guidelines to Medical Officers. [online] Available from: https://nhsrcindia.org/sites/default/files/2021-05/medico_legal.pdf. [Last accessed December, 2023].
12. Pravat Kumar Mukherjee versus Ruby General Hospital and Ors National Consumer. Disputes Redressal on 25 April, 2005 original petition no. 90 of 2002
13. 201st Law Commission Report on Emergency Medical Care To Victims Of Accidents And During Emergency Medical Condition And Women Under Labour 2006.
14. American Medical Association. "Pharma-ceutical Expiration Dates". Report 1 of the Council on Scientific Affairs (A-01). July 25, 2001.
15. Khanchandani R, Srivastava B, Sinha A, Gaur S, Gaur S, Bharat S. Efficacy, safety concern and disposal practices followed for expired drug preparations among medical personnel. Eur J Biomed Pharm Sci. 2015;2(1):463-5.
16. Simons FE, GU X, Simons KJ. Outdated EpiPen and EpiPen Jr auto injectors: past their prime? J Allergy Clin Immunol. 2000; 105:1025-30.
17. Cantrell L, Suchard JR, Wu A, Gerona RR. Stability of active ingredients in long-expired prescription medications. Arch Intern Med. 2012;172(21):1685-7.
18. Drugs past their expiration date. Med Lett Drugs Ther. 2015;57(1483):164-5.
19. FDA. How to Safely Dispose of Unused or Expired Medicine. [online] Available from: https://www.fda.gov/drugs/safe-disposal-medicines/disposal-unused-medicines-what-you-should-know. [Last accessed December, 2023].
20. Radley DC, Finkelstein SN, Stafford RS. Off-label prescribing among office-based physicians. Arch Intern Med. 2006; 166(9):1021-6.
21. Shah SS, Hall M, Goodman DM, Feuer P, Sharma V, Fargason C Jr, et al. Off-label drug use in hospitalized children. Arch Pediatr Adolesc Med. 2007;161(3):282-90.
22. Qureshi ZP, Liu Y, Sartor O, Chu YH, Bennett CL. Enforcement actions involving Medicaid fraud and abuse, 1996-2009. Arch Intern Med. 2011;171(8):785-7.
23. Lat I, Micek S, Janzen J, Cohen H, Olsen K, Haas C. Off-label medication use in adult critical care patients. J Crit Care. 2011;26(1):89-94.
24. Friedman WF, Hirschklau MJ, Printz MP, Pitlick PT, Kirkpatrick SE. Pharmacologic closure

of patent ductus arteriosus in the premature infant. N Engl J Med. 1976;295(10):526-9.
25. Stafford RS. Regulating off-label drug use: rethinking the role of the FDA. N Engl J Med. 2008;358(14):1427-9.
26. Riley JB Jr, Basilius PA. Physicians' liability for off-label prescriptions. Nephrol News Issues. 2007;21(7):43-4, 46-7.
27. Wilkes M, Johns M. Informed consent and shared decision making: a requirement to disclose to patients off-label prescriptions. PLoS Med. 2008;5(11):1553-6.
28. Gota V, Divatia JV. Off-label use of drugs: an evil or a necessity? Indian J Anaesth. 2015; 59(12):767.
29. Canterbury versus Spence, 464 F2d 772 (DC Cir 1972).
30. Klein versus Biscup, 109 Ohio App3d 855 (Ohio Ct App 1996).
31. State Board of Registration for the Healing Arts versus McDonagh, 123 SW3d 146 (Mo 2003).
32. Pirozzi versus Blue Cross-Blue Shield, 741 F. Supp. 586, 590 (D. Va. 1990).
33. Rheims S, Cucherat M, Arzimanoglou A, Ryvlin P. Greater response to placebo in children than in adults: a systematic review and meta-analysis in drug-resistant partial epilepsy. PLoS Med. 2008;5(8):e166.
34. Available from: http://www.research.uci.edu/Placebo Controlled Studies.htm. Last accessed on 9.11.2023
35. EMEA European Guidelines, 2008.
36. 2000 (1) CPR 405 (Uttar Pradesh SCDRC).
37. Kum Sakshi Satyajeet S versus Ashwini Prasad Hospital (MSCDRC): 2013(4) CLT 169: 2013(10) R.C.R. (Civil) 640.

SUGGESTED READING

1. Baldwa M, Baldwa V, Padvi N, Baldwa S. Legal Issues in Critical Care, 1st edition. New Delhi: CBS Publishers and Distributors Pvt. Ltd.; 2022.
2. Baldwa M, Baldwa V, Padvi N, Baldwa S. Legal Issues in Medical Practice, 2nd edition. New Delhi: CBS Publishers and Distributors Pvt. Ltd.; 2023.

Legalities in Developmental Pediatrics

Samir Hasan Dalwai, Atanu Bhadra, Abraham Paul, Pranjal Agarwal

Keywords: Developmental disabilities, Developmental disorders, Developmental pediatrics, Persons with disabilities

Aim: Healthcare providers in developmental pediatrics can adeptly navigate legal considerations and uphold ethical principles to manage the intricate medical and social facets of child development, ensuring optimal care for their patients.

Objective: In developmental pediatrics, a niche medical domain addressing developmental disorders in children, healthcare providers face a spectrum of legal considerations intricately tied to the ethical and social complexities of child development. Navigating these involves deftly managing issues such as informed consent, maintaining the delicate equilibrium between respecting patient autonomy, and fulfilling legal obligations.

■ INTRODUCTION

While it is commonly misunderstood that delving into the intricacies of law is a burdensome endeavor, it is crucial for doctors to recognize that the legal domain is more rational than one might initially perceive. Just as physicians readily go the extra mile for their patients in the medical realm, a similar commitment is required when navigating the complexities of the law. Both fields demand a dedicated pursuit of justice and well-considered actions in the interest of those being served.

To illustrate, one of the authors, a member of the Expert Panel of the Maharashtra State Commission for Protection of Child Rights in 2013 was called upon to assist in the case of a child with autism spectrum disorder. The facts of the case are that the parents of this child were asked by the school to remove their child from the school and seek admission in a special school as they thought the child was a threat to himself and others due to this condition. The parents approached the Courts against the school and also the Maharashtra State Commission for Protection of Child Rights. He was appointed as the Chairperson of the Committee to study the matter and provide a report to the Commission. After a few months of clinical observation as well as participating in the Commissions proceedings, the Commission accepted the Committee's report and issued an order reinstating the child in school with a Shadow Teacher.[1] The Commission's report along with the Committee's recommendations were accepted by the Hon'ble High Court of Bombay and a similar order in line with the Commission's order was duly passed by the Court. The impact of this order was that not only children with special needs could not be arbitrarily removed from schools by the management, but Shadow Teachers could be legally appointed to assist the child.

CHAPTER 20: Legalities in Developmental Pediatrics

Given their distinctive role in society, doctors have the potential to serve as invaluable advocates for children with developmental disabilities, championing their rights and aiding in their integration into the fabric of society. This chapter endeavors to acquaint readers with key legal provisions that are essential for doctors to grasp, thereby enhancing their comprehension of the legal landscape surrounding special-needs children. While legal disputes pertaining to negligence and other issues are addressed elsewhere in this book, the focus here is on providing doctors with the necessary knowledge to navigate the legal framework in the specific context of developmental disabilities.

LAW AND CHILDREN WITH DEVELOPMENTAL DISABILITIES

Over the past three decades, India has witnessed significant advancements in the legal framework concerning the well-being of individuals with special needs. Prior to these developments, the absence of a robust legal system subjected parents of children with special needs to emotional, economic, and practical hardships, hindering their ability to secure the legal rights of their children.

In response to these challenges, the Indian Parliament took a commendable step by enacting the Mental Health Act of 1987. While this legislation marked a positive beginning, it fell short of offering a comprehensive legal recourse for individuals in need. The Act, though addressing mental health concerns, inadequately tackled the pervasive stigma associated with mental illness and left considerable gaps in providing redressal for individuals with various other disabilities.

Recognizing these limitations, the Indian legislature embarked on a transformative journey spanning three decades. The objective was to adopt a modern, scientific, and humanitarian approach to address the multifaceted needs of society. Consequently, a series of legislative measures were introduced to bridge the gaps and create a legal framework that aligns with contemporary values.

These legislative interventions reflect a commitment to empowering individuals with special needs, aiming to facilitate their pursuit of an independent and successful life. The overarching goal is to establish a comprehensive support system through public institutions, ensuring that the legal framework not only protects but also promotes the well-being and autonomy of individuals with special needs.[2]

LAWS RELATED TO CHILDREN WITH DEVELOPMENTAL DISORDERS IN INDIA

The Indian legal regime seeks to protect the rights of persons with both specific and general disabilities.

Legal rights and remedies related to children with developmental disorders are provided in multiple places.[3] These include:
- Constitution of India
- Family law
- Health law
- Education law
- Succession law
- Guardianship law
- Income tax law
- Various Special Acts of Parliament:
  - The Persons with Disabilities (PWD) Act, 1995
  - The Mental Health Act, 1987
  - The Rehabilitation Council of India, 1992
  - The National Trust for Welfare of Persons with Autism, Cerebral Palsy
  - Mental Retardation, and Multiple Disabilities Act, 1999

The Safeguards in the Constitution for Children with Disabilities

- Article 15(1) enjoins on the Government not to discriminate against any citizen of India (including disabled) on the ground of religion, race, caste, sex or place of birth.
- Article 15(2) states that no citizen (including the disabled) shall be subjected to any disability, liability, restriction in the matter of their access to shops, public restaurants, hotels and places of public entertainment.
- There shall be equality of opportunity for all citizens (including the disabled) in matters relating to employment or appointment to any office.
- Every disabled person can move the Supreme Court of India to enforce his fundamental rights.
- The right to move the Supreme Court is itself guaranteed by Article 32.

Educational Law and Children with Disabilities

- The right to education is available to all citizens including the disabled.
- Article 29(2) of the Constitution provides that no citizen shall be denied admission into any educational institution maintained by the State or receiving aid out of State funds on the ground of religion, race, caste, or language.
- Article 45 of the Constitution directs the State to provide free and compulsory education for all children (including the disabled) until they attain the age of 14 years.

Health Law and Children with Disabilities

The health laws of India have many provisions for the disabled, largely included under the Mental Health Act, 1987.

Succession Law and Children with Disabilities

- The Hindu Succession Act, 1956, specifically provides that physical disability or physical deformity would not disentitle a person from inheriting ancestral property.
- Similarly, in the Indian Succession Act, 1925 which applies in the case of intestate and testamentary succession, there is no provision which deprives the disabled from inheriting an ancestral property.
- The position with regard to Parsis and the Muslims is the same.

Guardianship Laws

The Hon'ble Supreme Court of India states that a guardian is, *"a person invested with the power, and charged with the duty, of taking care of the person, managing the property and rights of another person, who, for defect of age, understanding, or self-control, is considered incapable of administering his/her own affairs"*.[4]

While the attributes of a guardian form an important part of a guardianship application, the Hon'ble apex Court has held that paramount consideration must be given to the welfare of the child, taking into account not only the child's ordinary contentment, health, education, intellectual development, and favorable surroundings, but also physical comforts, and moral and ethical values.[5]

The existence of an appropriate mechanism becomes even more necessary in cases of guardianship of individuals with special needs, so that parents, siblings, or relatives can continue making decisions on behalf of the individual, even after he/she/they attain the age of majority.

Income Tax Laws and Children with Disabilities

- *Section 80 DD*: This provides for a deduction in respect of the expenditure incurred by an individual on the medical treatment (including nursing), training and rehabilitation, etc., of handicapped dependents up to a limit of ₹20,000/-.
- *Section 80 V:* This ensures that the parent in whose hands income of a permanently disabled minor has been clubbed under Section 64, is allowed to claim a deduction up to ₹20,000/-.
- *Section 88B:* This provides for an additional rebate from the net tax payable by a resident individual who has attained the age of 65 years. The rebate has been increased from 10 to 20% in the cases where the gross total income does not exceed ₹75,000/-.

The Persons with Disabilities (Equal Opportunities, Protection of Rights and Full Participation) Act, 1995

- This Act ensures equal opportunities for the people with disabilities and their full participation in the nation building.
- Provides for both the preventive and promotional aspects of rehabilitation like education, employment and vocational training, reservation, research and manpower development, creation of barrier-free environment, rehabilitation of persons with disability, unemployment allowance for the disabled, special insurance scheme for the disabled employees, and establishment of homes for persons with severe disability.

Provisions of the Act Related to Children

- Prevention and early detection of disabilities
- Education
- Employment
- Nondiscrimination
- Research and manpower development
- Affirmative action
- Social security
- Grievance redressal.

Education Law

- Every child with disability shall have the rights to free education till the age of 18 years in integrated schools or special schools.
- Appropriate transportation, removal of architectural barriers, and restructuring of modifications in the examination system shall be ensured for the benefit of children with disabilities.
- Children with disabilities shall have the right to free books, scholarships, uniform, and other learning material.
- Special schools for children with disabilities shall be equipped with vocational training facilities.
- Nonformal education shall be promoted for children with disabilities.
- Teachers' training institutions shall be established to develop requisite manpower.
- Parents may move to an appropriate forum for the redressal of grievances regarding the placement of their children with disabilities.

Equal before Law

- Public building, rail compartments, buses, ships, and aircrafts will be designed to give easy access to the disabled people.
- In all public places and in waiting rooms, the toilets shall be wheel chair accessible. Braille and sound symbols are also to be provided in all elevators (lifts).
- All the places of public utility shall be made barrier-free by providing the ramps.

The Mental Health Act, 1987

- A right to be admitted, treated, and cared in a psychiatric hospital or psychiatric nursing home or convalescent home established or maintained by the Government or any other person for the treatment and care of mentally ill persons (other than the general hospitals or nursing homes of the Government).
- Even mentally ill prisoners and minors have a right of treatment as above.
- Minors under the age of 16 years, persons addicted to alcohol or other drugs which lead to behavioral changes, and those convicted of any offence are entitled to admission, treatment, and care in separate psychiatric hospitals or nursing homes established or maintained by the Government.

The Rehabilitation Council of India Act, 1992

This Act ensures the good quality of services rendered by various rehabilitation personnel as mentioned here:

- To have the right to be served by trained and qualified rehabilitation professionals whose names are borne on the Register maintained by the Council.
- To have the guarantee of maintenance of minimum standards of education required for recognition of rehabilitation qualification by universities or institutions in India.

The National Trust for Welfare of Persons with Autism, Cerebral Palsy, Mental Retardation and Multiple Disabilities Act, 1999

- The Central Government has the obligation to set up, in accordance with this Act, the National Trust for Welfare of Persons with Autism, Cerebral Palsy, Mental Retardation and Multiple Disability at New Delhi.
- The National Trust has to ensure that the objects for which it has been set up as enshrined in Section 10 of this Act have to be fulfilled.
- To make arrangements for an adequate standard of living of any beneficiary named in any request received by it, and to provide financial assistance to the registered organizations for carrying out any approved program for the benefit of disabled.
- Disabled persons have the right to be placed under guardianship appointed by the "Local Level Committees" in accordance with the provisions of the Act. The guardians so appointed will have the obligation to be responsible for the disabled person and their property and required to be accountable for the same.

Laws Related to Violence Against Children

Violence takes place in all settings: At home, school, childcare institutions, work, and in the community. Often violence is perpetrated by someone known to the child. The child protection legislation for children is established in four main laws:

1. The Juvenile Justice (Care and Protection) Act (2000, amended in 2015)
2. The Prohibition of Child Marriage Act (2006)
3. The Protection of Children from Sexual Offences Act (2012, amended in 2019)
4. The Child Labor (Prohibition and Regulation) Act (1986, amended in 2016).

Notable efforts have been made to set up fast track courts and deal with cybercrime against children.

CONCLUSION

In the dynamic landscape where ethical and legal standards in health care are in a perpetual state of evolution, practitioners in developmental pediatrics must engage in a continuous process of scrutinizing and enhancing their methodologies. This necessitates the seamless integration of contemporary guidelines into the fabric of informed consent procedures, the agile adaptation of assessment and intervention methodologies to harmonize with evolving ethical considerations, and a vigilant awareness of emerging legal prerequisites. This proactive approach ensures that healthcare providers in developmental pediatrics not only remain compliant with prevailing standards but also proactively contribute to the advancement and refinement of ethical and legal practices in their field.

LEARNING KEY POINTS

Key learning points for dealing with developmental disabilities:
- *Caution in diagnosis:* Label developmental problems cautiously; thorough assessments and documentation are essential.
- *Comprehensive care:* Avoid overlooking other medical conditions in children with developmental disabilities; provide comprehensive healthcare.
- *Stay informed:* Keep updated on relevant laws to effectively assist and advise parents of children with special needs.

TAKE-HOME MESSAGES

The Constitution of India and various Acts have addressed the issue of and provided relief to children with developmental disabilities. An adequate working knowledge of the same and fortifying the care of children with developmental disorders with appropriate documentation and certification would go a long way in enabling these children. Hence, get proper documentation and certification done to the advantage of child having developmental problems.

MUST AVOID THINGS

Resist the impulse to shun proper protocols and legalities while dealing with children with developmental concerns.

DO NOT DO

Do not treat beyond one's knowledge and skill.

WARNINGS

Do not brush away other medical conditions or comorbidities in children with developmental problems. For instance, a child with autism may have an acute abdominal perforation or acute tonsillitis or dental caries that needs medical care.

MESSAGES WHICH THE READER MUST BE AWARE

Doctors with their unique position in society can be excellent and much needed advocates for children with developmental disabilities, fighting for their rights and helping them achieve their rightful position in society.

MUST DO THING

Refer developmental problems to appropriate specialist with appropriate documentation.

MEDICAL NEGLIGENCE PEARLS

- Never label developmental problems without appropriate documentation and/or evaluations.
- Never overlook other medical conditions and comorbidities in children with developmental disabilities.

ONLY ONE FACT TO REMEMBER

It is always beneficial to keep oneself updated with these laws in order to help or offer advice to parents of children with special needs.

REFERENCES

1. Sarkar A. (2013). Panel asks Jamnabai to allow autistic kid to continue school. Mumbai Mirror. [online] Available from: https://mumbaimirror.indiatimes.com/mumbai/other/panel-asks-jamnabai-to-allow-autistic-kid-to-continue-school/articleshow/24641185.cms?utm_source=contentofinterest&utm_medium=text&utm_campaign=cppst [Last accessed December, 2023].
2. Sharma A, Singh V. Guardianship of Individuals with Special Needs: India's Evolving Legal Regime. 2023. SCC OnLine Blog Exp 37. [online] Available from: https://www.scconline.com/blog/post/2023/04/24/guardianship-of-individuals-with-special-needs-indias-evolving-legal-regime/ [Last accessed December, 2023].
3. Vikaspedia. Legal rights of the disabled in India. [online] Available from: https://vikaspedia.in/education/parents-corner/guidelines-for-parents-of-children-with-disabilities/legal-rights-of-the-disabled-in-india#:~:text=Appropriate%20transportation%2C%20removal%20of%20architectural,uniform%20and%20other%20learning%20material [Last accessed December, 2023].
4. Roxann Sharma v. Arun Sharma, (2015) 8 SCC 318 (5).
5. Gaurav Nagpal v. Sumedha Nagpal, (2009) 1 SCC 42.

SUGGESTED READING

1. Baldwa M, Baldwa V, Padvi N, Baldwa S (Eds). Legal Issues in Medical Practice, 2nd edition, 2 volume set. New Delhi, India: CBS Publishers & Distributors Pvt Ltd.; 2023.

CHAPTER 21

Medicolegal Aspects for Pediatric Surgery

Mahesh Baldwa, Namita Padvi, Varsha Baldwa, Sushila Baldwa

Pediatric surgeon should have sharp eyes to observe, soft hands to operate, and a lion's heart to care for pediatric patient.

Keywords: Anesthesia fitness, Expertise of super-specialty, Indemnity policies, Pediatric surgeon, Qualifications and skills

Aim: Medicolegal considerations are an integral part of pediatric surgery practice in India. By understanding the legal framework, maintaining proper documentation, adhering to the standard of care, and practicing open communication, pediatric surgeons can minimize the risk of legal complications and provide safe and effective care for their young patients.

Objective: Pediatric surgery is a specialized branch of medicine that deals with the surgical care of infants, children, and adolescents. While it is a rewarding field, it also carries significant medicolegal implications. In India, where the legal framework governing medical practice is evolving, understanding these aspects is crucial for pediatric surgeons to practice safely and effectively.

INTRODUCTION

Every person is prone to making mistakes, and making errors is a natural part of being human so are pediatric surgeons. Even the most reputable, knowledgeable, and experienced pediatric physicians and surgeons can face unexpected complications or delays in diagnosing and treating patients. Occasionally, unusual changes in the progression of a disease or unexpected anatomical variations can catch pediatric surgeons off guard, leading to challenging situations and alterations in the usual surgical procedures. In some cases, the family of a child patient may interpret these situations as negligence.[1,2]

QUALIFICATIONS AND SKILLS OF PEDIATRIC SURGEONS

Continuous updating of knowledge and equipment, as well as the retention of certificates by filing them properly from conferences, seminars, workshops, and similar events, is essential. Holding a recognized degree, MCh in Pediatric Surgery, recognized by the National Medical Commission (NMC) is crucial.

QUALIFICATIONS, SKILLS, AND EXPERTISE OF SUPERSPECIALTY PEDIATRIC SURGEONS

Super-specialty pediatric surgeons specializing in areas such as cardiac, neuro, urology, and gastro surgery, along with their respective teams, must possess a high level of expertise within their field, surpassing that of general pediatric surgeons. Legal expectations dictate that super-specialty pediatric surgeons deliver a more advanced and refined level of medical care, commensurate with their claim of super-specialization. The law courts require anticipatedly a higher degree of expertise from these super-specialty practitioners.

INDEMNITY POLICIES FOR SURGEONS AND ANESTHETISTS

Surgeons, across all surgical specialties, including anesthesiologists, face a higher susceptibility to litigation. As a result, they are required to pay a premium for their professional indemnity coverage that is 3 times higher than that of physicians. You can find a more comprehensive discussion of this topic in Chapter 25.

APPROPRIATELY EQUIPPED HOSPITAL/DAY CARE CLINICS

The surgical needs for various pediatric procedures differ significantly, ranging from minor day care surgeries such as abscess drainage, circumcision, fissure and fistula treatment, hydrocele repair, to moderate surgeries such as pyloric stenosis correction, hernia repair, appendectomy, and laparotomy. Complex procedures such as diaphragmatic hernia repair and the correction of anogenital malformations demand advanced anesthetic and surgical equipment in a sequential or parallel manner. Furthermore, specialized fields within pediatric surgery, such as pediatric cardiac surgery, pediatric urology, and pediatric orthopedic surgery, require specific and distinct sets of equipment and instruments. Even the setup for laparoscopic surgeries in day care facilities differs from that needed for minor surgeries. Therefore, the selection of a healthcare facility should align with the specific requirements of the pediatric surgical procedure in question.

Equipment, Gases, Drugs, and Blood

Ensure that all systems and equipment are in good working order and that you have competent and qualified personnel available. Check the functionality of equipment such as oxygen supply, pulse oximeter, Boyle's apparatus, suction apparatus, cautery tools, alternative power sources such as generators or inverters, and other necessary gadgets. It is important to book blood and blood products that may be required. Always perform a double check to verify the accuracy of labels on drugs, blood products, including blood group and expiry dates, to prevent errors.

Indication for Surgery

The pediatric surgeon evaluates the necessity of surgical intervention and discusses with the child's family why surgery is the most suitable course of action. Informed consent is obtained from the child's family. They should be informed about the expected duration of the surgery, the current surgical condition, potential benefits, and any potential post-surgical improvements or deteriorations namely complications. Ensuring a valid indication for any surgical procedure is a fundamental requirement. Performing surgery without a proper indication can lead to challenges for the pediatric surgeon.[1-3]

Anesthesia Fitness

The anesthetist must assess the pediatric patient's suitability for anesthesia through a preanesthetic examination. This involves gathering information about any prior surgeries, drug allergies, as well as any existing conditions related to the liver, kidneys, heart, and lungs. Additionally, the anesthetist conducts a clinical evaluation of the patient and reviews various reports, including blood tests, bleeding time and clotting time, renal function tests, liver function tests, electrocardiogram, and chest X-rays, among others. In a male child, one should avoid halogenated gas anesthesia with succinylcholine if malignant hyperthermia is one of the complications one wants to avoid.

Pediatric Physician Fitness/Clearance

The pediatric physician assesses the patient's fitness and provides clearance by reviewing various factors. These include the patient's surgical history, drug allergies, and the presence of any liver, kidney, heart, or lung conditions, as well as the control of any concurrent comorbidities such as asthma, seizures, bleeding tendencies, or jaundice. The pediatric physician conducts a clinical examination of the child patient and recommends specific tests, ideally to be completed within 2–7 days before clearing the patient for surgery. These tests may include a complete blood count, white blood cell (WBC) count (total and differential), platelet count, urinalysis, prothrombin time (PT), partial thromboplastin time (PTT) or bleeding/clotting time, chest X-ray, pulmonary function tests (PFTs), serum creatinine or renal function tests, serum glutamic-pyruvic transaminase (SGPT) or liver function tests, and an electrocardiogram. Additional tests such as human immunodeficiency virus (HIV) testing (following patient and family counseling guidelines) and screening for hepatitis B and C may also be considered.

Planned Pediatric Surgical Procedure

It is advisable to delay a scheduled pediatric surgical procedure until any underlying illness or metabolic issues, created by any infections, asthma, or fluid-electrolyte imbalances, are adequately managed or corrected before surgery.

Emergency Pediatric Surgical Procedure

An emergency pediatric surgical procedure refers to a critical situation in which a surgical intervention is necessary to save the child's life. Examples include emergencies such as the rupture of the spleen, where internal bleeding cannot be controlled without a splenectomy. Other life-threatening emergencies include testicular torsion and obstructed hernias.

Identification of Child Patient

Confirming the identity of a pediatric patient is crucial in healthcare settings. In a smaller pediatric hospital, for children aged ≥4 years, staff may verbally verify the patient's identity before surgery and cross-check this information with the documents provided. In larger hospitals, it is advisable to establish patient identity using wristbands or QR/barcoding before the patient enters the operating room. This practice helps prevent the occurrence of incorrect surgeries on the wrong patients.

Marking of Surgical Site and Side of Operation

Before proceeding with the actual surgery, it is essential to mark the surgical site and the correct side of the operation on the child patient's body using ink marker pen.

This marking should be confirmed by cross-referencing with the patient's medical records to prevent any errors in performing the surgery on the wrong site or side of the child patient.

Precounseling and Communication Prior to Obtaining Consent

Effective and thorough communication with both the child and their parents or guardians is crucial. It is essential to engage in a detailed discussion about the advantages and disadvantages of the chosen pediatric surgical procedure, all while maintaining a balanced approach that does not unnecessarily increase anxiety. It is important to avoid making absolute assurances of 100% cure, as there are no guarantees against surgical complications or recurrences. Furthermore, the expected cost of the surgery should be transparently discussed with material risks from patient point of view, for example, disability causing blindness, lameness, etc., along with the need for potential blood transfusions. Before a larger child patient, their parents, or an authorized individual signs the written consent, the contents of the consent form should be reviewed thoroughly. This process should involve at least 2 witnesses. In complex or challenging nonemergency situations, such as the removal of digits, testes, amputations, eye evisceration, or the removal of a diseased kidney, seeking an additional opinion from a pediatric surgical colleague is advisable.

Consent

Obtaining informed consent is an integral aspect of pediatric surgical management. It is important to note that a valid consent obtained by competent patient party does not absolve the need for due care and necessary precautions. It should never be seen as a justification for any negligence on part of support staff or as a way to bypass infrastructure deficiencies. Failing to obtain written consent is a clear lapse in the responsibilities of a pediatric doctor.

Detailed information about consent and related concepts can be found in Chapters 5 and 6.

At a minimum, the consent form should include the names of the pediatric surgeon and anesthetist, the name of chosen procedure, a discussion of its benefits and associated risks or limitations, as well as any common and known material complications. Additionally, alternative methods from patient point of view should be discussed, such as conservative versus operative treatment for conditions such as acute appendicitis, tracheoesophageal fistulas, pyloric stenosis, diaphragmatic hernia, or anogenital anomalies, as appropriate to the case.

Resurgery or 2–3 stage surgery requires fresh new consent each time: For subsequent surgeries or multiple stages of a surgical procedure, it is recommended to obtain a new and updated fresh consent for each additional stage or any modifications to the surgical plan.

Refusal of Your Advice Needs to be Documented

It is essential to record any instance where a patient or their parents decline or refuse medical advice. The refusal should be documented in the outpatient department (OPD) or inpatient department (IPD) records, as well as in the discharge case document or sheet. This documentation should include the signatures of the patient's parents and 2 witnesses. This practice is to avoid situation

CHAPTER 21: Medicolegal Aspects for Pediatric Surgery

like in Kerala High Court ruling in the case of Dr TT Thomas versus Smt Elisa and Others on 11 August 1986, as cited in I (1987) ACC 445 and AIR 1987 Ker 52.[4] (see below in case laws).

Emergency Surgery

In situations requiring immediate life-saving surgery, such as roadside accidents, it is imperative not to delay treatment while waiting for consent or any other prior formalities in hospital such as depositing of money, filling form, etc. Prioritizing life-saving measures in emergencies takes precedence over legal prerequisites, guided by the fundamental principle of acting in "good faith." This principle is supported by the ruling of the National Consumer Disputes Redressal in the case of Pravat Kumar Mukherjee versus Ruby General Hospital and Others on 25 April 2005, Parmanand Katara versus Union of India and Ors. Citations: 1989 Air 2039, 1989 Scr (3) 997, 1989 Scc (4) 286, Jt 1989 (3) 496 1989 Scale (2) 380, Paschim Banga Khet Mazdoor Samity and Ors. versus State of West Bengal (1995 3 SCC 42).

Documents are Irrefutable Evidence and Defense

The significance of comprehensive documentation is extensively discussed in Chapters 3 and 4.

Well-maintained documents serve as your primary support in the event of a medicolegal crisis. Conversely, inadequate documentation leads to weak evidence and defense, and the absence of documentation equates to no evidence or defense whatsoever.

It is imperative to thoroughly document case history; clinical examinations; investigative reports; consent forms; fitness certificates or assessment notes from pediatricians, surgeons, and pediatric anesthetists; anesthesia records; and drug administration details, including doses, records of gases employed, and volumes of intravenous fluids or blood administered. Additionally, meticulous records of vital signs, such as temperature, pulse rate, and blood pressure, input and output charts, and notes regarding pediatric surgical procedures performed are essential.

Operative notes should encompass a comprehensive range of details, including the time of arrival and departure from the operating theater, the patient's level of consciousness during transfer to the recovery room, intensive care unit (ICU), or ward, intravenous access details (site, initiation time, solution administered, etc.), aseptic techniques utilized, incision specifics, procedural findings, the use of prostheses or implants, specimens sent for histopathology or culture, irrigation solutions employed, the presence of drains or catheters, wound closure and dressing procedures, any unusual events or complications encountered, and the subsequent steps taken. These documents must be meticulously maintained, ensuring they are clean, clear, chronological, correct, comprehensive, and complete. Additionally, all paperwork, including reports, X-rays, CT scans, and referral notes, should be part of the documentation. Operative notes should include:

- Time of arrival and departure from operation theater and condition of transfer to recovery room/ICU/ward
- Level of consciousness at the time of such a transfer
- IV—site, time started, solution given, etc.
- Asepsis–chemical and the method used
- Incision details
- Procedural details and findings
- Prosthesis and implants

- Specimens of tissue, cultures, etc. sent
- Irrigation solution used
- Drains, catheters, etc.
- Closure of wound; dressing
- Any unusual event or complication and further step taken
- Document must be clean, clear, chronological, correct, comprehensive, and complete
- All the paper work along with reports, X-rays, computed tomography (CT) scans, etc. and referral notes form document.

According to legal requirements, IPD documents must be preserved for a minimum of 3 years. Following the NMC 2019 guidelines approved by the Medical Council of India (MCI), this duration applies to the pediatric age group as well. Optionally, individual pediatric surgeons may choose to maintain documents though not mandatory up to the child's age of 21 (3 years after reaching majority at 18 years) for added security. While not mandatory, in medicolegal cases involving accidents, head injuries, child abuse, etc., it is advisable to retain records for up to 30 years to safeguard the surgeon/physician. However, it is not legally obligatory or mandatory.

Documents serve as a reflection of the actions and conduct taken (or not taken) to fulfill the legal duty of care and cautions along with consent. It is often said that documents speak for themselves very loud and clear. Documents are considered to challenge substituted evidence of res ipsa loquitur, particularly in cases involving foreign objects left in the body. The documents show careful medical care provided by pediatric physicians, surgeons, and anesthetists to child patients. Medical care given should be accurately documented in OPD, IPD, and discharge records, as well as in other documents, serving as written evidence to ensure a strong defense in a court of law or in cases of sudden, unexpected deaths, such as those occurring during surgery or on the operating table.

Unforgivable Errors

Certain mistakes are considered unpardonable in the field of pediatric surgery. Leaving items such as mops, swabs, artery forceps, or cannula tips inside a patient's abdomen or body is legally indefensible, as the principle of res ipsa loquitur applies. Failing to achieve effective hemostasis, removing the wrong organ, or performing surgery on the wrong side is also regarded as negligence and speaks for itself—res ipsa loquitur in terms of liability.

Calm and Considerate Approach

A confident, reassuring, composed, and unhurried demeanor is vital when caring for child patients. Pediatric physicians and surgeons must convey their genuine concern for the welfare of the child patient through both their verbal and nonverbal communication and approach. Even when the prognosis may be uncertain or unfavorable, it is crucial to explain the situation compassionately using effective communication skills when addressing the parents of the child patient. Detailed information on communication skills is provided in Chapter 2.

Postoperative Care

The care provided to pediatric patients after surgery is just as critical as the surgical procedure itself. Attention to detail is essential in areas such as wound care, nutrition, administration of antibiotics, pain management, and maintenance of fluid balance. These aspects should be thoroughly documented in the pediatric patient's medical records, including OPD and IPD records, discharge cards, and case sheets, with comprehensive notes.

A well-documented discharge card should include detailed instructions regarding further care and management, as well as information about follow-up appointments. Such documentation serves as evidence of the pediatric surgeon's diligence and commitment to the patient's well-being.

It is crucial not to conceal or minimize mishaps, complications, failures, or recurrences from the patient's family or when recording them in medical documents. The disclosure of all adverse events in OPD/IPD records, discharge cards, or case sheets is not only ethically responsible but also serves as a clear and transparent explanation. This documentation practice is generally well-received by the judiciary and helps establish a record of honest and responsible medical care.

Pediatric Surgical Care More Important than Surgical Cure

It is imperative not to categorize pediatric surgery as either "Minor" or "Major." Mishaps can occur in what are often referred to as minor surgeries, possibly due to reduced vigilance or an assumption of simplicity. In reality, the surgical theater's equipment and personnel must remain current and alert, regardless of the perceived complexity of the procedure.

The pediatric anesthetist is an integral part of the surgical team. While the patient may not have directly selected the anesthetist and typically receives anesthesia at the recommendation of the pediatric surgeon, there is no master-servant relationship involved. The anesthetist is an independent specialist governed by their own knowledge, skill, and experience and is not under the control of the pediatric surgeon. Consequently, the anesthetist bears separate liability and accountability for their competence and actions, as highlighted in the case of Karam Veer Singh versus Garg Nursing Home (MPSCDRC), 2007 (3) C.P.J. 131.[5]

A recovery room or an equivalent facility is essential to provide careful monitoring of the patient as they emerge from the effects of anesthesia. This environment is conducive to the prevention of potential issues such as falls, extravasations, and airway obstructions, especially when overseen by an anesthesiologist.

By adhering to these guidelines, one can navigate the challenging waters of the increasing number of medicolegal cases with confidence and ensure a smoother journey.

Congenital heart disease—death—no negligence

P.S. Karunakar versus Narayana Hrudayalaya (KSCDRC) (Bangalore), 2007(2) C.P.J. 363:2007(53) R.C.R.(Civil), Appeal No. 955 of 2005. D/d. 19.1.2007[6]

A 16-month-old child with a heart defect could not undergo surgery due to an unstable health condition and sadly passed away. Negligence was alleged, but the evidence on record indicates that the hospital (OP-1) provided the best available treatment and conducted numerous tests. No negligence was established, and the complaint was rightfully dismissed. The appeal has also been dismissed.

Intussusception and Meckel's diverticulum, surgery not responsible for missing kidney— Ultrasonologists are liable for their casual approach while reporting the USG (ultrasonogram) in reporting missing left kidney

Master Hari Om Sharma (Minor) versus Indraprastha Apollo Hospital, (NCDRC), 2023 (2) C.P.R. 183:2023(2) C.P.J. 487, Consumer Case No. 381 of 2013. D/d. 29.03.2023[7]

Alleged due to the negligent removal of a minor's kidney without the consent of the complainant's parents sought compensation of ₹1.55 crore. The child underwent surgery at the age of 5 years for intussusception and Meckel's diverticulum. It is medically impossible to remove the left kidney from an incision in the right iliac fossa. Allegedly ultrasonologists were negligent in not reporting missing left kidney. While medical negligence is not, a mere lack of care, an error in judgment, or an accidental occurrence does not necessarily constitute proof of negligence on the part of a medical professional.

Nonreferral of birth defect of "Imperforate anus" to pediatric surgeon

West Bengal State Consumer Disputes Redressal Commission, Dr Susmita Bhattacharya versus Marzina Bibi Alias Begum and Others on 16 September, 2022[8]

Opposite parties (OPs) No. 1 to 3 from which it can be ascertained that the newborn baby was examined by the pediatric doctor and that the child has "Imperforate anus" was brought to the notice of the complainant, which is adequate enough to prove collective negligence of the OPs. Respondents No. 2 and 3 have failed to give proper explanation as to why they kept the newborn baby endangering his life even after alleged detection of the birth anomaly. In case, if the patient party ignoring the referral given by the doctor and wants to stay with given treatment, in that event, the nursing home authorities must take a bond from the patient party, but surprisingly, no such document has been produced neither before this commission nor before the learned district forum. ₹19 lakhs was reduced to 18 lakhs.

Cleft palate surgery—vegetative state after anesthesia—negligence

Karam Veer Singh versus Garg Nursing Home (MPSCDRC), 2007(3) C.P.J. 131:2008(1) CLT 138:2007(1) CLT 319:2006(46) R.C.R. (Civil) 398, Original Case No. 88 of 2000. D/d. 21.9.2006[5]

Coma caused by anesthesia overdose in cleft palate surgery: 3 instances of negligence by respondents: First, for failing to conduct essential preoperative and preanesthetic tests; secondly, for performing the operation without any immediate emergency, despite the established medical knowledge that anesthesia can lead to adverse reactions in patients with recent respiratory tract infections; and thirdly, for not exercising due care in the administration of anesthesia. Due to this negligence, the child has entered a vegetative state with no potential for recovery, and therefore, the respondents were required to jointly or severally compensate the complainants with a sum of ₹3 lakh.

Acute abdomen due to subacute obstruction due to gallbladder empyema which left a scar on the abdomen can be construed as a case of medical negligence

Baby Preeti Goel (Minor) versus Batra Hospital & Medical Research Centre (NCDRC) 2007(2) All. LJ 578:2007(3) C.P.J. 133:2007(2) CLT 480:2006(38) R.C.R.(Civil) 599[9]

Preeti Goel was experiencing persistent fever and severe abdominal pain accompanied by distention, resulting in an abdominal girth of 49 cm. The child had been unwell for the past 10–12 days, displaying symptoms of fever, an overall ill appearance, tenderness in the right hypochondrium, and a palpable spleen. An abdominal surgery was performed by the surgeon due to the child's acute abdominal pain and prolonged fever, following certain tests, including an X-ray, which indicated subacute intestinal obstruction caused by gallbladder empyema. This procedure left a scar on the abdomen, prompting considerations of medical negligence. However, the answer to this question is no. A right paramedical incision was made, and upon exploration, peritoneal fluid was discovered. An AIIMS Medical Board report stated that there was no negligence in the management of the case. It is evident that the doctors and hospital authorities made all possible efforts to save the critically ill child. There was no evidence to suggest that the child experienced any relapse after the surgery, aside from the presence of a scar on the abdomen. Consequently, the complaint was dismissed since scar on the abdomen is not negligence, and the complainants were instructed to pay ₹10,000 as costs to the hospital for filing a baseless complaint.

14-02-2018, Private hospital had engaged a doctor as a pediatric surgeon, who possesses degrees like MS, but was not recognized West Bengal Medical Council

On February 14, 2018, a private hospital engaged a doctor as a pediatric surgeon, possessing degrees like MS but was not recognized by the West Bengal Medical Council (WBMC). The WBERC (West Bengal Clinical Establishment Regulatory Commission) imposed a fine of ₹10 lakh on the Calcutta Medical Research Institute (CMRI) after discovering irregularities. During the investigation, it was revealed that the private hospital had employed a doctor as a pediatric surgeon who had received training abroad and possessed degrees like MS, but did not hold a pediatric surgery degree recognized by the WBMC. This doctor had conducted 3 surgeries on a newborn with certain complications, including issues related to stool passage, over the span of a few months. Compensation is required to be paid in this case.[10]

Complex supravalvular defect in heart—operated—death—no negligence

Prafulla Kumar Das versus Apollo Hospitals (NCDRC). 2002(2) C.P.J. 106[11]

The child had a complex and uncommon form of congenital cardiac anomaly, suffering from a supravalvular defect and diffuse hypoplasia of the aortic arch. The medical team explained to the child's family that the more severe supravalvular defect could be surgically repaired, while the less amenable diffuse hypoplasia of the aortic arch would be left untreated. The surgery was successful, and the child was on a path to recovery, receiving appropriate care and attention. The family was informed that the child would need to return for a balloon dilation procedure to alleviate the obstruction in the remaining underdeveloped portion of the aorta. Dr Reddy had advised them to bring the child back in case of any issues. Unfortunately, when the child experienced pain on May 18, 1992, they could have brought the child to Madras for medical attention, which might have saved him. Complainant Das failed to substantiate any allegations of medical negligence, and there was no valid basis for the complaint. As a result, the complaint was dismissed.

Cataract surgery in a 3-year-old child—later developed eye cancer—no negligence

S. Nirmala versus Dr A Govindarajan Eye Hospital, (TNSCDRC) (Circuit Bench) (Madurai), F.A. No. 153 of 2013 (Against the order made in C.C. No. 132/2010, dated

08.05.2012 on the file of the District Forum, Tiruchirappalli) D/d. 20.7.2022[12]

In 2006, the child developed eye cancer in the left eye. However, there was no concrete proof to establish the existence of eye cancer at that relevant time. The child's subsequent cancer diagnosis cannot be used as evidence of its presence in 2006 itself. Therefore, the doctor who initially diagnosed cataract in 2006 and performed the removal procedure cannot be held responsible. The District Commission correctly concluded that there was no medical negligence by the OPs, a decision we also endorse. The child was treated by the second OP for a brief period and subsequently recovered. There was no medical negligence, neither in diagnosis nor in treatment. Consequently, the appeal is dismissed, affirming the District Commission's decision.

Meconium plug confused with anal canal atresia—no negligence

Mr Nandkishor Chhaganlal Shah versus Kashiba Gordhandas Patel Children Hospital & Jajodia Research Institute, (GSCDRC), Appeal No. 1038 of 2013. D/d. 26.04.2023[13]

The newborn did not pass stool for 17 hours, and Dr Shah admitted that the invertogram X-ray did not definitively confirm rectal atresia. Dr Chitralekha Dave, a pediatric surgeon, also examined the child before surgery but did not recommend additional tests, relying on the previous ones. She believed colostomy surgery was necessary and administered a colon wash after the procedure. Two days post the surgery, the child passed stool naturally, confirming there was no rectal atresia. Mr Shah argued that a confirmed diagnosis should have preceded surgery, especially since the child passed stool naturally, indicating surgery was unnecessary. He suggested that doctors should have considered the possibility of a meconium plug, which could have been treated with an enema without surgery. Dr Dave recommended a distal loopogram after the hospital discharge, which showed the intestinal tube was intact. Mr Shah contended that if this diagnostic procedure had been performed earlier, surgery might have been avoided. However, it was clarified that a distal loopogram is performed through the colostomy opening and requires colostomy surgery first. Thus, the doctors' actions were reasonable in discharging their duties. The doctors used their skills and considered various factors, including symptoms, medical history, and surrounding circumstances, which led them to believe rectal atresia was probable. Even if there was an error in judgment, it cannot be considered negligence warranting compensation. The doctors' actions align with medical science, and therefore, the appeal failed.

Appendicitis surgery without bothering about malaria—death—negligence

Mrs Ragini Premnath versus Dr Prema Shankar, on 24 November, 2009[14]

Shamitha, the complainant's daughter, was diagnosed with chronic appendicitis before her medical examinations in October 2001. Despite her fever and suspicion of malaria, the 2nd OP, a doctor, performed a nonemergency appendectomy. The surgery occurred in a poorly equipped hospital that rented equipment externally. An expert witness suggested that the surgery could have waited for blood test results to confirm malaria, as surgical procedures on malaria patients carry higher risks. After the surgery, Shamitha experienced complications, including stomach bleeding. The hospital's lack of proper infrastructure became evident when they could not provide a needed

CHAPTER 21: Medicolegal Aspects for Pediatric Surgery

ventilator due to all ventilator units being occupied. Tragically, these complications resulted in Shamitha's demise. The verdict found the 2nd OP (doctor) and the 3rd OP (hospital) negligent, and the complainant was awarded ₹5,00,000 in compensation from these parties, along with a 9% annual interest rate.

Pain in abdomen—no diagnosis—death—no negligence

Sri Jalandhar Shah versus ESI Hospital Diamond Harbour Road, (WBSCDRC) (Kolkata), Complaint Case No. CC/241 of 2013. D/d. 10.03.2023[15]

On February 9, 2013, at 11:00 AM, the complainant took her 6-year-old son, Abhijit Kumar Shah, to hospital no. 1 due to acute abdominal pain and vomiting. Dr Pritam Banerjee, the attending doctor, administered 2 injections and instructed the complainant to return if the symptoms persisted after 2 hours. When the child's condition did not improve, the complainant contacted Dr Banerjee, who referred Abhijit to the surgery department at 1:00 PM. Two days later, the child passed away.

The West Bengal Medical Council submitted a report stating that the cause of death was difficult to ascertain without a postmortem examination. The child had severe metabolic abnormalities, including electrolyte imbalances and elevated urea and creatinine levels, possibly due to dehydration from vomiting and abdominal pain. The report noted that acute appendicitis is challenging to diagnose quickly, and ultrasound is used as a screening test.

The Council also considered observations from an Enquiry Committee at ESIC, Joka, which pointed out poor documentation, lack of communication with specialists, and insufficient information provided to the patient's family. The Council ultimately concluded that while the patient may not have received optimal treatment due to the absence of a definitive diagnosis, there was no evidence of medical negligence. Therefore, the case was closed without any findings of negligence.

Not referring the child to higher burn center immediately after administration of preliminary treatment—negligence

Muthu Vijayan versus De Viswanathan M.S. (K.C.D.R.C.) (Thiruvananthapuram) 2012(1) C.P.J. 43:2012(2) CLT 556:2011(48) R.C.R. (Civil) 408, O.P. No. 50 of 2001. D/d. 5.11.2011[16]

The child suffered severe burn injuries and was initially treated at OP-2 hospital by doctor OP-1. However, the child's health deteriorated, leading to transfer to another hospital where surgery was performed. A compensation claim was filed based on the child's third-degree burns. Another doctor who treated the child at the second hospital stated that the burns were infected, showing signs of septicemia, and discoloration on the third day indicated wound infection. Third-degree burns are serious and warrant referral to a specialized burn center. OP's failure to promptly refer the child to such a center after initial treatment was a clear case of negligence.

A plastic surgeon confirmed that the treatment provided at OP-2 hospital did not meet standard practices. Compensation of ₹3,00,000 with 7% interest per annum was granted.

Cancel FIR filed against pediatric surgeon

On February 14, 2023, an additional sessions judge named Dheeraj Mor in Delhi reversed a previous order that had called for the cancellation of an FIR against a pediatric surgeon, Dr YK Sarin. Dr Sarin had been contesting a decision made by a Magistrate court.[17]

National Consumer Disputes Redressal Commission grants compensation of ₹1 crore to the parents who lost their only child in a corrective surgery for squint eye

Dr Reba Modak versus Sankara Nethralaya, (NCDRC) 2022(5) ALL MR 44:2022(4) C.P.J. 72:2023(2) Andh LD 23[18]

Severe medical negligence and service deficiency led to the tragic death of a 6-year-old child during a surgery for squint correction. The discharge summary provided insufficient details about the cardiopulmonary resuscitation (CPR) and the events in the operating room. The failure to diagnose an intraoperative oculocardiac reflex (OCR) resulted in a cardiac arrest, causing the child's demise. Patients at risk for OCR require particular attention, and in this case, the child's mother had undergone a hysterectomy, leaving no possibility of having another child. To address this medical negligence, a just and substantial compensation of ₹1 crore is warranted for the grieving parents who lost their child, as it should not be a mere token amount.

Congenital esophageal atresia not operated in one of the twins—no negligence

National Consumer Disputes Redressal in Dr Ishita Tikkha v/s Managing Director, Apollo Cradle on 20 March, 2023[19]

Dr Ishita Tikkha (the patient), during her pregnancy, was under antenatal care (ANC) of Dr Neera Kripal, it was a twin pregnancy delivered by lower segment cesarean section (LSCS). The complaint, filed by the complainant who was a gynecologist and her husband, a pediatrician, alleged negligence in the treatment of their newborn with congenital esophageal atresia. However, the evidence presented failed to prove any negligence or deficiency in service, resulting in the dismissal of the complaint.

Congenital heart disease as bronchopneumonia was treated first but death occurred—no negligence

Ruben Banerjee versus Ehirc Heart Ins. & Research Centre (NCDRC) 2008(1) CLT 705:2008(1) C.P.J. 239:2008(1) C.P.C 487:2007(53) R.C.R.(Civil) 489[20]

Child was suffering from congenital heart disease, initial treatment for bronchopneumonia was provided, but the child ultimately passed away. Medical negligence was alleged, but it was determined that the child died due to bronchopneumonia, which became fatal. No expert evidence or postmortem examination was presented to support the claim of negligence. Surgery had been deferred in the best interest of the child, and no negligence on the part of the doctors was established, leading to the dismissal of the complaint.

Circumcision—postoperative respiratory distress aspiration—vegetative state—negligence

Shilaben Ashwinkumar Rana versus Bhavin K. Shah (SC) 2019(2) R.C.R. (Civil) 184:2019(2) ALT 12:2019(2) JT 289:2019(1) Law Herald (SC) 552:2019(2) ICC 133:2019(2) C.P.R. 839:2019(2) Apex Court Judgments (SC) 313:2019 NCJ 577:2019(4) TAC 363:2019(3) ACC 639:2019(4) C.P.J. 4:2019 ACJ 3020:2020 All SCR 755:2020(18) SCC 652[21]

In a circumcision case, a child developed respiratory distress after aspiration and ended up in a vegetative state. Negligence was claimed, and it was found that aspiration of vomit material occurred soon after surgery, a known complication to the surgeon and anesthetist. Their failure to take adequate precautions was deemed a clear case of medical negligence. The doctor's affidavit admitted that the child suffered severe mental retardation and brain hypoxic ischemic encephalopathy. Consequently, the supreme court enhanced the compensation to ₹7,00,000 at a rate of 6% due to the child's future nursing care, medical needs, and other requirements.

Diaphragmatic hernia surgery—blood transfusion—HIV—negligence

Government of India versus Master Akash, (NCDRC) (New Delhi) 2022(3) C.P.R. 48:2023(1) C.P.J. 389[22]

Master Akash, who had a history of HIV exposure through a wrong blood transfusion at the age of 3 days, underwent surgery for diaphragmatic hernia with intestinal obstructions and adhesions. He continued to experience health issues, including fever, pneumonia, and cough. Following concerns from well-wishers, HIV testing was performed at VMMC & Safdarjung Hospital, confirming him as HIV positive with AIDS. He received treatment at Safdarjung Hospital and AIIMS, eventually leading to a medical negligence claim. The State Commission held the appellants responsible for medical negligence, leading to this appeal. The appellants failed to provide evidence, such as the blood bank register and test reports, to establish that the blood units used were HIV negative. Other potential sources of HIV infection could not be ruled out, especially if blood donors were in the window period where HIV tests may yield negative results. As a result, the appellants were directed to pay ₹10 lakh in compensation to the complainant, and the appeal was dismissed.

Herniotomy—burn injuries leaving permanent scar on both legs—negligence

Master PM Ashwin versus Manipal Hospital, Bangalore (KSCDRC), 1997(1) C.P.J. 238: 1997(1) C.P.C 540[23]

The complainant, who was diagnosed with a right-sided hernia, was advised to undergo immediate surgery. During the surgery while the patient was under anesthesia, a nurse placed an excessively hot water bag under the patient's legs, resulting in burn injuries that left permanent scars on both legs. The respondents did not exercise reasonable care in performing their duties, and the possibility of the patient facing future disabilities was not ruled out.

As a result, the OPs were collectively and individually held liable and were instructed to pay a compensation of ₹5 lakh.

Micro stitches on the minor injury on his forehead—death—negligence

Madhu Sudan versus Dr Suresh Gupta (DSCDRC), 2006(2) C.P.J. 348 Complaint Case No. C-405 of 1992. D/d. 20.3.2006[24]

A 2½-year-old child was brought to the OPs for minor stitches on a forehead injury. However, after being administered anesthesia, the child never regained consciousness and passed away within 3 days. A lump-sum compensation of ₹2 lakh, payable jointly and severally by OP No. 1 and OP No. 2 was awarded.

Fracture of bone in the left elbow—anesthesia—hypoxia—brain damage—negligence of anesthetist

Kumari Mariyam Kousar versus State of Karnataka, (KSCDRC) (Bangalore), Consumer Complaint No. 53 of 2014. D/d. 06.04.2023[25]

While playing with her friends outside, complainant suffered a fall from her bicycle, resulting in a left elbow bone displacement and subsequent open reduction and internal fixation (ORIF) surgery. The complainant has alleged medical negligence against OPs No. 1 to 11. OP No. 8, an anesthetist, detected hypoxia and brain injury (bradycardia). OP No. 7 and 11 provided immediate care after the hypoxia incident and ensured the complainant regained consciousness before transferring her to Manipal Hospital for further treatment. There is no evidence of negligence on the part of OP No. 7 and 10, as determined by the inquiry officers. Even OP No. 9, who performed the closed reduction procedure, was not found to be negligent. The hypoxia incident occurred during the plaster of Paris application after the successful surgery and was promptly addressed by OP No. 8. Expert opinion is not necessary to establish medical negligence on the part of OP No. 8, as the Doctrine of Res Ipsa Loquitur applies. Dr Surangamma Thripati (OP No. 8) was directed to pay an award of ₹30,00,000/-, while the complaints against OPs No. 1 to 7 and OPs No. 9 to 11 were dismissed.

Adenoidal hypertrophy with nasal septal deviation surgery—operating table (OT) death—postmortem done—negligence

Krishna Khatri versus Shri Balaji Hospital Pvt. Ltd., (DSCDRC) (New Delhi) 2020(1) C.P.J. 19, Complaint No. 88 Of 2005. D/d. 20.11.2019[26]

A child reported experiencing slight breathing difficulties and was taken to Apollo Hospital for examination. The diagnosis revealed "Adenoidal hypertrophy," a minor issue. The medical professionals recommended a minor ENT surgery, emphasizing that it carried no significant risks or dangers. Unfortunately, the 11-year-old, a bright child, tragically passed away during this minor procedure. A postmortem examination was conducted. As a result, OP-1, 3, and 4 were instructed to collectively or individually compensate the amount of ₹20 lakhs, along with applicable interest.

Urinary infection due to vesicoureteral (VU) reflux—removal of kidney—leaving of the cotton gauze is per se negligence

Acharya Vinoba Bhave Rural Hospital versus Samiksha, (NCDRC)[27] 2019(4) C.P.R. 96:2020(1) CLT 48, Revision Petition No. 251 of 2015, Revision Petition No. 1361 of 2015 and Revision Petition No. 905 of 2015 (Against the Order dated 04.12.2014 in Appeal No. 477 of 2008 of the State Commission Maharashtra). D/d. 20.9.2019.

A 3-year-old patient experienced a urinary infection caused by VU reflux, treated surgically, ultimately resulting in the removal of a kidney. The total medical bills for the patient did not exceed 50,000. The responsibility now falls on the treating doctor and the hospital to clarify the specific course of treatment provided. Negligence per se can be inferred from the inadvertent leaving of cotton gauze. The patient was just 6 years old when she lost her kidney, leading to an awarded amount of ₹18,00,000/-.

Hypoxic encephalopathy during intussusceptions surgery—negligence

V Ganesh versus Dr KS Shanmuga Sundaram (Madras), 2010(1) MLJ 1351:2009(17) R.C.R. (Civil) 352, A.S. No. 147 of 2002. D/d. 13.10.2009[28]

On April 3, 1989, a child suffering from acute gastroenteritis was referred to Pediatrician Dr K Manonmani, who diagnosed intussusceptions as the underlying issue. Upon referral back to him, immediate surgery was recommended. Expert ophthalmologist Dr N Radhakrishnan, an Assistant Professor of Ophthalmology at Medical College Hospital, Coimbatore,

CHAPTER 21: Medicolegal Aspects for Pediatric Surgery

offered a certified opinion suspecting cortical blindness resulting from cortical damage following abdominal surgery due to hypoxic encephalopathy. Hypoxic encephalopathy, causing both mental and physical disabilities at a 100% level, was attributed to a faulty administration of anesthesia. Neither the surgeon nor the anesthetist provided a valid explanation for this occurrence. This situation was considered negligence, and an award of ₹5,00,000 was granted.

Head injury in child—death—no negligence

Namita Nursing Home versus Anita, (PSCDRC) (Chandigarh), 2000(1) C.P.C 170, Appeal No. 26 of 1998. D/d. 30.6.1999[29]

A child sustained a head injury after falling on the road and was admitted to the OP's clinic. Despite the doctor's best efforts, the child could not be saved. The District Forum ordered the appellant to pay compensation of ₹2 lakh along with ₹1,000. This case does not demonstrate apparent negligence on the surgeon's part during the operation. The decision of whether the child needed immediate burr-hole surgery for safety, considering the risk of a potentially fatal fracture, rested with the surgeon. The timing of the CT scan, whether it could be performed while the child was unconscious or if waiting until the patient's condition stabilized was necessary, was also at the discretion of the surgeon. There is no postmortem report available. Expert opinion is required to determine whether the doctor followed conventional and traditional treatment standards while providing medical care to the patient. Thus, the burden falls on the complainant to prove medical negligence, which is lacking in this case. The doctor made every effort to save the child, but unfortunately, the outcome was not successful despite the best treatment. Given these circumstances, the impugned order cannot be upheld and is hereby set aside.

Accidental injury—suturing—infection—no negligence

Ku. Anuja Dubey versus Superintendent, Bombay Hospital, (MPSCDRC) (Bhopal), First Appeal No. 814 of 2008 (Arising out of order dated 01.01.2008 passed in C.C. No. 371 of 2007 by the District Forum, Indore). D/d. 23.6.2016[30]

The complainant contends that there was a deficiency in service. Accidental injury occurred, and the complaint alleges improper suturing, leading to pain and pus formation. However, the District Forum dismissed the complaint, prompting an appeal. In this case, a tetanus toxoid injection was administered, and the wound was sutured using local anesthesia. The complainant did not provide any medical literature or expert opinion to support the argument that the wound should have been sutured with thinner thread instead of 2-0 Ethilon suture. It is important to note that without proper postoperative care, infection can affect any patient. In this instance, the appellant did not return for follow-up care after the suturing. As a result, negligence was not proven, and the appeal was dismissed.

Appendicitis—not operated in time of emergency—held negligent

In *Dr TT Thomas versus Elisa,* AIR 1987 Ker. 52:1987 ACJ 192 (Kerala HC)[31]

The doctor did not conduct an emergency operation due to the lack of the patient's consent in emergency, resulting in the patient's unfortunate demise. The patient initially complained of severe abdominal pain, and after examination by a general practitioner, it was diagnosed as appendicitis.

The patient was admitted to the hospital, but the operation was not performed on the same day in emergency. Tragically, on the following day, the patient passed away due to a perforated appendix. The defendant-surgeon claimed that the patient had refused to consent to the operation, which was the reason for the delay in performing the emergency surgery. However, both the trial court and the High Court did not accept this explanation, as there was no mention in the patient's refusal on case sheet that consent had been sought and refused by the patient. It was determined that the burden of proof for claiming that consent was sought and refused rested with the party making that assertion, especially when the patient had passed away. Consequently, the doctor was found negligent for not performing the emergency operation and a compensation of ₹37,000 was awarded.

Improper postoperative care—postoperative treatment by homoeopathy doctors, typhoid perforation developing severe complications including fecal fistula in Ch. Padma versus Sudha Nursing Home, 2002 (1) CPJ 53 (Andhra Pradesh SCDRC)[32]

The complainant did not raise any concerns about the typhoid perforation operation itself. However, the postoperative treatment was primarily administered by doctors who were not qualified in allopathy. PW1 testified that the duty doctors were trained in homeopathy and that her postoperative care suffered from infections and a lack of proper attention in the OP's nursing home. PW2 corroborated this statement, mentioning that after the operation, nonallopathic doctors attended to the patient. RW1, in his testimony, admitted that routine tasks such as monitoring pulse, recording blood pressure, and temperature were carried out by other doctors under his supervision. He also acknowledged that homeopathy doctors assisted him in the nursing home and assessed the patients' general conditions in the ward. Given this admission, PW1's claims find support in RW1's own statements.

Although RW1 limited his responsibilities to his department and overseeing patients' general conditions in the ward, he engaged homeopathy doctors to oversee the postoperative care of PW1, as alleged by PW1. This constitutes a deficiency in service. Consequently, PW1 developed fecal fistula and bedsores, which were not adequately addressed by qualified nursing home doctors. These shortcomings amount to a service deficiency on the part of the OP.

SUMMARY

Even the most qualified, knowledgeable, and experienced pediatric surgeons can encounter unexpected mishaps and complications in their practice. These issues may be diagnosed or addressed belatedly. Occasionally, unusual deviations in the disease process or anomalous anatomical conditions can catch pediatric surgeons off guard, leading to perplexing situations and necessitating adjustments to routine surgical procedures. Patients and their families may perceive these situations as instances of negligence.[1-3]

Before proceeding with any surgical intervention, a pediatric surgeon must carefully assess the need for surgery, explain to the patient's family why surgery is the best option, and obtain informed consent. The patient's family should be informed about the expected duration of the surgery, the current surgical condition, and the potential benefits or complications that may arise after the procedure. Ensuring that there is a clear and valid medical indication for any surgical procedure is an essential prerequisite. Performing surgery without a proper indication can lead to challenges and difficulties for the surgeon.

Equally important is the evaluation of the patient's anesthesia fitness by the anesthetist through a thorough preanesthetic examination. This examination includes a review of the patient's history of previous surgeries, drug allergies, denture use, and any heart or lung disorders. The anesthetist also conducts a clinical examination and reviews various reports, such as hemogram, renal function tests, liver function tests, cardiogram, and chest X-rays.

In many cases, the patient's overall medical fitness and clearance for surgery are assessed by a pediatric physician. This evaluation involves obtaining a history of previous surgeries, drug allergies, heart and lung conditions, asthma control, seizure history, bleeding tendencies, and jaundice. The physician conducts a clinical examination and may request additional reports, including hemogram, WBC counts, platelet count, urinalysis, PT, prothrombin index (PI), PTT or bleeding/clotting time, chest X-ray, blood sugar levels, PFTs, serum creatinine or renal function tests, and SGPT or liver function tests. These tests should ideally be performed within 7 days before clearing the patient for surgery. In some cases, additional tests such as HIV testing (after counseling the patient's family) and screening for hepatitis B and C may be necessary.

In certain situations, the disease process may distort the patient's anatomy to an extent that complications occur inadvertently.

LEARNING KEY POINTS AND TAKE-HOME MESSAGES

- No pediatric surgeon should leave mops, swabs, scissors artery forceps, tips of cannula inside abdomen.
- Pediatric surgeon should achieve good hemostasis.
- Pediatric surgeon should never removal of wrong organ.
- Pediatric surgeon should never operate on wrong side.

MUST AVOID THINGS

Never ever take consent on a blank/unfilled form.

ONLY ONE FACT TO REMEMBER

A pediatric surgeon is the captain of the ship, hence vicariously liable for all assistants working and helping in doing surgery.

DO NOT DO

For any surgery never do coercion, misrepresentation for getting consent form signed.

WARNINGS

Never ever give 100% guarantee or warrantee for cure.

MEDICAL NEGLIGENCE PEARLS

Informed/real consent requires signature of competent parent/guardian. This is known as proxy/surrogate consent.

MUST DO THING

Before closing the abdomen, count all the mops and instruments so that nothing is left in the abdomen to scare surgeon of Res ipsa loquitur postoperatively.

MESSAGES WHICH THE READER MUST BE AWARE

Consent is autonomy given to patient party to decide whether to undergo any suggested surgery. Consent for doctor is a document that protects him from allegation of battery and assault (based on the principle of volunti non fit injuria).

MCQs

Choose one correct answer

1. Consent for emergency life-saving surgical procedure:
   a. Is mandatory
   b. Is not mandatory
   c. Is irrelevant
   d. None of the above
2. Planned surgical procedure requires:
   a. Consent
   b. Pre anesthetic checkup
   c. Physician checkup and clearance
   d. All of above

Answers

1. b   2. d

REFERENCES

1. Baldwa M, Baldwa V, Padvi N, Baldwa S. Legal Issues in Medical Practice. New Delhi: CBS Publishers & Distributors Pvt Ltd; 2023.
2. Baldwa M, Baldwa V, Padvi N, Baldwa S. Legal Issues in Critical Care. New Delhi: CBS Publishers & Distributors Pvt Ltd; 2022.
3. Baldwa M, Baldwa V, Padvi N, Baldwa S. Legal Issues in Dermatology. New Delhi: CBS Publishers & Distributors Pvt Ltd; 2018.
4. Kerala High Court. Dr TT Thomas versus Smt. Elisa and Ors. on 11 August, 1986. Equivalent citations: I (1987) ACC 445, AIR 1987 Ker 52.
5. Karam Veer Singh versus Garg Nursing Home (MPSCDRC), 2007(3) C.P.J. 131.
6. PS Karunakar versus Narayana Hrudayalaya (KSCDRC) (Bangalore), 2007(2) C.P.J. 363:2007(53) R.C.R. (Civil), Appeal No. 955 of 2005. D/d. 19.1.2007.
7. Master Hari Om Sharma (Minor) versus Indraprastha Apollo Hospital, (NCDRC), 2023(2) C.P.R. 183:2023(2) C.P.J. 487, Consumer Case No. 381 of 2013. D/d. 29.03.2023.
8. WB State Consumer Disputes Redressal Commission, Dr Susmita Bhattacharya versus Marzina Bibi Alias Begum & Others on 16 September, 2022.
9. Baby Preeti Goel (Minor) versus Batra Hospital & Medical Research Centre (NCDRC) 2007(2) All. LJ 578:2007(3) C.P.J. 133:2007(2) CLT 480:2006(38) R.C.R. (Civil) 599.
10. Millenium Post. (2018). CMRI to pay Rs 10 lakh as fine for negligence over child's death. [online] Available from https://www.millenniumpost.in/kolkata/cmri-to-pay-rs-10-lakh-as-fine-for-negligence-over-childs-death-331873 [Last accessed December, 2023].
11. Prafulla Kumar Das versus Apollo Hospitals (NCDRC), 2002(2) C.P.J. 106.
12. S Nirmala versus Dr A Govindarajan Eye Hospital, (TNSCDRC) (Circuit Bench) (Madurai), F.A. No. 153 of 2013 (Against the order made in C.C. No. 132/2010, dated 08.05.2012 on the file of the District Forum, Tiruchirappalli). D/d. 20.7.2022.
13. Mr Nandkishor Chhaganlal Shah versus Kashiba Gordhandas Patel Children Hospital & Jajodia Research Institute (GSCDRC), Appeal No. 1038 of 2013. D/d. 26.04.2023.
14. Mrs Ragini Premnath versus Dr Prema Shankar, on 24 November, 2009.
15. Sri Jalandhar Shah versus ESI Hospital Diamond Harbour Road, (WBSCDRC) (Kolkata) Complaint Case No. CC/241 of 2013. D/d. 10.03.2023.
16. Muthu Vijayan versus De Viswanathan M.S. (K.C.D.R.C.) (Thiruvananthapuram) 2012(1) C.P.J. 43:2012(2) CLT 556:2011(48) R.C.R. (Civil) 408, O.P. No. 50 of 2001. D/d. 5.11.2011.
17. Times of India. (2023). Delhi court relief for paediatric surgeon over 'negligence'.

[online] Available from: http://timesofindia.indiatimes.com/articleshow/97959159.cms?utm_source=contentofinterest&&&utm_medium=text&utm_campaign=cppst%25257B17%25257D&utm_source=contentofinterest&utm_medium=text&utm_campaign=cppst [Last accessed December, 2023].
18. Dr Reba Modak versus Sankara Nethralaya, (NCDRC) 2022(5) ALL MR 44:2022(4) C.P.J. 72:2023(2) Andh LD 23.
19. Dr Ishita Tikkha versus Managing Director, Apollo Cradle, on 20 March, 2023.
20. Ruben Banerjee versus Ehirc Heart Ins. & Research Centre (NCDRC), 2008(1) CLT 705:2008(1) C.P.J. 239:2008(1) C.P.C 487: 2007(53) R.C.R. (Civil) 489.
21. Shilaben Ashwinkumar Rana versus Bhavin K. Shah (SC)2019(2) R.C.R.(Civil) 184:2019(2) ALT 12:2019(2) JT 289:2019(1) Law Herald (SC) 552:2019(2) ICC 133:2019(2) C.P.R. 839:2019(2) Apex Court Judgments (SC) 313:2019 NCJ 577:2019(4) TAC 363:2019(3) ACC 639: 2019(4) C.P.J. 4:2019 ACJ 3020:2020 All SCR 755:2020(18) SCC 652.
22. Government of India versus Master Akash, (NCDRC) (New Delhi) 2022(3) C.P.R. 48: 2023(1) C.P.J. 389.
23. Master PM Ashwin versus Manipal Hospital, Bangalore (KSCDRC), 1997(1) C.P.J. 238: 1997(1) C.P.C 540.
24. Madhu Sudan versus Dr Suresh Gupta (DSCDRC), 2006(2) C.P.J. 348 Complaint Case No. C-405 of 1992. D/d. 20.3.2006.
25. Kumari Mariyam Kousar versus State of Karnataka, (KSCDRC) (Bangalore), Consumer Complaint No. 53 of 2014. D/d. 06.04.2023.
26. Krishna Khatri versus Shri Balaji Hospital Pvt. Ltd., (DSCDRC) (New Delhi) 2020(1) C.P.J. 19, Complaint No. 88 Of 2005. D/d. 20.11.2019.
27. Acharya Vinoba Bhave Rural Hospital versus Samiksha, (NCDRC) 2019(4) C.P.R. 96:2020(1) CLT 48, Revision Petition No. 251 of 2015, Revision Petition No. 1361 of 2015, and Revision Petition No. 905 of 2015 (Against the Order dated 04.12.2014 in Appeal No. 477 of 2008 of the State Commission Maharashtra). D/d. 20.9.2019.
28. V Ganesh versus Dr KS Shanmuga Sundaram (Madras), 2010(1) MLJ 1351:2009(17) R.C.R. (Civil) 352, A.S. No. 147 of 2002. D/d. 13.10.2009.
29. Namita Nursing Home versus Anita, (PSCDRC) (Chandigarh), 2000(1) C.P.C 170, Appeal No. 26 of 1998. D/d. 30.6.1999.
30. Ku. Anuja Dubey versus Superintendent, Bombay Hospital, (MPSCDRC) (Bhopal), First Appeal No. 814 of 2008 (Arising out of order dated 01.01.2008 passed in C.C. No. 371 of 2007 by the District Forum, Indore). D/d. 23.6.2016.
31. Dr TT Thomas versus Elisa, AIR 1987 Ker. 52: 1987 ACJ 192 (Kerala HC).
32. Ch. Padma versus Sudha Nursing Home, 2002 (1) CPJ 53 (Andhra Pradesh SCDRC).

CHAPTER 22

Legalities in Neonatology

Anurag Pangrikar, Hemant R Gangolia, Jyoti Kumar Gupta, Mahesh Baldwa

Keywords: Documentation, Do not resuscitate, High-risk newborn screening, Infant milk substitute, National rare disease policy, Negligence in neonatology

Aim: Enhance neonatal welfare by mitigating medicolegal risks amidst rising survival rates, parental expectations, and healthcare costs.

Objectives: (1) Quantify and explain long-term sequelae of advanced care to parents and optimize resource allocation. (2) Foster open communication and shared decision-making between providers and parents. (3) Support research, advocate for equitable access, and address medicolegal challenges collaboratively.

INTRODUCTION

Neonatal period (first 28 days of life) is the most critical period of life. Globally 2.4 million children died in the first month of life, amounting to 47% of all child deaths under the age of 5 years. Most neonatal deaths (75%) occur during the first week of life.[1] Global statistics shows that despite of best care, mortality in newborn period is the highest. Preterm birth, perinatal asphyxia, infections, and birth defects are the leading causes of most neonatal deaths. Due to advances in neonatology and intensive newborn care, survival rate of more preterm and sick babies is increasing, thus raising the level of expectation of the parents from baby-care system. Advance health care on one end raising the survival rate of neonate but on another end it is giving rise to significant morbidity and neurodevelopmental sequelae in survived sick newborns. High cost of newborn care along with high expectations of the parents is leading to increasing number of medicolegal litigations.

CHALLENGES IN NEONATOLOGY PRACTICE

Chances of mortality and morbidity are maximum in neonatal period and the cost of the treatment is also high in neonatal intensive care unit (NICU), so there are fair chances that medicolegal may arise in treating sick neonate. As compensation is traditionally calculated as per life expectancy rule and degree of disability, so the largest speculated lifespan for neonate clubbed with residual neurodevelopmental sequelae has led to mammoth compensation ever for pediatricians, which is major cause of concern for pediatrician community. High-risk newborn screening is mandatory for every high-risk babies and failure to advise appropriate high-risk screening and refer them has been costing maximum to pediatricians. Medicolegal challenges in neonatology may be categorized as related to resuscitation, related to intensive care in NICU and high-risk newborn screening.

CATEGORIZATION OF ERRORS IN NEONATAL INTENSIVE CARE UNIT

- *Treatment error or delay (48%):* Delayed referral to medical team once diagnosis made, not investigated or managed as per protocol.
- *Missed/delay in diagnosis (16%):* Cerebral palsy/birth asphyxia, respiratory distress syndrome, sepsis, seizures, jaundice, and procedure-related complications.
- *General improper care (30%):* Improper handling of neonates, lack of observation, and failure to appropriately monitor glucose levels despite risk factors.
- Equipment misuse (6%).
- *Medical management error:* Lost or tampered medical records, poorly documented notes, clinician without proper qualification, untrained staff, infrastructure-related issues including space, staff and equipment, and early discharge without feeding support.
- Issues related to consent, communication, and documentation of communication.
- *Issues related to transport of sick newborn:* Vehicle, temperature, oxygen, fluids, glucose, and person trained to manage emergency.
- Post discharge follow-up not communicated, risk factors not explained.

MEDICOLEGAL ISSUES IN NEONATOLOGY PRACTICE

Medicolegal issues in neonatology practice can be categorized in three heads: Medical, which involves actual medical management; Ethical, which involves taking right decisions while maintaining patient's interests in all aspects, and lastly important one Legal, which involves maintaining a standard care of practice and providing honest and actual information to parents and caretakers. Following are the medicolegal problems, which may give rise to medicolegal implications:

- *Neonatal jaundice:* Common allegation are picking late of neonatal jaundice. Rh and ABO-Rh incompatibility may be missed in case of miscommunication and poor history taking.
- *Respiratory distress:* This may arise in various conditions, including prematurity, meconium aspiration, perinatal asphyxia, diaphragmatic hernia, pneumonia, septicemia, and aspiration. It may be missed when baby is wrapped and is with mother.
- *Infections:* Common allegations are picking late, catching infection from hospital setting, inability to manage properly, and use of wrong antibiotics in wrong doses.
- *Birth injuries:* Injuries may be caused at birth and may be missed in initial examination. Missing may give rise to allegation of sustaining injury in NICU. These injuries are to be checked properly and to be explained very cautiously.
- *Congenital defects:* Searching and documenting congenital defects is very important as this may deteriorate the baby very rapidly and missing may create medicolegal liability.
- *Hypoglycemia:* Low blood sugar levels can occur in newborns, especially in those born to mothers with diabetes and preterm low birth weight babies. Hypoglycemia can lead to seizures and must be treated promptly. Missing hypoglycemia may give rise to medicolegal implications.

- *Gastrointestinal issues:* Conditions like necrotizing enterocolitis (NEC) and pyloric stenosis can affect the gastrointestinal system of newborns and require surgical intervention in some cases and should be picked early.
- *Inborn errors of metabolism:* Some infants are born with metabolic disorders that can lead to severe health problems if not diagnosed and managed early. One should have high index of suspicion for these and screening should be advised in neonatal period.
- *Hemorrhagic disorders:* Disorders of blood clotting, such as hemophilia or vitamin K deficiency bleeding, can result in abnormal bleeding in the newborn period. History of drug intake by mother and family history of such disease is very important.
- *High-risk newborn screening:* High-risk newborn screening is recommended for various high-risk conditions. So, one should not forget to advise and refer for screening. Remember mammoth compensations in neonatology practice are related to high-risk newborn screening
- *Neurological issues:* Seizures are frequently missed by attendants and presented late. These have to be managed judiciously and proper workup and management should be done.

POINTS TO PONDER AT THE TIME OF NEONATAL RESUSCITATION

Medicolegal implications start from the very moment of receiving a call for neonatal resuscitation. Whenever pediatrician receives a call for resuscitation of newborn baby, he should be prompt in attending the emergency call. He should note down the timing of attending the baby. Fact of resuscitation done by other person before him must be documented.

One should not forget to document resuscitation procedure performed, drug used during resuscitation, clinical condition of baby at birth and after resuscitation, APGAR (Appearance, Pulse, Grimace, Activity, and Respiration) score, gestational age, sex, weight of baby, antenatal and perinatal history, general examination of baby, vitals, congenital defects, birth injuries, history of cord around neck, fetal distress, loss of fetal movement, and risk factors involved.

Discussion with obstetrician and supporting operation theater (OT) staff regarding seeking important history is must. One should develop the habit of seeing antenatal ultrasound, mother's investigation, and case papers. Important maternal history like blood group of mother, indication of lower segment cesarean section (LSCS), history of leaking per vaginum (PV), progress of labor, history of medical condition like diabetes, hypertension, thyroid, HIV, hepatitis, hepatitis C, high-risk pregnancy, previous obstetric history, personal history, history of drug intake in pregnancy, X-ray exposure, blood transfusion, and antenatal steroid given to mother must be documented.

If baby is sick then he or she should be admitted in NICU immediately. If NICU is not well equipped with necessary apparatus trained staff, then baby should be shifted to appropriate set up with proper transfer protocol. In case of delay in admission, denial consent must be recorded.

CARE AND DOCUMENTATION IN NICU FROM MEDICOLEGAL PROSPECTIVE

Proper nursing care must be ensured to each baby. Strict monitoring should be done in NICU as a routine and impending complications should be picked up early. Vitals should be charted regularly as per consultant advice and NICU protocol. Proper nursing care such as vital monitoring, asepsis maintenance, temperature monitoring, daily weight charting, anthropometry at regular interval, observation of pain protocol, passing of meconium and stool, urine output, and blood sugar monitoring should be strictly done and charted. Remember oxygen saturation for preterm babies have to be kept in range of 92–95 to avoid hyperoxia. Baby should be kept dry; eye and genitalia must be covered in all baby during phototherapy. Photograph and video making in NICU by attendants should be discouraged as these may be used as evidence of poor care at the time of litigation. Changing the baby is big and common allegation in hospitals, so identification mark should be applied on each baby and foot print must be taken on bead head ticket i.e., indoor file.

Nosocomial infection is a big threat to admitted babies, and hospitals have been alleged for negligent in infection control. For this, asepsis protocol must be followed in NICU. Fumigation and NICU sterilization should be routinely done and record should be preserved. Microbiological analysis of NICU with culture and sensitivity report should be prepared routinely. NICU equipment must be routinely serviced and inspected by electricians and engineers, and record of these should also be maintained.

The highest amount of care is warranted to prevent accidental injury in NICU, such as burn, erosion of nose in continuous positive airway pressure (CPAP) application, and intravenous (IV) line-related injury. Birth injuries should be thoroughly inspected and documented. Never forget to give hepatitis B immunoglobulin to infant born to hepatitis B-positive mother, never forget to ask for direct Coomb test and bilirubin level in Rh-negative mother. Always monitor blood sugar as a routine practice in all preterm, intrauterine growth restriction (IUGR), and infant of diabetic mother. Hypoglycemia must be avoided by judicious blood sugar monitoring. All asphyxiated babies are at risk of multiorgan damage, so urine output, capillary filling time (CFT), and blood pressure monitoring should be done routinely and documented. Neonate must be suspected for having congenital birth defects and surgical problems. High index of suspicion and timely referral of pediatric surgeon is must to avoid medicolegal litigation. In case of prolong jaundice, hypothyroidism and neonatal obstructive jaundice must be suspected to avoid medicolegal issues.

Documentation at the Time of Discharge from Neonatal Unit

Discharge of newborn is a crucial event, and discharge card of newborn must be made with utmost seriousness. All the efforts in securing life of sick newborn may go in vain when discharge card is made hurriedly and leaving aside important necessary documentation may land up hardworking sincere pediatrician in troublesome medicolegal litigation. So, important points must be remembered and documented at the time of making of discharge card of a neonate.
- High-risk newborn screening must be performed in NICU whenever indicated in sick newborn and for the same in follow-up should be documented in discharge card.
- As per Facility Based Newborn Care (FBNC) guidelines, high-risk neonate should be documented in bold letters in

- discharge card, and address, timing, and contact number of high-risk newborn screening referral center should be documented.
- Prognosis and risk of neurodevelopmental delay should be documented in high-risk newborn discharge card.
- Anthropometry, especially weight, head circumference, length at discharge and at birth should be documented in discharge card.
- Exclusive breastfeeding till 6 month of age should be documented in discharge card.
- Advice for vaccine should be documented.
- Discharge card of all the babies whose weight is <2 kg or discharged on IV antibiotics should be documented with discharge against medical advice or discharge on persistent request, and consent of DAMA (discharged against medical advice) or DOPR (discharge on patient request) should be taken on BHT.
- If IV antibiotics are being advised on discharge card, then dilution, mode of administration with duration of infusion and to be given in hospital should be documented in discharge card.
- All investigations performed should be documented in discharge card with date.
- Condition at admission and at discharge along with course in hospital should be documented.
- Consent should be taken on BHT at the time of discharge regarding the fact that condition of baby is better and is accepting feed properly, and he has understood the treatment, high-risk newborn screening, risk factors, care at home, and follow-up advised.
- Follow-up date and schedule should be mentioned on discharge card.
- Care at home and risk factors should be explained and documented on discharge card. It is good practice to give information brochure for the same.

HIGH-RISK NEWBORN SCREENING

According to systemic review published in Lancet,[2] there is high prevalence of long-term neurodevelopmental sequelae after intrauterine and neonatal insults, which is as follows: sepsis 40%, meningitis 42%, hypoxic-ischemic encephalopathy (HIE) 31%, preterm birth 31%, jaundice 18%, tetanus 26%, and cytomegalovirus (CMV) infection 41%. Standard Treatment Guidelines 2022 published by Indian Academy of Pediatrics (IAP) Standard Treatment Guidelines Committee has mentioned the risk of neurodevelopment disability based on perinatal risk factors,[3] like gestation, birth weight, stage of HIE, hypoglycemia, neonatal jaundice, infection, seizures, circulation, ventilation, antenatal, and neuroimaging. All neonates with perinatal risk factors must go for high-risk newborn screening. Before discharge every high-risk neonate should be assigned for risk of neurodevelopmental sequelae, head circumference should be monitored, and follow-up schedule should be planned. Retinopathy of prematurity (ROP) screening should be advised at 4 weeks chronological age for all preterm (<2,000 g) subsequently as per recommendation of ophthalmologist and visual acuity at 6 months and 1 year. Thyroid screening should be performed in 1 week. Otoacoustic emission (OAE) should be done before discharge, if refer repeat at one and half month with first immunization and brainstem-evoked response audiometry (BERA) at 3 months. Neurosonogram should be performed first at day 3–5 and second at 40 weeks corrected age.

Newborn screening for common metabolic and genetic disorders should also be an integral part of neonatal care as early detection and treatment can help prevent intellectual and physical defects and life-threatening illnesses.[4] The Advisory Committee on Heritable Disorders in Newborns and Children recommends that every newborn screening program should include a Recommended Uniform Screening Panel that screens for 34 core disorders and 26 secondary disorders.[5]

Failure to assess high-risk neonate and refer it for high-risk screening is causing mammoth compensation award to pediatrician in today's time. In V Krishnakumar versus State of Tamil Nadu & Ors.[6] case, 1.38 crores compensation was awarded where referral for ROP was not documented in the discharge card. It was the case of the blindness in a girl child following the ROP.

CONSENT IN NEONATOLOGY PRACTICE

Admission in NICU should be done only after obtaining proper inform consent. Gravity of disease of baby, risk of life, risk of complications, and risk of neurodevelopmental sequelae must be disclosed to attendants. Daily prognosis must be explained to attendants, and daily inform consent should also be documented in case sheet in separate chart. Separate consent must be taken for procedure like artificial ventilation, CPAP, lumber puncture, central line, and intercostal drainage (ICD) with risk involved. Do not resuscitate (DNR) consent should be taken in video recording apart from written consent by parents with two witness along with endorsement from two consultant and superintendent of hospital.

Undertaking from attendants should be taken at the time of shifting baby to mother that they are receiving a healthy baby with apparently no ailments, baby is accepting feed properly and home care, high-risk newborn screening, vaccination, follow-up schedule, and risk factors have been explained to them. It is a good practice to give a brochure of Do's and Don'ts and risk factors.

Telemedicine is a new tool and may be quite helpful in managing neonates in NICU. As per telemedicine guidelines, consent is implied only in case when patient initiate teleconsultation. In all other cases inform consent has to be taken. So, it is prudent to take prior consent for procuring teleconsultation.

Is mother's consent necessary before initiating the Infant Milk Substitute?

A 31-year-old engineer, Jincy Verghese, resident of Panvel, gave birth to baby boy and was kept in the nursery for monitoring of sugar levels for 1 day. The newborn was given formula feed whereas the human milk bank was part of hospital. She said "But my wish was not respected by the hospital where I delivered my baby. Despite having a milk bank, they chose to give my baby formula feed. I want the government to tell all the hospitals to get prior consent of the mother before feeding a newborn formula milk". The online petition by Panvel mother champions right to breastfeed was initiated there on change.org.

In some countries, like Ireland, consent is taken before formula is administered, but India has no such legislation. The World Health Organization (WHO) says a child can be given formula only if he/she has a medical condition. In Australia, if formula is ordered for medical reasons, the "Mothers Consent Stamp" (kept on the ward) must be used in the baby's notes. All mothers whose breastfeeding babies receive formula must sign permission.

The Indian Academy of Pediatrics has taken a resolution on Infant Milk Substitutes (IMS) Act,[7] which suggests that a written consent should be taken from mother before starting infant formula in neonatal unit.

ETHICAL DILEMMA IN NEONATOLOGY PRACTICE: DO NOT RESUSCITATE

A pediatrician may face a situation where the birth weight and gestational age is such that survival, especially intact survival, may be almost impossible or baby is born with congenital anomaly or anomalies that are incompatible or may be compatible with life, but the expected quality of life may be poor or a big drain on resources of family/society. In these situations, resuscitation is not likely to lead to prolonged and useful survival and such babies are the candidates for DNR. DNR is a clear concept in most developed countries.[8] Whereas tertiary NICUs can use a gestational age criteria of 24 weeks, others like special care neonatal units being setup in district hospitals should use a gestational age cut-off of 28 weeks. Lesions incompatible with life or compatible with poor quality life are the criteria for all neonatal units to follow. It is strongly recommended that each unit should document its own criteria for DNR decisions.

End-of-life care: Consensus Statement by IAPs states following recommendations[9] for DNR: (1) DNR or end-of-life care should not be activated till consensus is achieved between treating team and the next of kin; (2) Consensus within healthcare team (including nurses) needs to be achieved before discussion with family members; (3) Discussion should involve the family members—next of kin and other persons who can influence decisions; (4) If family members want to include their family physician or a prominent person from the community, it should be encouraged. Similarly, if family members want a particular member of treating team, he/she should be included; (5) Treating doctors should have all the facts of the case including investigations available with them before discussion; (6) Unit in-charge or treating doctor should be responsible for achieving consensus and should initiate the discussion; (7) After presenting the facts of the cases, family members should be encouraged to ask questions and clear doubts (if any); (8) At the end of discussion, a summary of the discussion should be prepared and signed by the next of kin and the unit in-charge or treating doctors; (9) DNR orders should be reviewed in the event of unexpected improvement or on request of next of kin. Same should be documented; (10) DNR orders remain valid during transport.

CRIMINAL LIABILITY IN NEONATOLOGY PRACTICE

A pediatrician may be held criminally liable under Section 315 of IPC for causing death of newborn baby during neonatal resuscitation if DNR policy is not followed in proper way. Section 315 of IPC says that "Whoever before the birth of any child does any act with the intention of thereby preventing that child from being born alive or causing it to die after its birth, and does by such act prevent that child from being born alive, or causes it to die after its birth, shall, if such act be not caused in good faith for the purpose of saving the life of the mother, be punished with imprisonment of either description for a term which may extend to ten years, or with fine, or with both".

Similarly, where babies are changed due to negligence of hospital, pediatrician, and hospital management may be booked under Section 418 of IPC for which there is provision of imprisonment of either description for a term, which may extend to three years, or with fine, or with both.

Giving adoption to destitute or illegitimate newborn without performing legal formalities may attract Section 81 of Juvenile Justice Act, 2015 by which pediatrician or hospital management will be penalized with imprisonment for three to seven years.

NEWBORN WITH MULTIPLE CONGENITAL ANOMALY OR STILL BIRTH

Among live born infants 3–5% have major congenital abnormalities and a further 3% have minor abnormalities. The clinical assessment of a newborn with multiple congenital abnormalities must be thorough and accurate. Some abnormalities may be quite prominent or involve large areas while others may be rather subtle. The pediatrician should take care to continue to search for the less obvious anomalies even when a major malformation is present. Such babies should be properly worked up and hospitalized if needed and karyotyping should be advised. Pediatric surgeon and genetics specialist should be consulted. In case of still birth, pediatrician should examine and confirm the diagnosis of still birth and should refer for autopsy in indicated cases, thereby helping arrival at a final diagnosis. In government set-up still birth should be reported as per standard protocol prescribed by the Ministry of Health and Family Welfare.

Worldwide the most common cause of malpractice claim against radiologists is error in diagnosis, i.e., failure to diagnose congenital defects.[10] Doctors are under an obligation to disclose to their patients the risks of passing on a genetic condition to their prospective children. However, the doctor need not disclose all risks or recommend all available testing procedures. In the case of Munro versus Regents of the University of California[11], the court held that the doctor was not under an obligation to recommend a Tay-Sachs test when the doctor had no reason to suspect his patients were at any more at risk for Tay-Sachs than the general population.

The ultrasonography (USG) scans routinely advised are Dating scan and Anomaly scan. While the dating scan is done in the first trimester of pregnancy, the anomaly scan is done at 18–22 weeks to confirm the presence or absence of any structural defect in the baby. Not all congenital anomalies are detected by USG.

NATIONAL RARE DISEASE POLICY 2021

The Ministry of Health and family Welfare, Government of India formulated a National Policy for Treatment of Rare Diseases (NPTRD) in July, 2017. The WHO defines rare disease as often debilitating lifelong disease or disorder with a prevalence of 1 or less, per 1,000 population. Rare diseases in policy have been categorized in three groups.
- *Group 1:* Disorders amenable to one-time curative treatment
- *Group 2:* Diseases requiring long-term/lifelong treatment having relatively lower cost of treatment and benefit has been documented in literature and annual or more frequent surveillance is required.
- *Group 3:* Diseases for which definitive treatment is available, but challenges are to

make optimal patient selection for benefit, very high cost and lifelong therapy.

The policy recommends a screening and diagnostic strategy wherein those pregnant women in whom there is a history of a child born with a rare disease and that rare disease diagnosis has been confirmed, would be offered prenatal screening test(s) through amniocentesis and/or chorionic villi sampling. In cases where the diagnosis could not be established during the prenatal period, it would be imperative to offer to the newborn or the infant as the case may be and would include newborn screening. Nidan Kendras have been set up for genetic testing and counseling services. These Nidan Kendras will be performing screening, genetic testing, and counseling for rare diseases.

Financial support up to Rs. 20 lakh under the Umbrella Scheme of Rashtriya Arogaya Nidhi shall be provided by the Central Government for treatment, of those rare diseases that require a one-time treatment (diseases listed under Group 1). Beneficiaries for such financial assistance would not be limited to BPL families, but extended to about 40% of the population, who are eligible as per norms of Pradhan Mantri Jan Arogya Yojana, for their treatment in Government tertiary hospitals only. State Governments can consider supporting patients of such rare diseases that can be managed with special diets or hormonal supplements or other relatively low cost interventions (diseases listed under Group 2).

IMPORTANT DECIDED MEDICOLEGAL CASES

MBBS can practice neonatology

Dr P. Madanmohan Rao versus Kharja Moizuddin, 2004 (7) CLD 313 (Andhra Pradesh SCDRC)

"The treatment of newborn babies—qualifications—OP 1, possessing a medical degree (MBBS) and OP 2, holding an MBBS degree along with a diploma in pediatrics and a Fellowship in Neonatology, both duly registered with the Medical Council of India and the State Medical Council—The District Forum's decision to uphold the complaint, alleging a deficiency in service, based on the doctors' supposedly lacking qualifications, without any claims of service-related shortcomings in patient care or the proper treatment procedures—such a ruling is untenable as no evidence has been presented to demonstrate that the doctors were ineligible to practice pediatrics".

Newborn burn injury—two to three fingers and suffered permanent deformity of fingers in his right hand —negligence

Shri Naresh Gopalkrishna Vyas versus Care Hospital Nagpur Through its Managing Director, (MSCDRC) (Nagpur Circuit Bench)

The baby, weighing 2.8 kg, was born without any external abnormalities or signs of injury. However, it was later discovered that the baby had sustained burn injuries, resulting in the loss of nails on two to three fingers and permanent deformity in the right hand. As a result, the baby requires plastic surgery on the right hand. The OP nos. 2 and 3 did not provide an explanation for the cause of this injury when questioned. This negligence has led to a joint and several liability for OP nos. 1, 2, and 3, who are now required to pay compensation of Rs. 2000,000/-.

Delivery—premature child—death—no negligence

Dr Monika Chopra versus Resham Singh, (PSCDRC) (Special Bench), 2016(4) C.P.R. 42, First Appeal No.1205 of 2014, dated 8.8.2016[12]

A newborn child sadly passed away under circumstances involving low birth weight, bluish discoloration, mild breathing difficulties, and a low heart rate. The baby received continuous care and attention from a pediatrician and was later admitted to Ankur Hospital for a 15-day period. However, it is crucial to note that the medical professionals involved were not found negligent in their efforts to save both the mother and the child. As a result, the District Forum's initial decision to award compensation of Rs. 260,120/- along with Rs. 20,000/- as litigation costs was overturned on appeal. The complaint was dismissed, and the appeal filed by the opposing party (OP) was allowed, leading to the dismissal of the complainant's appeal".

Kernicterus—child becoming mentally handicapped—contributory negligence of parents—no negligence of doctor

Lalluram Meena versus Dr S. Mathur & Another, 2001 (3) CPJ 200 (Rajasthan SCDRC)

"Physiological jaundice, irreversible mental handicap, and convulsions emerged in a newborn child shortly after discharge from the hospital. The complainant did not consult a physician nor provide treatment to prevent the elevation of serum bilirubin to toxic levels, which could have averted kernicterus. As a result, the child developed mental handicaps. It is argued that the parent's contributory negligence played a role. The first sign of complications, convulsions, occurred 2-3 hours after discharge. Expert medical care at that moment could have prevented the bilirubin levels from reaching toxic levels capable of causing kernicterus. No negligence or failure to fulfill clinical duties on the part of the healthcare provider, opposite party no.1, has been established. Once discharged from the hospital, any alleged deterioration in the child's health or mental capabilities cannot be attributed to the opposite parties".

Kernicterus is avoidable

Dr Rakesh Lain versus Rakesh Kumar Khare & Others, 2003 (1) CPJ 27 (Madhya Pradesh SCDRC)

The case involves a newborn baby with jaundice. A serum bilirubin test conducted at a nursing home confirmed the child's condition. However, while under the care of OP 2, the serum bilirubin levels increased. The patient was subsequently referred to a children's hospital, where it was discovered that the child's bilirubin levels had risen significantly due to delays and negligence on the part of OPs. 1 and 2. Notably, no pathological tests or phototherapy were performed at the nursing home, and the treatment provided did not adhere to the medical code of conduct. Consequently, the child suffered permanent physical disability as a result of this negligence. The District Forum initially awarded compensation of Rs. 41 lakh and medical expenses of Rs. 75,000, a decision that was upheld by the State Commission.

Negligence and mistake both are different things—Prima facie, it is clear that both doctors were not negligent while discharging their duty as Medical Practitioners

Dr Pradeep versus State of Maharashtra, (Bombay HC) (DB) (Nagpur Bench) 2017[13]

On December 5, 2015, the complainant's wife gave birth to a son. On December 30, 2015, the complainant admitted the newborn child to Dr Bagade's hospital due to the child's deteriorating health. On January 1, 2016, following Dr Bagade's advice, the child was admitted to Dr Jaiswal's hospital. The child remained an indoor patient from January 1, 2016, to January 7, 2016, and showed signs of improvement. Consequently, Dr Jaiswal referred the child back to Dr Bagade's hospital, where the child was treated until January 10, 2016. On January 10, 2016, the complainant took his child home. However, on the night of January 11, 2016, the complainant observed deterioration in his child's health. In the early morning of January 12, 2016, at around 5:30 am, he rushed the child to Dr Jaiswal's hospital. Doctors on duty at Dr Jaiswal's hospital, Mr Prafulla Khobragade and Mr Wankhede, examined the child, provided a prescription for medication, and advised the complainant to take the child home. At approximately 9:10 am, the child's condition worsened significantly, prompting the complainant to seek help from Child Specialist, Dr Abhishek Sondawale. Dr Sondawale examined the child and advised the complainant to return to Dr Jaiswal's hospital as the child was in critical condition. The complainant took the child to Dr Jaiswal's hospital, where Dr Bhoot, the doctor on duty, examined the child and declared him dead. On May 16, 2016, the complainant filed a report, alleging that Dr Wankhede, who examined the child at Dr Jaiswal's hospital but did not admit him, and Dr Sondawale, who did not provide medical treatment, were responsible for his child's death.

Regarding the quashing of the FIR, it should be noted that, for doctors to be prosecuted, there must be evidence of gross negligence in their medical treatment. The report of the Medical Board did not indicate that both doctors had committed any negligence. Instead, the Medical Board stated that the doctors had made a mistake by not admitting the child and providing treatment. Negligence and mistake are distinct concepts. It is evident that both doctors were not negligent in carrying out their medical duties.

Therefore, there is no basis for an offense under Section 304A of the Indian Penal Code, and the FIR is quashed".

Neonatal Klebsiella infection—gangrene—amputation—no negligence

Sri Dipankar Das versus ILS Hospital, Agartala, (TSCDRC), Case No. CC. 4 of 2019. D/d. 17.05.2021[14]

Miss Divyashree Das, born on February 27, 2017, at Agartala Government Medical College and GBP Hospital, had a low birth weight. Due to the need for better incubator facilities and treatment, the baby was transferred to ILS Hospital in Agartala (referred to as opposite party no. 1) on the same day of her birth. The family was informed about the poor prognosis, resulting from a *Klebsiella* infection and was advised to move the baby to a higher level medical facility. The minor daughter had already developed gangrene, necessitating amputation. During cross-examination, it was explicitly mentioned that any infection, not just *Klebsiella*, could lead to gangrene. The witness voluntarily stated that he had specifically informed the patient's parents that there were very few chances of the limbs surviving and that amputation of the leg might be necessary. Subsequently, the complainant transferred his minor daughter to the "Institute of Child Health" (ICH) in Kolkata, where, after an examination, the doctors at ICH recommended amputation of the right leg up to the lower limb.

Death caused by infection and not due to hyaline membrane disease

Hogan versus Almand, 205 SE 2d 440, Ga 1974

"Medical Negligence Resulting in Undiagnosed Newborn Infection and Fatality—a pregnant woman was admitted to the hospital as her expected delivery date approached. She experienced significant bleeding and ultimately gave birth unassisted in her room. Tragically, her newborn passed away just one day after delivery. Laboratory tests had previously indicated a severe infection in the newborn, but the pediatrician overseeing the case failed to acknowledge these reports. Instead, the pediatrician incorrectly diagnosed the newborn with hyaline membrane disease, despite the baby not being premature, and administered treatment accordingly. Subsequent post-mortem examinations revealed that the true cause of death was the infection. The Court concluded that there was a valid basis for a negligence claim against the pediatrician".

Thalassemia major missed diagnosis on DNA exam—no negligence

In the case of Sailesh Munjal versus All India Institute of Medical Sciences (NCDRC), Original Petition No. 224 of 1994, dated 20.5.2004[15]

There was an error in the DNA diagnosis process, leading to the missed diagnosis of thalassemia major. The sequence of events involves the complainant, whose previous child had been diagnosed with thalassemia major, consulting regarding a second pregnancy. Following the diagnosis by the medical facility (OP), the complainant was advised to proceed with the pregnancy. The child was subsequently delivered, but their hemoglobin level was found to be low, and they were diagnosed with thalassemia major. The error in this case stemmed from a significant mistake in the extraction of DNA from chorionic villus samples, which ultimately impacted the test results.

The complainant alleged a deficiency in service due to this error. However, it is important to note that no scientific technology can claim to be entirely perfect. In prenatal tests based on DNA technology, there is typically a small margin of error (approximately 1–2%) in the results. While the test can reduce the risk of disease recurrence from 25% to 1%, it cannot completely eliminate the possibility. The court found no concrete evidence to demonstrate negligence during the DNA analysis process, and the doctrine of res ipsa loquitur (the thing speaks for itself) did not apply. As a result, the Court ruled that no compensation was payable as there is no negligence.

LSCS—meconium aspiration—no negligence of pediatrician

Mrs Pulkit Kapoor versus Handa Hospital, (PSCDRC) (Chandigarh), Consumer Complaint No. 599 of 2018. D/d. 19.04.2021[16]

A 24-year-old female patient, at 38^{+6} weeks of pregnancy, presented in an emergency state with early labor. An emergency cesarean section (LSCS) was performed. After a prolonged labor, a male baby was delivered through LSCS at 11:04 pm on the same day, July 26, 2016. The baby required resuscitation, and it was noted that the baby experienced respiratory distress and peripheral cyanosis due to meconium passage after birth. According to the complainants' own admission, opposite party no. 3, Dr Pardeep Handa, a pediatrician arrived at opposite party no. 1 hospital immediately after the delivery. The records from DMC and hospital, where the child was transferred, indicate that the child was intubated and receiving bag and tube ventilation upon admission, a procedure carried out by opposite party no. 3. The primary lapse appears to be on the part of opposite party no. 2, the obstetrician, who failed to take appropriate measures for the safe delivery of the child. Therefore, there is no evidence of service deficiency or medical negligence on the part of opposite party no. 3, and the complaint against him should be dismissed. The responsibility for compensation, amounting to Rs. 3500,000/- (Rupees Thirty-Five Lac only), falls upon opposite parties no. 1 (Hospital), No. 2 (Obstetrician), and No. 9 (Insurance Company)".

CONCLUSION

Neonatal and preterm care has evolved significantly over the past decades, with remarkable advancements and improved outcomes. This achievement is reflected in increased survival of sick newborn but at the same time morbidity remains with such babies in form of sequelae and neurodevelopmental delay. Hard work of pediatrician in ensuring intact survival may go in waste in absence of high-risk newborn screening, explanation of prognosis and documentation, and inform consent. As preterm and neonatal care becomes increasingly complex, understanding and addressing medicolegal issues are essential for healthcare providers and institutions dedicated to delivering optimal care while upholding legal and ethical standards. This comprehensive approach of documenting and communicating the real prognosis and risk factors will not only benefit themselves but also to families of newborn.

LEARNING KEY POINTS AND TAKE-HOME MESSAGES

- High-risk newborn screening advice is the most crucial event in neonatal care; failure of which may land the treating pediatrician in medicolegal litigation.
- Hard work of paediatrician in ensuring intact survival may go in waste in absence of high-risk newborn screening, explanation of prognosis and documentation and inform consent.
- Inform consent and documentation of risk of life, complication and neuro-developmental sequelae is must for all paediatricians.
- Exclusive breast feeding must be advised to all neonates.
- Breast feeding formula should be offered only after written consent of mother in neonatal units.

MUST AVOID THINGS—DO NOT DO

- Never forget to refer preterm baby for ROP screening.
- Never forget to perform TSH after 1 week age.
- Never stop resuscitating a newborn without DNR consent in prescribed way.

MUST DO THINGS

- Newborn and preterm may suffer kernicterus so monitor jaundice and manage.
- High-risk newborn screening should be advised to all high-risk newborn.
- Take care of iatrogenic injuries and infection in NICU.
- OAE screening should be performed in all babies.

MESSAGES WHICH THE READER MUST BE AWARE

Sudden unexpected deaths are common, manage or transfer accordingly.

WARNINGS

Avoid iatrogenic burn injuries.

MEDICAL NEGLIGENCE PEARLS

Use expressed breast milk or directly promote breastfeeding and avoid problems related to IMS act.

ONLY ONE FACT TO REMEMBER

Always treat a sick preterm or newborn in NICU.

MCQs

Choose one correct answer

1. Congenital anomaly USG scan is done in:
   a. First semester
   b. Third semester
   c. 18–22 week GA
   d. None of the above
2. ROP screening of preterm baby has to be carried on:
   a. 4 week chronological age
   b. Before discharge from NICU
   c. Either of the above
   d. None of the above
3. In high-risk newborn, essential documentation on discharge card is:
   a. High-risk newborn screening advice
   b. Mentioning the address and contact number of screening referral center
   c. Noting in discharge card in Bold letters "**High-Risk Neonate**"
   d. All of the above
4. Mammoth compensations in medical negligence in neonatology practice are attributed to:
   a. Maximum life span of patient
   b. Chances of neurodevelopmental sequelae are high
   c. Sympathy of the court
   d. All of the above

Answers

1. c   2. c   3. d   4. d

REFERENCES

1. WHO. Newborn Mortality. [online] Available on https://www.who.int/news-room/fact-sheets/detail/levels-and-trends-in-child-mortality-report-2021 [Last accessed December, 2023].
2. Mwaniki MK, Atieno M, Lawn JE, Newborn CR. Long-Term neurodevelopmental outcomes after intrauterine and neonatal insults: A systemic review. Lancet. 2012; 379(9814):445-52.
3. Chapter 123: Early Detection and Intervention of a High-risk Neonate, Standard Treatment Guidelines 2022. [online] Available from: https://iapindia.org/pdf/Ch-123-Early-Detection-and-Early-Intervention-of-a-High-risk-Neonate.pdf [Last accessed December, 2023].
4. Boyle CA, Bocchini Jr JA, Kelly J. Reflections on 50 years of newborn screening. Pediatrics. 2014;133:961-3.
5. Advisory Committee on Heritable Disorders in Newborns and Children recommends that every newborn screening program include a Recommended Uniform Screening Panel. [online] Available from: https://www.aafp.org/pubs/afp/issues/2017/0601/p703.html [Last accessed December, 2023].
6. V Krishnakumar vs State of Tamil Nadu & Othrs [online] Available from: https://indiankanoon.org/doc/152852131/ [Last accessed December, 2023].
7. IAP Resolution on IMS Act. [online] Available from: https://iapindia.org/news.php?news=54&title=_IAP_Resolution_on_IMS_Act [Last accessed December, 2023].
8. Chen J, Flabouris A, Bellomo R. The medical emergency team system and not-for-resuscitation orders: results from the MERIT study. Resuscitation. 2008;79:391-7.
9. Mishra S, Mukhopadhyay K, Tiwari S, Bangal R, Yadav BS, Sachdeva A, et al. End-of-Life Care: Consensus Statement by Indian Academy of Pediatrics. Indian Pediatr. 2017; 54:851-9.

10. Whang JS, Baker SR, Patel R, Luk L, Castro A 3rd. The causes of medical malpractice suits against radiologists in the United States. Radiology. 2013;266:548-54.
11. Munro v. Regents of the University of California 1989, at 884-885.
12. Dr Monika Chopra v. Resham Singh, (PSCDRC) (Special Bench), 2016(4) C.P.R. 42, First Appeal No. 1205 of 2014, dated 8.8.2016
13. Dr Pradeep v. State of Maharashtra, (Bombay HC) (DB) (Nagpur Bench), 2017 ALL MR (Cri) 3430: 2017(3) AIR Bom.R (Cri) 133: 2017(5) Mh.LJ (Crl.) 486: 2018(1) Bom.C.R (Cri.) 178, Criminal Application (Apl) No. 503 of 2016 with Criminal Application (Apl) No. 505 of 2016. D/d. 06.07.2017.
14. Sri Dipankar Das v. ILS Hospital, Agartala, (TSCDRC), Case No. CC. 4 of 2019. D/d. 17.05.2021.
15. Sailesh Munjal v. All India Institute of Medical Sciences (NCDRC), Original Petition No. 224 of 1994, dated 20.5.2004.
16. Mrs Pulkit Kapoor v. Handa Hospital, (PSCDRC) (Chandigarh), Consumer Complaint No. 599 of 2018. D/d. 19.04.2021.

Legal Hurdles of Police, RTI, Labor and Drug Inspectors, Fire NOC, Bio-Waste in Medical Practice etc.

Hemant R Gangolia, Satish Agrawal, Sameer Sadawarte, C Nirmala

Keywords: Bio-waste management, Drug inspector, Police calling, RTI

Aim: To address the legal hurdles faced by medical practitioners in India, measures such as streamlining right to information act (RTI) procedures, clarifying police calling guidelines, rationalizing drug inspector visits, providing training on biomedical waste management, simplifying administrative procedures, and fostering open communication between healthcare stakeholders should be considered.[1,2]

Objective: Medical practitioners in India face a multitude of legal hurdles that can hinder their ability to provide care effectively. These hurdles can range from administrative complexities to legal challenges, and they can have a significant impact on the quality and accessibility of healthcare services.

INTRODUCTION

In today's era of consumerism, the medical practice is challenging and it requires the thought full mind for the promptness in the unexpected situations in day-to-day practice. There are too many laws covering the medical profession and having the stressful impact on the pediatric practice for that matter any medical practice.

It is beyond the scope of this chapter to cover all the legal hurdles during the medical practice in view of so many legalities and liabilities related to the existing laws of the land, therefore, we will try to cover common practical unexpected scenarios, hurdles seen in our day-to-day practice where one has to be calm and act appropriately.

Let us go through the scenarios where one should learn to anticipate and act accordingly.

RTI IN MEDICAL PRACTICE

Sometimes in practice, we do not find solutions to some medicolegal issues in the law books and we need the relevant information related to the issue, for example, the period of keeping the medical records. RTI is the best method to get the information, therefore, one should be aware of how to go about it and learn the methodology of RTI.

RTI Act 2005 gives the right to each and every citizen of India to know about the requisite information. For the details of the act, one can search *https://rti.gov.in/rtiact.htm*.[3]

Every citizen of India has a right to free speech and expression under Article 19(1)(a) of the Constitution of India. The right to know and seek information is an integral part of the fundamental right enshrined under Article 19(1)(a), and this right was made available to citizen of India via Right to Information Act which came into force on October 12th, 2005. Section 2(f) of RTI Act provides access to records held by private bodies through regulatory public authority as ordained by any law in force. As per clinical establishment act, clinics and hospitals are obliged to preserve medical records for 3 year and these need to furnish district health authorities on demand. So, this provides legal access to health record of clinical establishments through district health authorities under RTI Act 2005. Records can be asked for prescribed retention period only as per ruling by Chief Information Commission in TV Varghese versus BSNL case in case of nonavailability of record after prescribed retention period.[6-8] Subjudice information relating to pending proceeding should be asked through court or tribunal as per ruling by Chief Information Commission in R K Moraraka versus Central Bank of India.[11]

As doctors, we can file RTI to get the relevant information related to the medical practice. One should try to learn the process of filing RTI.

As well sometimes, the relatives or patient or third party files RTI to get the information about the treatment and management.

The issue is whether to respond to the RTI and to provide the requisite information or not.

The states where the Clinical Establishment Act has been implemented, it is legally binding on the clinical establishment to answer and provide the information as asked through RTI.

In the states where the Clinical Establishment Act is not implemented, one should know the Central Information Commission ruling.

One can file RTI to Private hospital for a copy of one's medical report.[4] In the decision passed by the Central Information Commission in a case titled Prabhat Kumar versus Directorate of Health Services GNCTD,[5] Delhi bearing no. CIC/SA/A/2014/000004,[5] it has been held that the medical records of a patient both for private and government hospitals have to be provided under the RTI Act to the patient and/or to their family members. It has also been held that nonfurnishing of medical records especially by private hospitals shall amount to violation of Article 14 of the Constitution of India which shall also imply levying a penalty on such hospitals.

Since it has been held in the CIC order that the medical records of a patient both for private and government hospitals have to be provided under the RTI Act.[8-10]

Hence, one can file RTI to Private hospital for a copy of one's medical report. So, it is clear that information can be asked from private hospitals and medical practitioners through regulating public authority and all clinical establishments are obliged to issue medical record or information pertaining to preservation period as per various statutes applicable to them.

The way out in the states where the Clinical Establishment Act has not been implemented, provision of medical records can be denied to the third party, relatives in view of the Right to confidentiality unless and until the applicant is patient himself or parents/guardian in case of minor.

FIR AND POLICE STATION

In an important decision Honorable Supreme Court of India said, that if the advice of a lawyer and Doctors goes wrong in some way, even than no case under section 420 IPC or something like that can be registered against him/her. Though Supreme Court also said that Lawyer and Doctors should take care of the interests of his/her clients (Justice P Sthasivam and Justice Ranjan Gogoi bench).[12]

CHAPTER 23: Legal Hurdles of Police, RTI, Labor and Drug Inspectors, Fire NOC, Bio-Waste...

Court also said that in professions like lawyers and doctors, the professionals cannot guarantee for the success of the case. Courts said that the advocate cannot provide guarantee to his/her client that he would definitely win the case and nor doctor can tell his patient that is operations are always successful. And though this professions doctor and lawyer can only say that they are experienced in their work and they would do their best efforts so that they are successful.

But practically, FIR that is First Information Report can be lodged by anyone, the citizen of India at the Police Station against the one having allegations/grievances. FIR is done online at the police station by the police and is registered always under IPC sections and Acts. If a patient or his relations feel that there has been criminal negligence in treating causing simple/grievous injury/death, one can file First Information Report (FIR) or noncognizable (NC) in the police station. If death is caused, the case is usually registered under IPC section 304-A and for the grievous injury caused by surgery/treatment, case may be registered under IPC sections 337, 338. All above three IPC sections are cognizable, hence as cognizable offences are serious ones, police can arrest the doctor without warrant but at the same time these offences are bailable. Therefore, one gets the bail outright at the police station.

One of the important Supreme court of India judgment, Martin D'Souza versus MohIshfaq I (2009) CPJ 32 (SC)[13] states, "We, therefore, direct that whenever a complaint is receive against a doctor or hospital by the consumer for a (whether District, State or National) or by the Criminal Court then before issuing notice to the doctor or hospital against whom the complaint was made, the consumer forum or criminal court should first refer the matter to a competent relating to which the medical negligence is attributed, and only after that doctor or committee reports that there is a prima facie case of medical negligence should notice be issued to the concerned doctor/hospital. This is necessary to avoid harassment to doctors who may not be ultimately found negligent. We further warn the police officials not to arrest or harass doctors unless the facts clearly come within the parameters laid down I Jacob Mathew's case[14] (supra), otherwise the policemen will themselves have to face legal action". Jacob Mathew Petitioner versus State of Punjab and Anr. Respondent 2005(3) CPR 70 (SC) defines the standard treatment and states that practitioner must bring to his task a reasonable degree of skill and knowledge, and must exercise a reasonable degree of care and stick to standard care and standard protocols. Most of the Police department of the states have issued the circulars to the police stations of not to arrest doctors but to follow the Supreme Court judgment guidelines".

On the other hand, in case of any mishap, untoward incidence doctor should lodge the FIR, before the concerned patient approaches the police station. When FIR is lodged by doctor as it is online to take care that it is registered under Doctor Protection Act and the relevant IPC sections.

Mishaps are part and parcel of medical practice; therefore, in any case of mishap calling/informing the police is the best option. How does one inform the police? The staff/assistants should always have the telephone number of the police station so that one can call immediately the police station in anticipation of any mishap or any untoward incidence. One may dial 100 also which is documented, registered call.

Later on, it is better to inform officially by a letter explaining the incidence.

In case of any complaint received by the police station, if police officials call, one should always attend the call and get all the information regarding the purpose of the call. If police officials ask to come to the police station, one may refuse it in view of the busy OPD or any if existing emergency politely and to inform about the time to attend it. It is always better to go to police station in the morning rather evening in view of any arrest, the police have to produce the accused in judicial First Class Magistrate within 24 hours so that minimizes the chance of being behind the bars as most likely to get the bail by Magistrate as most of the sections related to medical negligence are bailable.

When police officials come to the clinic/nursing homes/hospitals with the summons, do not keep them waiting unless and until one is busy with dire emergency, attend them respectfully. One should receive the summons and one should write the date and time of its receipt duly signed. One may ask the time to come and can address the issues of OPD timings and the availability. Sometimes, the police officials can come for an enquiry or in emergency on the receipt of telephonic call of the complaining patient. One has to cooperate with them and can answer their queries and in case of sudden death/mishaps to cooperate for the panchnama if carried out. The police may come to investigate the case and collect evidence to prove the negligence of the doctor. The evidence may include the medical records of the patient, the prescription of the doctor, the postmortem report, the statements of the witnesses, the expert opinion of other doctors, etc.

The rights of the doctor if they are arrested for the charge of medical negligence in India are as follows:

- The doctor has the right to be informed of the grounds of arrest and the nature of the offence by the police officer who arrests him.
- The doctor has the right to consult and be defended by a legal practitioner of his choice. He can also seek the assistance of the Indian Medical Association or other professional bodies to defend his case.
- The doctor has the right to be produced before a magistrate within 24 hours of his arrest, excluding the time necessary for the journey from the place of arrest to the court.[1] He can also apply for bail before the magistrate or the high court, depending on the gravity of the offence.
- The doctor has the right to be treated with dignity and respect by the police and the court. He cannot be subjected to any torture, cruelty, or inhuman treatment during his arrest, detention, or trial.

WHEN DRUG INSPECTOR ARRIVES?

Drug inspector is responsible for monitoring and ensuring the quality, safety, and efficacy of drugs from the production stage to the selling stage. A drug inspector may work under the Drug Controller General of India (DCGI) or the State Drug Controller (SDC) or FDA depending on their posting.

When a drug inspector arrives for a medical malpractice case to a doctor, they may have to perform the following tasks:
- Inspect and audit the doctor's clinic, laboratory, pharmacy, or other establishment that deals with drugs.
- Collect and analyze samples of drugs, medicines, cosmetics, or other substances used or prescribed by the doctor.

CHAPTER 23: Legal Hurdles of Police, RTI, Labor and Drug Inspectors, Fire NOC, Bio-Waste...

- Check the records, licenses, prescriptions, invoices, and other documents related to the drugs.
- Verify the compliance of the doctor with the Drugs and Cosmetics Act, 1940 and the rules and regulations made thereunder.
- Report any violations, adulterations, spuriousness, misbranding, or other irregularities in the drugs or their usage.
- Initiate legal action against the doctor if found guilty of medical malpractice or negligence.
- Educate and advise the doctor and the public about the safe and proper use of drugs.

The Drugs and Cosmetics Act, 1940 and the Drugs and Cosmetics Rules, 1945 are the main legal framework for regulating the manufacture, sale, and distribution of drugs and cosmetics in India. The Act and the Rules have various provisions and sections that deal with the responsibilities and liabilities of doctors and other medical practitioners who keep or use drugs and cosmetics in their clinics or hospitals.

SCHEDULE K (See Rule 123 of drugs and cosmetic rules 1945).[15]

Drugs supplied by a registered medical practitioner to his own patient or any drug specified in Schedule C supplied by a registered medical practitioner.

That means, in short, the distributors must supply drugs to private practitioners and hospitals who have the right to buy and stock, dispense, or sell any drug without a license, provided the drugs are dispensed to their own patients within the premises and not sold to outsiders under the sign of "Pharmacy", "Pharmacist", "Dispensing Chemist" or "Pharmaceutical Chemist" or any other sign that indicates sale of medicines. The latest amendment to Schedule K was made in 2020, which added some new drugs and substances to the list. One can find the full text of Schedule K in the Cosmetics Rules, 2020 or the Drugs and Cosmetics Rules, 1945.[16,17]

National Medical Commission, Ethics and Medical Registration Board, Notification, New Delhi, August 2nd, 2023 states under Chapter 1, Professional Conduct of RMPs at point number 12 as follows:

12. Responsibility of RMP regarding the sale of drugs:[18,19]
- RMP shall not run an open shop to sell medicines prescribed by RMPs other than himself or for the sale of medical or surgical appliances. They are allowed to sell medication only to his/her own patients (L2).
- RMP can prescribe or supply drugs, remedies, or appliances as long as there is no exploitation of the patients. Drugs prescribed by RMP or bought from the pharmacy for a patient should explicitly state the generic name of the drug (L2).
- RMP shall not administer, dispense or prescribe secret remedial agents of which he does not know the composition or action in the body. The manufacture or promotion or use of these remedies is prohibited (L3).

L2 and L3 are the levels of disciplinary action as per breach of conduct as follows:
- *Level 2:* This penalty may be awarded even when the role of the doctor in causing direct harm was not conclusively proved but the doctor was found to have breached any of the codes listed above. The maximum action is a suspension of the license to practice for up to one month (30 days).
- *Level 3:* This penalty may be awarded when the role of the doctor in causing

direct harm was conclusively proved and the doctor was found to have breached relevant regulation. This maximum action is a suspension of the license to practice for a maximum period of 3 months. Holding suspension can be given in this level as per regulations.

In short, doctors should keep the invoices related to the purchase, disposal of the drugs used in practice for its patients only with due attention to the storage of medicines as per storage conditions recommendations.

WHEN LABOR INSPECTOR ARRIVES?

In India, the labor inspectors are responsible for enforcing various labor laws and ensuring that employers comply with them. They may inspect the premises of factories, shops, and other establishments to ensure that they are following the necessary regulations and guidelines.

According to the Clinical Establishments Act of 2010 in India,[19] doctors running a clinic or hospital must maintain some mandatory records under the law. These records include:
- Record of employment of adults, letters of employment issued and hours of work
- Records regarding the treatment of patients.

According to the Employees' Provident Funds and Miscellaneous Provisions Act, 1952 in India, the applicability of the act depends on the number of employees working in an establishment. The act is applicable to all factories wherein:
- 10 or more persons are/were employed with the aid of power
- 20 or more workers are/were employed without the aid of power, on any day in the preceding 12 months.

The Code on Wages, 2019[20] has standardized the definition of wages, based on which employers deduct provident fund contributions. The Code of Wages is a part of four labor codes that resulted from the merging 29 out of the 44 central government labor laws.

Some of the labor laws that are to be followed in India by a nursing home or a hospital are:
- *The Minimum Wages Act, 1948:*[21] This act sets the minimum wages for different categories of employees, such as sweepers, ward boys, ayahs, peons, nurses, technicians, etc. The wages consist of basic wages and special allowance, which vary every 6 months depending on the consumer price index.
- *The Industrial Disputes Act, 1947:*[22] This act regulates the settlement of industrial disputes, such as strikes, lockouts, layoffs, retrenchments, etc. It also provides for the constitution of works committees, conciliation officers, boards of conciliation, courts of inquiry, labor courts, industrial tribunals, and national tribunals.
- *The Payment of Gratuity Act, 1972:*[23] This act provides for the payment of gratuity to the employees who have completed 5 years of continuous service in an establishment employing twenty or more persons. The gratuity is calculated at the rate of 15 days' wages for every completed year of service or part thereof in excess of 6 months, subject to a maximum of 20 lakh rupees.
- *The Payment of Bonus Act, 1965:*[24] This act provides for the payment of bonus to the employees who have worked for not less than thirty working days in an accounting year in an establishment employing ten or more persons. The bonus is calculated at the rate of 8.33% of the salary or wage

earned by the employee during the accounting year or one hundred rupees, whichever is higher, subject to a maximum of 20% of such salary or wage.
- *The Employees' Provident Fund Act, 1952:*[25] This act provides for the establishment of provident fund, pension fund, and deposit-linked insurance fund for the employees in factories and other establishments employing twenty or more persons. The act requires the employer and the employee to contribute a certain percentage of the basic wages, dearness allowance, and retaining allowance to the funds. The act also provides for the administration, inspection, and audit of the funds.
- *The Bombay Shops and Establishments Act, 1948:*[26] This act applies to the shops and establishments in the state of Maharashtra, including hospitals and nursing homes. The act regulates the working hours, weekly offs, holidays, leave, overtime, health, safety, and welfare of the employees. The act also requires the registration and renewal of the shops and establishments with the local authorities.

In short, doctors have to keep the relevant records, registers as attendance register, salary register, etc. as per the relevant acts applicable to the clinical establishment. The best way out is to appoint the person having the knowledge of the labor laws or the retired drug inspector to look after the requisites of the employees.

POLLUTION CONTROL COMPLIANCE

The biomedical waste management rules and regulations for doctors in India are the legal framework for ensuring the safe and proper handling and disposal of the waste generated from the diagnosis, treatment, or immunization of human beings or animals, or in research activities pertaining to such fields. The rules aim to protect the health and environment of the people and prevent the spread of diseases and infections.

The main rules and regulations for doctors in India are:
- The Biomedical Waste Management Rules, 2016,[27] as amended in 2018, which are issued by the Ministry of Environment, Forest and Climate Change under the Environment (Protection) Act, 19861. These rules specify the duties and responsibilities of the occupier (the person who has the control over the institution that generates biomedical waste), the operator (the person who owns or operates a common biomedical waste treatment facility), and the prescribed authority (the State Pollution Control Board or the Pollution Control Committee). The rules also define the categories, standards, procedures, and guidelines for the segregation, collection, storage, transportation, treatment, and disposal of biomedical waste. The rules also mandate the use of barcodes, global positioning system, and online reporting system for tracking and monitoring the biomedical waste. The rules also prescribe the penalties and offences for noncompliance with the rules.
- The Clinical Establishments (Registration and Regulation) Act, 2010, which is enacted by the Ministry of Health and Family Welfare to provide for the registration and regulation of all clinical establishments in the country. The act defines a clinical establishment as any facility that offers services or facilities relating to diagnosis, treatment, or care

for illness, injury, deformity, abnormality, or pregnancy in any recognized system of medicine. The act requires all clinical establishments to obtain a certificate of registration from the district registering authority and comply with the minimum standards of facilities and services, as prescribed by the Central Government or the State Government. The act also empowers the Central Government or the State Government to make rules and regulations for the implementation of the act, including the management of biomedical waste.

- The State-specific laws and regulations, which are enacted by the respective State Governments or Union Territories to supplement or modify the central laws and regulations, as per their local needs and conditions. For example, some states have their own acts or rules for the registration and regulation of hospitals, nursing homes, or other health care facilities, such as the Bombay Nursing Home Registration Act, 1949, the Delhi Nursing Homes Registration Act, 1953, or the Karnataka Private Medical Establishments Act, 2007. Some states also have their own guidelines or manuals for the management of biomedical waste, such as the Maharashtra Bio Medical Waste Management Manual, 2017, or the Tamil Nadu Bio Medical Waste Management Guidelines, 2018.

Biomedical waste means any waste, which is generated during the diagnosis, treatment, or immunization of human beings or animals or research activities pertaining thereto or in the production or testing of biological or in health camps. Biomedical waste includes all the waste generated from the Health Care Facility which can have any adverse effect to the health of a person or to the environment in general if not disposed properly. All such waste which can adversely harm the environment or health of a person is considered as infectious and such waste has to be managed as per BMWM Rules, 2016. The health care waste comprises 15% biomedical waste and 85% general waste.

The quantity of such waste is around 10–15% of total waste generated from the Health Care Facility. This waste consists of the materials which have been in contact with the patient's blood, secretions, infected parts, biological liquids such as chemicals, medical supplies, medicines, laboratory discharge, sharps metallic and glassware, plastics, etc.

Bio Medical Waste Management Rules, 2016 categorizes the bio-medical waste generated from the health care facility into four categories based on the segregation pathway and color code. Various types of biomedical waste are further assigned to each one of the categories, as detailed below:

1. *Yellow category:*
   - *Human anatomical waste:* Human tissues, organs, body parts and fetus below the viability period (as per the Medical Termination of Pregnancy Act 1971, amended from time to time).
   - *Animal anatomical waste:* Experimental animal carcasses, body parts, organs, tissues, including the waste generated from animals used in experiments or testing in veterinary hospitals or colleges or animal houses.
   - *Soiled waste:* Items contaminated with blood, body fluids like dressings, plaster casts, cotton swabs and bags containing residual or discarded blood and blood components.
   - *Discarded or expired medicine*: Pharmaceutical waste like antibiotics,

cytotoxic drugs including all items contaminated with cytotoxic drugs along with glass or plastic ampoules, vials, etc.
- *Chemical waste:* Chemicals used in production of biological and used or discarded disinfectants.
- *Chemical liquid waste:* Liquid waste generated due to use of chemicals in production of biological and used or discarded disinfectants, silver X-ray film developing liquid, discarded Formalin, infected secretions, aspirated body fluids, liquid from laboratories and floor washings, cleaning, house-keeping and disinfecting activities, etc.
- *Discarded linen, mattresses, beddings contaminated with blood or body fluid, routine mask and gown: Microbiology, biotechnology, and other clinical laboratory waste (pretreated): Microbiology, biotechnology, and other clinical laboratory waste:* Blood bags, laboratory cultures, stocks or specimens of microorganisms, live or attenuated vaccines, human and animal cell cultures used in research, industrial laboratories, production of biological, residual toxins, dishes and devices used for cultures.

2. *Red category:* Wastes generated from disposable items such as tubing, bottles, intravenous tubes and sets, catheters, urine bags, syringes without needles, fixed needle syringes with their needles cut, vacutainers, and gloves.

3. *White category:*
    - Waste sharps including metals
    - Needles, syringes with fixed needles, needles from needle tip cutter or burner, scalpels, blades, or any other contaminated sharp object that may cause puncture and cuts. This includes both used, discarded and contaminated metal sharps.

4. *Blue category:* Broken or discarded and contaminated glass including medicine vials and ampoules except those contaminated with cytotoxic wastes.

General waste consists of all the waste other than biomedical waste and which has not been in contact with any hazardous or infectious, chemical, or biological secretions and does not includes any waste sharps. This waste consists of mainly:
- Newspaper, paper, and card boxes (dry waste)
- Plastic water bottles (dry waste)
- Aluminum cans of soft drinks (dry waste)
- Packaging materials (dry waste)
- Food containers after emptying residual food (dry waste)
- Organic/bio-degradable waste—mostly food waste (wet waste)
- Construction and demolition wastes.

These general wastes are further classified as dry wastes and wet wastes and should be collected separately.

This quantity of such waste is around 85–90% of total waste generated from the facility. Such waste is required to be handled as per Solid Waste Management Rules, 2016 and Construction and Demolition Waste Management Rules, 2016, as applicable.

It is mandatory for each doctor to register with the State Pollution Control Board for authorization to generate the biomedical waste. The registration is valid for 3 years and has to be renewed every 3 years on payment of the prescribed fees. Then one has to register with or to appoint the agency as the service provider for the collection and disposal of biomedical waste as per the recommended norms. The fees for the service provider are to be negotiated as per the nature of the clinical establishment along with the help of local medical associations. The requisites certificates and documents related to the state pollution control board and the agency service provider to be kept in the establishment which will be needed while renewal of the clinical establishment registration.

Is clinical establishment commercial activity?
This is a debatable issue and often comes while paying the premises tax to the local bodies as well for the electricity and water bills. Many times, conflicts occur at the local level with the concerned local governing authorities and electricity providers. Therefore, it is an attempt to discuss here about the court rulings to say on this and to be used as the references to solve the local conflicts.

Marked difference in treatment and discrimination with medical professionals with others like lawyers, have been apparent since long in government policies. So, few pertinent questions have become relevant once again; one whether Medical Profession is profession or commerce, second is there any legal basis of such discrimination. Answer of these questions have been given by the Supreme Court Precedents which are binding on all subordinate courts under article 141 and on government bodies under article 144 of Indian Constitution. The only need is to be aware of these important judicial verdicts.

PROFESSIONAL ESTABLISHMENT OF A DOCTOR IS NOT COMMERCIAL ACTIVITY: SUPREME COURT

In Dr Devendra M Surti versus State of Gujarat[28] on May 2, 1968 Equivalent citations: 1969 AIR 63, 1969 SCR (1) 235, honorable Supreme Court held that Professional Establishment of a doctor cannot be held commercial in character. It was held that:

We are therefore of opinion that the professional establishment of a doctor cannot come within the definition of S.2(4) of the Act unless the activity carried on was also commercial in character. As to what exactly is meant by "Commerce" it may be difficult to define but in an early case—McKav versus Rutherfurd(3), Lord Camp-bell gave a useful definition: "Commerce is that activity where a capital is laid out on any work and a risk run of profit or loss; it is a commercial venture".

It is therefore clear that a professional activity must be an activity carried on by an individual by his personal skill and intelligence. There is a fundamental distinction therefore between a professional activity and an activity of a commercial character and unless the profession carried on by the appellant also partakes of the character of a commercial nature, the appellant cannot fall within the ambit of S. 2 (4) of the Act.

SUPREME COURT DECLARED LAWYER'S OFFICE AS NONCOMMERCIAL CITING IN DR DEVENDRA M SURTI VERSUS THE STATE OF GUJARAT

Supreme Court of India on August 24, 2005 declared lawyer's office as noncommercial in Chairman, M.P. Electricity Board versus Shiv Narayan and Anr Appeal (civil) 1065 of 2000. Supreme Court held:

A professional activity must be an activity carried on by an individual by his personal skill and intelligence. There is a fundamental distinction, therefore, between a professional activity and an activity of a commercial character. Considering a similar question in the background of Section 2(4) of the Bombay Shops and Establishments Act (79 of 1948), it was held by this Court in Dr Devendra M Surti versus The State of Gujarat (AIR 1969 SC 63) that a doctor's establishment is not covered by the expression "Commercial establishment".... Even if it is accepted that the user was not domestic, it may be nondomestic. But it does not automatically become "commercial". The words "nondomestic" and "commercial" are not interchangeable.

Law propounded by Supreme Court in Dr Devendra M Surti versus State of Gujarat[28] has been followed by various high courts as follows:

- *In Dr DV Chug versus State and Anr CRL.M.C.No.1474/2007 and Crl.M.A. 5115-16/2007 case*, Delhi High court enunciated principals enunciated by Supreme Court in Dr Devendra M Surti versus State of Gujarat 1968 case and held: On considering the submissions of ld. counsel appearing for the parties, I am of the considered view that the professional establishment of a doctor cannot come within the definition of commercial activity.... Commerce is that activity where a capital is put into; work and risk run of profit or loss. If the activities are undertaken for production or distribution of goods or for rendering material services, then it comes under the definition of commerce. The word "profession" used to be confined to the three learned professions; the Church, Medicine, and Law. There is a fundamental distinction between the professional activities and commercial activities.
- *In Dr (Smt) Shubhada Motwani versus The State of Maharashtra and Ors.* Criminal Writ Petition No.1731 of 2002, Bombay High Court in its Judgment on June 12th, 2014 said:
We have heard the learned counsel for the petitioner and the counsel on behalf of the State. The Apex Court in "Devendra M Surti, Dr versus State of Gujarat" (supra) has, after examining the provisions of the "Gujarat Shops and Establishments Act", which are identical to the provisions of Bombay Shops and Establishments Act, 1948 come to the conclusion that "private dispensary of doctor is not commercial establishment".
- *In Kavita Pravin Tilwani versus The State of Maharashtra and Others* Criminal Writ Petition No.3989 of 2013, Bombay High Court in its judgment on July 10th, 2014 said that:
The Apex Court in the case of Devendra M Surti (supra) has held that private dispensary of a doctor is not a commercial establishment ... A similar issue had arisen before the Division Bench of this Court in the case of Narendra Keshrichand Fuladi (supra). The Division Bench held that a legal practitioner having an office cannot be said to be carrying on commercial activity and would not fall within the definition of the expression "commercial establishment..." The writ petition is accordingly allowed in terms of prayer clauses (a) and (b) and is accordingly disposed of.
- *In Dr Pradeep Arora versus The State of Maharashtra Writ Petition No. 7590 of 2017*, Nagpur Bench, Bombay High Court in its Judgment on November 2nd 2018 said that:
The notification declared any hospital to be an establishment and the explanation was to define "hospital" mean, inter alia, any maternity home. This Court held that

the said notification insofar as it seeks to include a maternity home run by the medical practitioner within the Act was beyond the powers conferred by the Act and, therefore, it was held to be invalid. The reliance was placed upon several previous decisions, including the decision in the case of wp7590.17.odt Dr Devendra Surti, cited supra.

- *In Satya Prakash Singh versus State of UP and Ors.*, Civil Misc Writ Petition no 16843 of 2011, Allahabad High Court in its judgment on 29th May 2012 held that:

The work of a doctor, chartered Accountant or a Lawyer or a matter of fact any consultant is a profession which is distinct from any trade or business. Generally, profession is an activity which is created by an individual by his personal skill, intelligence depending upon his character. It is not in the nature of any trade or business. It is vocation or occupation requiring special advance education, knowledge and skill predominantly of an intellectual nature rather than physical or manual.

The profession of lawyer and that of a doctor stand on equal footing as both are professionals and so is the lawyer's office and of doctor's clinic/dispensary or even pathology laboratory. The building in question is recognized by the respondents themselves partial as residential nature, therefore the portion of the doctor's clinic/dispensary or laboratory situated therein would be a part of the residential premises ... Authorities have erred in treating the ground floor portion of the building in question to be commercial in nature for the reason that at one point of time a doctor's clinic or pathology was being run there. It is a part of residential building.

So, it can be seen that the law propounded by Honorable Supreme Court in Dr Devendra M Surti versus State of Gujarat 1968 has been enunciated again and again by Supreme Court itself and various High Courts and principle remains the same that profession cannot be equated with commerce and doctor's clinic cannot be rendered commercial establishment. Need of the hour is to be aware of these and to apprise government bodies about these judicial precedents which are binding on them related to premise tax, electricity, and water bills. Our Medical Associations have great role to play in this matter.

▪ POCSO ACT AND PEDIATRICIANS

Sexual crimes against minors are a serious violation of human rights and a grave offence under the law. Doctors in India have a duty to prevent and respond to such crimes in their hospital or clinic, as per the following guidelines:

The Protection of Children from Sexual Offences (POCSO) Act, 2012[29] is the main legal framework for safeguarding children from sexual abuse and sexual offences in India.[1] The Act defines a child as any person below the age of 18 years and provides punishment as per the gravity of the offence. The Act also mandates the reporting of such cases by any person who has knowledge or apprehension of such offences, including doctors.

Doctors should be aware of the signs and symptoms of sexual abuse and sexual offences in children, such as physical injuries, behavioral changes, emotional distress, sexualized behavior, etc. Doctors should also be sensitive and empathetic while dealing with such cases and provide appropriate medical care and counseling to the child and the family.

Doctors should follow the protocol for reporting such cases to the authorities, such as the police, the child welfare committee, or the special juvenile police unit, as per the POCSO Act and the local laws and regulations. Doctors should also maintain the confidentiality and privacy of the child and the family, unless required by law.

As a pediatrician, one should read the POCSO Act in true spirit, word by word and to anticipate the issues pertaining to the sexual abuse when we see the children in the OPD. Some of the important sections of the act pertaining to our practice are:

- Section 19 of the Protection of Children from Sexual Offences Act, 2012 (POCSO Act) mandates the reporting of sexual crimes against children. It requires every person who suspects or has knowledge of a sexual offence being committed against a child to report it to the local police or the Special Juvenile Police Unit. The term "any person" also includes a child who may report an offence.
- Section 21 of the Protection of Children from Sexual Offences Act, 2012 (POCSO Act) provides for a punishment for failure to inform the Special Juvenile Police Unit (SJPU) or Local Police or record a case if she/he/they come across any material or object which is sexually exploitative of the child. The punishment for such failure is either imprisonment up to 6 months or with fine or both. Any person in charge of a company or an institution who fails to report the commission of a sexual offence relating to a subordinate under their control is liable to be punished with imprisonment and a fine under Section 21 of the act.

If you or someone you know is a victim of sexual abuse or exploitation, you can report it to the POCSO e-box by pressing the e-box button available at the Commission's website, *www.ncpcr.gov.in*. You can also register your complaints on email id: pocsoebox-ncpcr@gov.in or mobile number: +91-9868235077.

In addition, you can contact CHILDLINE 1098, a national 24-hour toll-free emergency phone service for children in distress.

FIRE PREVENTION COMPLIANCE

Fire safety is a crucial aspect of healthcare facilities such as clinics, nursing homes, and hospitals. Here are some general fire safety tips that can be followed to ensure the safety of patients and staff:

- Ensure all exit doors, evacuation routes, and essential pathways are not blocked and are free of clutter. Follow local regulations on locking doors and maintaining fire doors.
- Train personnel in the use of fire extinguishers.
- Make sure staff members know where fire alarms are and how to activate them.
- Know where oxygen and compressed gas shut-off controls are and how to use them.

In addition, the National Building Code of India—2005[30] provides detailed guidelines for fire prevention and life safety in relation to fire and fire protection of buildings. The code specifies construction, occupancy, and protection features that are necessary to minimize danger to life and property from fire. Hospitals have been classified as sub-division C-1 under Group C for Institutional Buildings with some specific requirements applicable for this category in addition to the general requirements common for all occupancies.

The NBC gives detailed guidelines for Construction Materials, General Requirements for all buildings, Life Safety,

Fire Protection, Specific Occupancy wise Requirements, and specific requirements for buildings above 15 meters.

It is mandatory for all hospitals to obtain No Objection Certificate from the concerned Fire Department before the building can be occupied.

The NOC is to be renewed every year.

SUMMARY

Private hospitals and medical practitioners in India are subject to a complex web of legal requirements, including transparency through the RTI Act, cooperation with police in case of mishaps, adherence to drug regulations, employment record maintenance, regulatory compliance for renewal, awareness of judicial precedents, reporting child sexual offences, and obtaining a No Objection Certificate from the Fire Department. By adhering to these regulations, healthcare providers can ensure ethical, accountable, and patient-centric care.

LEARNING KEY POINTS

- As per RTI Act 2005, the information can be asked from private hospitals and medical practitioners through regulating public authority and all clinical establishments are obliged to issue medical record or information pertaining to preservation period as per various statutes applicable to them.
- Informing and calling Police is the best option in the mishaps, untoward incidences. One has to cooperate with the police officials in case of FIR, arrival of them in clinical establishments with the knowledge of the rights of doctors during police official intervention.
- To follow Drugs and Cosmetics Rules, 1945 (and the amendments) and National Medical Commission, Ethics and Medical Registration Board, Notification related to sell and storage of medicines.
- According to the Clinical Establishments Act of 2010 in India, doctors running a clinic or hospital must maintain records of employment of adults, letters of employment issued and hours of work.
- The requisites certificates and documents related to the state pollution control board and the agency service provider to be kept in the establishment which will be needed while renewal of the clinical establishment registration.
- Need of the hour is to be aware of the court rulings and to apprise government bodies about these judicial precedents which are binding on them related to premise tax, electricity, water bills in view of the activities being not commercial.
- Section 19 of the Protection of Children from Sexual Offences Act, 2012 (POCSO Act) mandates the reporting of sexual crimes against children.
- It is mandatory for all hospitals to obtain No Objection Certificate from the concerned Fire Department before the building can be occupied. The NOC is to be renewed every year.

TAKE-HOME MESSAGES

In instances of mishaps or untoward incidents, hospitals are obligated to inform and cooperate with the police.

MUST AVOID THINGS

Always answer to police investigations.

ONLY ONE FACT TO REMEMBER

Follow labor laws, as they are partners in success of you clinic and hospitals.

CHAPTER 23: Legal Hurdles of Police, RTI, Labor and Drug Inspectors, Fire NOC, Bio-Waste... 303

DO NOT DO
Do not destroy document and records before 3 years of mandated preservation of records as per law.

WARNINGS
Clinics to follow schedule K and Private hospitals must strictly follow these regulations, ensuring that medications are dispensed and stored appropriately, maintaining detailed records of their movement.

MEDICAL NEGLIGENCE PEARLS
Under the Protection of Children from Sexual Offences Act, 2012, hospitals are mandated to report any suspected or confirmed cases of sexual crimes against children.

MUST DO THING
Fire Department Clearance is important.

MESSAGES WHICH THE READER MUST BE AWARE
Always segregate bio waste before giving to transporter.

REFERENCES
1. Baldwa M, Baldwa V, Padvi N, Baldwa S. Legal issues in Medical Practice, 1st edition. New Delhi: CBS Publishers & Distributors; 2019.
2. Tiwari S. Textbook on Medicolegal Issues, 2nd edition. New Delhi: Jaypee Brothers Medical Publishers; 2018.
3. RTI Act, 2005. [online] Available from: https://rti.gov.in/rtiact.htm. [Last accessed December, 2023].
4. File No. CIC/AD/A/2013/001681SA File decided on 23 July 2014.
5. File No. CIC/SA/A/2014/000004 order dated 03.11.2014.
6. Appeal No. 251/ICPB/2006, dated. 2.1.2007.
7. Appeal No CIC/AT/A/2006/00588, dated 9th July 2007.
8. CIC/MA/2006/003636 Order dated September 11 2006.
9. CIC/AT/A/2009/000351-Order dated June 19 2009.
10. CIC/AT/A/00061 Order dated May 01 2007.
11. Appeal no 908/ICPB/2007/F.No.PBA/07/211 on 17th September 2007.
12. Law Corner. (2018). No Direct FIR against a advocate or doctor – Supreme Court. [online] Available from: https://lawcorner.in/no-fir-against-advocate-or-doctor/. [Last accessed December, 2023].
13. Katju M. (2009). Martin D'Souza v. MohIshfaq I (2009) CPJ 32 (SC). [online] Available from: https://indiankanoon.org/doc/1092676/. [Last accessed December, 2023].
14. Lahoti R. (2005). Jacob Mathew Petitioner V. State of Punjab & Anr. Respondent 2005(3) CPR 70 (SC). [online] Available from: https://indiankanoon.org/doc/871062/. [Last accessed December, 2023].
15. SCHEDULE K (See Rule 123 of drugs and cosmetic rules 1945) {3}. [online] Available from: https://pharmafranchisehelp.com/wp-content/uploads/2020/08/Schedule-K.pdf. [Last accessed December, 2023].
16. Central Drugs Standard Control Organisation. Drugs Rules, 1945. [online] Available from: https://cdsco.gov.in/opencms/opencms/en/Acts-and-rules/Drugs-Rules/. [Last accessed December, 2023].
17. Central Drugs Standard Control Organization. *THE DRUGS RULES, 1945. [online] Available from: https://www.drugscontrol.org/pdf/schedule_k.pdf. [Last accessed December, 2023].
18. National Medical Commission. National medical commission registered medical practitioner professional conduct regulations 2023. [online] Available from: https://www.nmc.org.in/rules-regulations/national-medical-commission-registered-medical-practitioner-professional-conduct-regulations-2023-reg/. [Last accessed December, 2023].
19. Clinical Establishments Act of 2010.

20. The Code on Wages, 2019.
21. The Minimum Wages Act, 1948.
22. The Industrial Disputes Act, 1947.
23. The Payment of Gratuity Act, 1972.
24. The Payment of Bonus Act, 1965.
25. The Employees' Provident Fund Act, 1952.
26. The Bombay Shops and Establishments Act, 1948.
27. The Biomedical Waste Management Rules, 2016, (amended in 2018).
28. Dr. Devendra M. Surti vs State of Gujarat on 2 May, 1968 Equivalent citations: 1969 AIR 63, 1969 SCR (1) 235.
29. The Protection of Children from Sexual Offences (POCSO) Act, 2012.
30. National Building Code of India, 2005.

SECTION 4

Miscellaneous

- **Understanding National Medical Commission Act 2019 and Professional Conduct, Etiquette and Ethics and CEA 2010**
  Namita Padvi, Mahesh Baldwa, Varsha Baldwa, Sushila Baldwa

- **Professional Indemnity and Out-of-Court Settlement**
  Satish Tiwari

Miscellaneous

CHAPTER 24

Understanding National Medical Commission Act 2019 and Professional Conduct, Etiquette and Ethics and CEA 2010

Namita Padvi, Mahesh Baldwa, Varsha Baldwa, Sushila Baldwa

"The patient will never care how much you know, until they know how much you care."

Keywords: CEA, Medical Council of India, National Medical Commission, Professional conduct

Aim: The National Medical Commission (NMC) is India's apex regulatory body for medical education and practice. Established in 2019 to replace the Medical Council of India (MCI), the NMC aims to improve access to quality and affordable medical education, ensure adequate and high-quality medical professionals across the country, promote equitable and universal healthcare, encourage community health perspectives, enforce high ethical standards in medical services, and maintain a medical register for India.

Objective: The NMC also grants recognition to medical institutions, prescribes minimum qualifications for medical professionals, conducts examinations, enforces ethical standards, and investigates complaints. It can prescribe regulations with each and every aspect including ethical code of conduct.

INTRODUCTION

The National Medical Commission (NMC) as an umbrella regulatory body with certain other bodies under it. The NMC will subsume the Medical Council of India (MCI) and will regulate medical education and practice in India.

NATURE OF THE MEDICAL PROFESSION AND MEDICAL PRACTICE

The medical profession is comprised a motley group of practitioners each subscribing to a different system of medicine. Allopaths constitute 43.3% of the profession, homeopaths 16%, and practitioners of Indian systems of medicine (viz., *Ashtang Ayurveda, Unani Tibb, and Siddha*) account for 35.7% of all trained medical personnel. Most of these professionals conduct private practice in urban areas and in an individual capacity. The urban concentration is particularly indicated for allopaths (72.8% of them were found in towns and cities) and to a lesser extent for practitioners of the *Ayurveda* and *Unani* (42.7% and 61.2% of whom were in urban areas).

ETHICS

The word "ethics" is derived from the Greek word "ethos" which means customs and habits. It means something in conformity with moral norms or standard of professional conduct. The word relates to the precepts which should control moral behavior. Ethics is that science of knowledge, which deals with the nature and grounds of moral obligations, distinguishing what is right from what is wrong.

Basics of Ethics

Since the dawn of the civilization, by trial and error, it has become established that a society and more so it is medical profession, a publicly oriented and noble profession, cannot survive and thrive without observance and practice of certain rules of conduct guided by ethical, moral, legal, and social values of the land. Human culture is built upon the foundation of value system formed on the basis of society ethical fabric of honesty, integrity, respect to each other, pursuit of excellence, happiness by adhering to civic duties, accountability, and loyalty to one and all elements of society. If one reads the history of human civilization, it becomes evident that the evolution of ethical concepts preoccupied philosopher's attention. Apart from ethicists even sociologists, theologians, almost all professional of the society stressed on ethical concepts. The prime object of the medical profession is to render service to humanity with full respect and dignity to all human beings. A doctor's role is to cure when possible and to relieve pain and suffering always. Sometimes, physician may fail not in his duties but effect cure but even when cure is not possible he must demonstrate to public and family at large that while he could not effect, cure even though he tried his best. The science and practice of medicine has continued to change with the times and advancement of knowledge but the fundamental principles of professional behavior have remained unchanged.

Conflicts between Old Ethos and New Changing Values

Even in the presence of conflict between traditional age old ethos and customs and changing values and orientations, the code of conduct, rules, and obligations coined together as "medical ethics" still upholds, fosters, and guarantees the mode of conduct and behavior of the members of medical profession, as to the obligation of the doctor to the (1) patient, (2) fellow doctors, (3) state through the health professionals, and (4) the society. Though, ethics differs from written "law" or "legislation" or "rules" or "regulations" as in general ethics is governed and guided by moral sense and conscience and not by any statute or an act of legislation. India has a written ethical code duly legislated in 2002[1] and adopted by NMC. Ethical code, though legislated does not have equal force as general laws have. Ethics and laws share the social purpose of encouraging right conduct. Laws including codified and written legislated ethics in India achieve this purpose through the sovereign power of government. All over world medical professional actions and conduct is governed by good conscience, it tells the doctor to do what is good and what is bad, if done to his patient.

Four Ethical Principles of Importance in Brief

There are four basic ethical principles underlying good medico-ethical practice in Western countries. These are *autonomy, justice, beneficence,* and *nonmaleficence.* They sound tongue twisters and also of little help in day today practice yet we shall discuss the age old principles in brief to benefit our insight about ethics.

The first principle is *autonomy:* The right of a fully informed patient to choose out of the treatment offered to the patient.

The second principle is called *justice:* The right to receive what is recommended by doctor.

The third principle is *beneficence:* The obligation of doctor to do good in a given situation before, during, and after the administration of treatment. This does not necessarily imply to preserve life at all costs. In situations, where outcome in a given situation is living a poor quality life, that it is considered less beneficial for the patient than death itself.

The fourth and final principle we shall discuss is *nonmaleficence:* The obligation to avoid doing harm while giving treatment (Latin—*primum non nocere*).

Conflict Within

Autonomy can come into conflict with beneficence when patients disagree with recommendations that healthcare professionals believe are in the patient's best interest. When the patient's interests conflict with the patient's welfare, different societies settle the conflict in a wide range of manners. In general, Western medicine defers to the wishes of a mentally competent patient to make their own decisions, even in cases where the medical team believes that they are not acting in their own best interests. However, many other societies prioritize beneficence over autonomy.

PROFESSION

The term profession is derived from the original Latin *profiteor*. For the medical professional, this public commitment is to the welfare of patients and for improving health status of people. This medical morality, avowal, the public commitment has been behind it as tradition for many centuries.

Since the dawn of the civilization, by trial and error, it has become established that a society and more so it is medical profession, a publicly oriented and noble profession, cannot survive and thrive without observance and practice of certain rules of conduct guided by ethical, moral, legal, and social values of the land.

Human culture is built upon the foundation of value system formed on the basis of society ethical fabric of honesty, integrity, respect to each other, pursuit of excellence, happiness by adhering to civic duties, accountability, and loyalty to one and all elements of society.

NATIONAL MEDICAL COMMISSION ACT 2019[1]

The NMC Act 2019 replaced the 63-year-old MCI Act-1956. The president dissolved the MCI in 2018 and a Board of Governors was appointed to perform its functions. The NMC act repeals the Indian Medical Council Act 1956. It has eight chapters encompassing 61 sections. Section 31 provides for national and state medical register. National Medical Council rules are yet to be framed. The rules are framed and the NMC is constituted for development and regulation of all aspects of medical education, profession, and institutions. NMC is progressive legislation which will reduce the burden on medical students. It will ensure probity in medical education, bring down costs of medical education, simplify procedures, ensure quality education, and provide wider access to people to quality healthcare. The bill which has received president's accent and is notified on 25th of September 2020. The MCI Act 1956 stands dissolved. The NMC has 33 members.

National Exit Test under National Medical Commission

It has provision for making national standards in medical education uniform by proposing that the final year MBBS examination be treated as an entrance test for PG and a screening test for students who graduate in medicine from foreign countries. This examination, called the National Exit Test (NEXT), under the NMC moves away from a system of repeated inspections of infrastructure and focuses on outcomes rather than processes. Once a candidate clears NEXT, he can register himself and obtain a license to practice. NEXT shall also be applicable to Institutes of National Importance (INIs) like All India Institute of Medical Sciences (AIIMS) to have common standards in the country. The NMC provides that the Medical Assessment and Rating Board (MARB) will conduct an assessment to the medical college and develop a system of ranking medical colleges which would enable the students to choose the medical college wisely.

How many pediatricians are there in India?
There are a total of 23,663 pediatricians in India as of December 05, 2023.

Summary of the Amendments Done in NMC Act in March 2022

- One single entrance examination for MBBS (all entrance examination including AIIMS entrance scrapped)
- Final Professional Examination all over the country will be one
- The examination will provide for:
  - MBBS Degree
  - Registration and License to practice
  - Postgraduate entrance merit. If one fails one will have to write supplementary. If one wants merit to be improved one can write it again.
- NEET UG 2023 offers admission to a total of 101,043 MBBS seats in the country. Out of the total number, 48,265 are seats from private medical colleges. Apart from the MBBS seats, 27,868 BDS seats, 603 BVSc and AH seats, and 52,720 AYUSH seats.
- No Medical College in a state can be set up without an essentiality certificate from the Concerned State Government.
- Ratings of all Medical Colleges will be done by the Rating Board of the Commission and ranks will be allotted.
- The State Medical Councils will continue to work as they are presently working.
- One year imprisonment and INR 5 lakh fine for quackery.
- *No bridge course* for graduates of any other pathies of medicine.
- The same final year examination for foreign degree holders also to license them to practice in India.
- Mid-level Community Health Providers (CHPs) like pharmacists/nurses and other paramedicals (as decided by the commission after formation) will be eligible to be registered in a separate register and allowed to dispense a few notified primary healthcare medicines to patients. There will be no PG NEET, Nationwide single examination of final MBBS which will serve as certificate exam and as PG eligibility test. Candidate can reappear in this NEXT examination as many times as he or she wishes. 50% PG seats fee in private colleges will be decided by center and 50% by MOU with state government. State government will look after and regulate all medical colleges in states and center will not intervene.
- There will be rating of medical colleges according to result of NEXT examination.

CHAPTER 24: Understanding National Medical Commission Act 2019 and Professional Conduct...

- 1 year imprisonment and fine for bogus degree holders.
- 21 out of 25 members will be senior medical professors, will be members of NMC and their membership will be for 4 years, and they will decide regarding healthcare workers.
- Bridge course is scrapped. There will be no bridge course for BAMS and BHMS degree holder.

The NMC of 2019 has four autonomous boards to take care of its different functions:
1. Undergraduate Medical Education Board to set standards and regulate medical education at undergraduate level
2. Postgraduate Medical Education Board to set standards and regulate medical education at postgraduate level
3. MARB for inspections and rating of medical institutions
4. Ethics and Medical Registration Board to regulate and promote professional conduct and medical ethics and also maintain national registers of (1) licensed medical practitioners and (2) CHPs.

ETHICS AND MEDICAL REGISTRATION BOARD SHALL REGULATE ETHICS

The word "ethics" is derived from the Greek word "ethos" which means customs and habits. It means something in conformity with moral norms or standard of professional conduct. The word relates to the precepts which should control moral behavior. Ethics is that science of knowledge, which deals with the nature and grounds of moral obligations, distinguishing what is right from what is wrong in healthcare. NMC has for time being adopted Indian Medical Council (Professional conduct, Etiquette, and Ethics) Regulations, 2002 as such.

Introduction to Ethics Code 2002 which is Currently Applicable Till NMC Reissues its Code of Conduct

The repealed MCI is empowered by Section 20A read with Section 33(m) of the Indian Medical Council Act, 1956 (102 of 1956)[2] to enact Regulations called the Indian Medical Council (Professional conduct, Etiquette and Ethics) Regulations, 2002 with approval of Central Government, gazetted on 6th April, 2002.[3] The NMC has adopted "2002 Professional conduct, Etiquette and Ethics" as for now.[4-8] Ethical code under NMC 2019 was rolled out on 02-08-23 and held in abeyance on 24-08-23 so situation is as it was till next Central Government, Gazette notification.

The regulations have eight Chapters as follows:
1. Chapter 1—code of medical ethics
2. Chapter 2—duties of Registered Medical Practitioner (RMP) to their patients
3. Chapter 3—duties of RMP in consultation
4. Chapter 4—responsibilities of RMP to each other
5. Chapter 5—duties of RMP to the public and to the paramedical profession
6. Chapter 6—unethical acts
7. Chapter 7—misconduct
8. Chapter 8—punishment and disciplinary action.

Who is a Medical Practitioner with Registration Number? Described in Chapter 1, 2, and 7 of Code

The Indian Medical Council Act defines a medical practitioner as practitioner of modern medicine duly registered with the "MCI" or state medical council by virtue of requisite prescribed qualifications. A medical practitioner is licensed to practice in the state or country by adhering to code of ethics-2002 by signing Declaration format of which is given in Appendix I.[1]

- RMP should obtain membership in Medical Society like the Indian Medical Association, etc. (1.2).
- RMP should complete least 30 hours continuing medical education (CME) programs every 5 years required for renewal of license (1.2).
- RMP should display the registration number in clinic and in all prescriptions, certificates, money receipts (1.4 and 3.7.2) otherwise commits misconduct under 7.4.
- RMP shall display as suffix only recognized medical degrees (1.4) otherwise commits misconduct under 7.4.

Consent in Eyes of Ethics is Described in Chapter 2 and 7 of Code

The first and foremost principle of ethics is autonomy. That means right to full disclosure of information to allow patient to choose out of the treatment modalities offered to the patient. Informed consent has pivotal role since it flows from the doctrine of autonomy in India and legal principle of volenti non fit injuria. The ethical code 2002 describes same as follow:

- "Consent" is not defined under ethics 2002 code specifically. Few places where it is referred are given here.
- When a physician who has been engaged to attend an obstetric case is absent and another is sent for and delivery accomplished, the acting physician is should secure the patient's consent to resign on the arrival of the physician engaged (2.5).
- RMP should obtain in writing the consent from the husband or wife, parent or guardian in the case of minor, or the patient himself as the case may be. In an operation which may result in sterility the consent of both husband and wife is needed (7.16).
- No act of in vitro fertilization (IVF) or artificial insemination (AI) shall be undertaken without the informed consent of the female patient and her spouse as well as the donor (7.21).
- RMP shall not publish photographs or case reports of patients without their permission, in any medical or other journal in a manner by which their identity could be made out. If the identity is not to be disclosed, the consent is not needed (7.17).
- Consent taken from the patient for trial of drug or therapy which is not as per the guidelines shall also be construed as misconduct (7.22).
- Code refers to consent in earlier mentioned regulations only.

Right of Patient to Receive Treatment and General Duties of RMP are Described in Chapter 1, 2, 6, and 7 of Code

The second and third principle is called *justice and beneficence. Justice means* the right to receive what is recommended by RMP and *beneficence* means obligation of RMP to do good in a given situation before, during, and after the administration of treatment. The ethical code 2002 has described same as follows:

- RMP is not bound to treat each and every person (2.1.1).
- RMP should be ever ready to respond to treat in emergency (2.1.1).

CHAPTER 24: Understanding National Medical Commission Act 2019 and Professional Conduct...

- RMP once having undertaken a case, the RMP should not neglect the patient, nor should he withdraw from the case without giving adequate notice to the patient (2.4).
- RMP should neither exaggerate nor minimize the gravity of a patient's prognosis (2.3).
- RMP should have patience while treating the patient (2.2).
- RMP should delicacy while treating the patient (2.2).
- RMP shall not refuse on religious grounds alone to give assistance in or conduct of sterility, birth control, circumcision, and medical termination of pregnancy (7.15). RMP shall not to refuse professional service on grounds of religion, nationality, race, party politics, or social status.
- RMP should maintain secrecy (2.2).
- Confidentiality and secrecy should be maintained unless revelation is required by the laws of the State (2.2). Otherwise it is misconduct (7.14).
- RMP should report communicable as duty to society (2.2).
- RMP is having any incapacity is not permitted to practice his profession though not specified under code may mean RMP is under influence of alcohol, sleeping pills, sleep deprived, overworked, emotionally unstable, anxiety neurosis, and may also mean RMP is human immunodeficiency virus (HIV), Au antigen positive, hepatitis C virus (HCV) positive, epilepsy, under effect of drugs, and disease which may compromise his performance. Whether it should be disclosed to patient or not is not specified in the code (2.1.2).
- RMP posted in rural area is found absent on more than two occasions during inspection same shall be construed as misconduct (7.23).
- RMP posted in a medical college/institution both as teaching shall remain in hospital/college during the assigned duty hours. If they are found absent on more than two occasions during this period, the same shall be construed as a misconduct (7.24).
- RMP should ensure rational prescription (1.5).
- RMP should prescribe drugs with preferably by generic names (1.5).
- All the drugs prescribed by a RMP should always carry a proprietary formula and clear name (6.5).

Duties of RMP's while Consulting other RMP is Described in Chapter 3, 4, and 7 of Code

- RMP should avoid unnecessary consultations (3.1).
- RMP should request consultation in case of serious illness and in doubtful or difficult conditions in interest of the patient (3.1.1 and 3.2).
- RMP should consult pathologists judiciously and not in a routine manner (3.1.2).
- RMP should consult radiologists judiciously and not in a routine manner (3.1.2).
- RMP should maintain utmost punctuality in making available for consultations (3.3).
- RMP should make all statements to the patient in presence of consulting RMPs (3.4 and 3.4.1).
- If two RMPs differ in opinion should not divulge such difference unnecessarily but when there is irreconcilable difference of opinion in a particular circumstance then it should be frankly and impartially explained to the patient party (3.4.2).

- Attending RMP refers to specialist RMP by preparing case summary and specialist RMP should communicate opinion in writing to the attending RMP (3.6).
- Role of attending RMP after specialist RMP consultation is to take routine care whereas consultant may change treatment if asked by attending RMP or in case of emergency (3.5).
- Consulting RMP should not show insincerity, rivalry, or envy (4.2).
- Visiting RMP should avoid remarks upon diagnosis or treatment that has been adopted by other RMP (4.5).
- When consulting RMP has been called should normally not take charge of the case (4.3).
- The consultant RMP shall not criticize the referring RMP (4.3).
- Consulting RMP shall discuss diagnosis treatment plan with the referring RMP (4.3).
- RMP shall not claim to be specialist unless he has a special qualification in that branch (7.20).
- RMP should appoint another RMP (locum) to attend his patients during his temporary absence (4.4).
- RMP should render gratuitous service to all RMPs and their immediate family dependents (4.1).
- RMP should not be averse to any suggestion of seeking a second opinion by patient party. RMP, who are open-minded and communicative are much less likely to be complained against by patient.

RMPs Fees is Described in Chapter 1, 2, 3, 4, and 7 of Code

- Prime object is to render service to humanity and reward or financial gain is a subordinate consideration (1.1).
- The usual commercial rule of caveat emptor (let the buyer beware) does not apply in the doctor patient relationship though it is the patient who seeks for physician's help for obtaining relief (1.8).
- RMP has right to be reimbursed but the Code does not prescribe any standard of charges nor does it say that charges must be reasonable. There is no capping of fees charged by RMP (1.8).
- RMP should display charges (1.8 and 3.7.1).
- RMP should announce his fees before rendering service and not after the operation or treatment is under way (1.8).
- It is unethical to enter into a contract of "no cure no payment" (1.8).
- RMP should expose incompetent or corrupt, dishonest, or unethical conduct on the part of members of the profession (1.7).
- RMP is engaged to attend an obstetric case is absent and another RMP is sent for delivering baby can charge his fees (2.5).
- RMP should display the registration number on money receipts (1.4 and 3.7.2) otherwise commits misconduct under 7.4.
- RMP should render gratuitous service to all RMPs and their immediate family dependents (4.1).

Maintenance of Medical Records are Described in Chapter 1, 3, and 7 of Code

- RMP does not maintain the medical records of indoor patients for a period of 3 years as per regulation 1.3 and Appendix 3, and refuses to provide the same within 72 hours when the patient or authorized representative makes a request for it as per the regulation 1.3.2 commits misconduct under 7.2.

- Code does not mention about outpatient department (OPD) records but says indirectly that RMP should display the registration number on all prescriptions, certificates (1.4 and 3.7.2) otherwise commits misconduct under 7.4. Generally OPD records are in custody of patient in India.
- Code does not mention how to destroy records. Signing professional certificates, reports, and other documents: RMP should sign documents as per format given in Appendix 4 otherwise liable for misconduct (7.7).
- There is no other law in India where documents by any other professional or officials are mandated to be provided within 72 hours. This is too harsh. In light of law of limitation for filing cases or prosecuting doctors, time period is 2 or 3 years along with discretionary power of law courts to allow condonation of delay for filing medical negligence cases.

ASSOCIATION WITH UNQUALIFIED PERSONS

A RMP shall not employ in connection with his professional practice any attendant who is neither registered nor enlisted under the Medical Acts (1.6), RMP running of a nursing home by employing assistants to help, the ultimate responsibility rests on the RMP (7.18).

Performing or enabling unqualified person to perform an abortion or any illegal operation for which there is no medical, surgical, or psychological indication (7.9).

A RMP shall not issue certificates of efficiency in modern medicine to unqualified or nonmedical person (7.10).

COMMISSION AND CUT PRACTICE

A RMP shall not indulge in cut practice for referring patients (6.4.1, 6.4.2, and 6.4).

RMP and Pharma Co.

A RMP shall not receive any gift, travel facilities, monetary grants, medical research from Pharma Co. and same is unethical if it is not as per clause 6.8 even endorsement of Pharma Co. is unethical.

ADVERTISING AND SOLICITING PATIENTS BY RMP

- RMP shall not do advertising (6.1).
- RMP shall not solicit patients directly or indirectly as a group of RMPs or by institutions or organizations (6.1.1).
- RMP shall not use touts or agents for procuring patients (7.19).
- RMP should not use unusually large sign board which should only mention name and qualifications otherwise it is advertising (7.13).
- RMP should not contribute to the lay press articles and talks on the radio/TV/internet chat and give interviews regarding diseases and treatments which amount to advertising. It is improper to affix a sign-board on a chemist's shop or in places where he does not reside or work (7.11).
- RMP or institutions or organizations shall not print self-photograph of RMP on any material of publicity otherwise it will amount to advertising (6.1.2).
- An institution run by RMP may be advertised in the lay press, but such advertisements should not contain anything more than the name of the institution, type of patients admitted, and fees (7.12 and 7.13).
- RMP is permitted to make a formal announcement in press regarding the following:
  - On starting practice
  - On change of type of practice

- On changing address
- On temporary absence from duty
- On resumption of another practice
- On succeeding to another practice
- Public declaration of charges.

Patent and Copyrights

A RMP may patent surgical instruments, appliances, and medicine or copyright applications, methods, and procedures (6.2).

Running an Open Shop (Dispensing of Drugs and Appliances by RMPs)

A RMP should not run shop for sale of medicine and surgical appliances (6.3).

SECRET REMEDIES

A RMP shall not indulge in secret remedial agents and their use is unethical and as such prohibited (6.5).

MEDICAL RESEARCH

Clinical drug trials or other research involving patients or volunteers as per the guidelines of the Indian Council of Medical Research (ICMR) can be undertaken (7.22).

EVADE LEGAL RESTRICTIONS

A RMP should not evade legal restrictions related to Drugs and Cosmetics Act, 1940 violation of this is misconduct under 7.8; Pharmacy Act, 1948, Medical Termination of Pregnancy Act, 1971; Bio-Medical Waste (Management and Handling) Rules, 1998 etc.

DUTIES OF RMP TO THE PUBLIC

A RMP, as good citizens, possessed of special training in medicine should disseminate preventive advice related to public health issues (5.1) to prevent prevention of epidemic and communicable diseases (5.2).

DUTIES OF RMP TO THE PARAMEDICAL PROFESSION

A RMP should seek cooperation of pharmacist and nurse (5.3).

HUMAN RIGHTS

A RMP shall not aid or abet torture (6.6).

EUTHANASIA

Practicing mercy killing or euthanasia shall constitute unethical conduct (6.7).

SOME MORE MISCONDUCTS

- Abuse of professional position by committing adultery or improper conduct with patient (7.4).
- *Conviction by Court of Law:* Conviction by a Court of Law for offences involving moral turpitude/criminal acts (7.5).
- On no account sex determination test shall be undertaken with the intent to terminate the life of a female fetus (7.6).

Annexed Guidelines Appended to NMC Code of Conduct 2022

There are 11 guidelines annexed to regulations.

PROCEDURE FOR DISCIPLINARY ACTION AND PUNISHMENT

- During the pendency of misconduct complaint, council may restrain the physician from performing the procedure or practice which is under scrutiny (8.5). Professional incompetence shall be judged by peer group as per guidelines prescribed by MCI (8.6).
- If found guilty punishment of removal on name of RMP from the register for temporarily or permanently may take place (8.3).

- Decision on complaint against delinquent physician shall be taken within time limit of 6 months (8.4) if not the complaint may abate.

Any person aggrieved by the decision of State Medical Council on any complaint against a delinquent physician, shall have the right to file an appeal to the MCI within a period of 60 days from the date of receipt of the order passed by the said Medical Council (8.8).

Ethics Board of NMC and Profession Practice

Ethics under NMC will be different. So far, even if MCI suspends a doctor, the decision is not binding state medical councils who can refuse to comply with it. In contrast, the new NMC clearly states that the ethics board will "exercise appellate jurisdiction with respect to actions taken by state medical councils".

Professional or Ethical Misconduct

The State Medical Councils will receive complaints relating to professional or ethical misconduct against a RMP. If the medical practitioner is aggrieved of a decision of the State Medical Council, he may appeal to the Ethics and Medical Registration Board.

The State Medical Councils and the Ethics and Medical Registration Board have the power to take disciplinary action against the medical practitioner including imposing a monetary penalty. If the medical practitioner is aggrieved of the decision of the Board, he can approach the NMC to appeal against the decision. Appeal of the decision of the NMC lies with the central government.

Offences and Penalties

No person is allowed to practice medicine as a qualified medical practitioner other than those enrolled in a State Register or the National Register. Any person who contravenes this provision will be punished with a fine between 1 and 5 lakh rupees.

CLINICAL ESTABLISHMENTS (REGISTRATION AND REGULATION) ACT, 2010

Introduction

The Clinical Establishments (Registration and Regulation) Act (CEA) is significant piece of healthcare legislation in India that was enacted to regulate and standardize clinical establishments across the country. This comprehensive law aims to ensure the provision of quality healthcare services, protect the rights of patients, and establish accountability within the healthcare sector. Private healthcare serves 72% of the population in rural areas and 79% in urban areas. The CEA 2010 is an important shall help to improve the quality and safety of healthcare services in India.

The key objectives of the Act are:
- To ensure that clinical establishments maintain minimum standards of facilities and services.
- To protect the safety and well-being of patients.
- To promote transparency and accountability in healthcare delivery.

Key provisions of the Act are:
- Mandatory registration of all clinical establishments with the designated authorities.
- Establishment of a system for periodic inspection and certification of clinical establishments.
- Prescription of minimum standards of facilities, equipment, and personnel for different categories of clinical establishments.

- Implementation of a system for redressal of patient grievances.
- Penalties for noncompliance with the provisions of the Act.

Clinical Establishments (Registration and Regulation) Act Application

The CEA has been embraced in 14 states and union territories, including Assam, Jharkhand, Arunachal Pradesh, Rajasthan, Uttar Pradesh, Bihar, Uttarakhand, and Sikkim. However, in general, no one has implemented CEA 2010 comprehensively thus far. This Act is applicable to all kinds of clinical establishments from the public and private sectors, of all recognized systems of medicine including single doctor clinics.

The CEA, 2010 is applicable in the following states and union territories across India: Arunachal Pradesh, Assam, Bihar, Chandigarh, Dadra and Nagar Haveli, Daman and Diu, union territory of Andaman and Nicobar Islands, Haryana, Himachal Pradesh, Jammu and Kashmir, Jharkhand, Karnataka, Lakshadweep, Maharashtra, Manipur, Meghalaya, Mizoram, Nagaland, Puducherry, Rajasthan, Sikkim, Telangana, Tripura, Uttar Pradesh, and Uttarakhand.

The CEA, 2010 is not applicable in several states, including Goa, Gujarat, Kerala, Madhya Pradesh, Odisha, Punjab, Tamil Nadu, and West Bengal, and the union territory of Delhi. These states have not adopted the Act or have chosen not to implement it. The states have the choice of passing a similar bill. u/a 251(1) of constitution.

The following states have their own acts with the specified names:
- *Odisha:* Odisha Clinical Establishments (Registration and Regulation) Act, 2013
- *Puducherry:* Puducherry Clinical Establishments (Registration and Regulation) Act, 2010
- *Punjab:* Punjab Clinical Establishments (Registration and Regulation) Act, 2010
- *Rajasthan:* Rajasthan Clinical Establishments (Registration and Regulation) Act, 2010
- *Sikkim:* Sikkim Clinical Establishments (Registration and Regulation) Act, 2010
- *Tamil Nadu:* The Tamil Nadu Clinical Establishments (Registration and Regulation) Act, 2017
- *Telangana:* Telangana Private Medical Establishments Act, 2010
- *Tripura:* Tripura Clinical Establishments (Registration and Regulation) Act, 2010
- *Uttar Pradesh:* Uttar Pradesh Private Medical Establishments Act, 2011
- *Uttarakhand:* Uttarakhand Clinical Establishments (Registration and Regulation) Act, 2010
- *West Bengal:* West Bengal Clinical Establishments (Registration and Regulation) Act, 2013
- *Andaman and Nicobar Islands:* Andaman and Nicobar Islands Clinical Establishments (Registration and Regulation) Act, 2010
- *Delhi:* Delhi Healthcare Services (Regulation) Act, 2007.

Another exception will be establishments run by the *Armed forces*.

Constitutionality of the Clinical Establishments Act of 2010

It has been a subject of inquiry. In the case of Dr Ashwani Goyal versus Union of India, which was heard in the Delhi High Court (DB), the petitioner, Dr Ashwani Goyal, who is a medical practitioner, filed a writ petition. This petition was framed as a Public Interest Litigation (PIL) and aimed to challenge the validity of various provisions within the CEA of 2010. The fundamental question before the court was whether the CEA 2010 holds constitutional validity. After due consideration of the matter, the court arrived at a conclusion. The court found no merit in the claims put forth by the petitioner and, as a result, chose to summarily dismiss the petition, affirming the constitutionality of the CEA of 2010.

The question of whether the CEA violates the fundamental rights of medical professionals practicing their profession has been the subject of legal scrutiny. In the case of "Dr Yashbir Singh Tomar versus State of Uttarakhand", which was heard in the Uttarakhand High Court, the validity of various provisions of the Parliamentary Statute known as the CEA was challenged. This case focused on examining whether the Act encroached upon the fundamental rights of medical professionals.

Specific Provisions of the Clinical Establishments Act were Challenged

In a separate legal case titled "Dr Ashwani Goyal versus Union of India and Anr". on July 31, 2012, specific provisions of the CEA were challenged. These provisions included Sections 1(3), 2(c), 2(d), 2(h), 2(o), 3, 10(1), 11, 12, 13, 25, and 41, and their compliance with constitutional standards was under scrutiny.

From a legal perspective, the freedom to practice a trade and profession is considered a fundamental right and is subject to reasonable restrictions as outlined in clause (6) of Article 19 of the Constitution of India. These restrictions ensure a balance between individual rights and societal interests.

Furthermore, it is important to note that Article 47 of the Constitution places a responsibility upon the State to aim at improving public health. This underscores the constitutional imperative to regulate and standardize clinical establishments to ensure the well-being of the public and the quality of healthcare services.

The application of the CEA of 2010 in India is not uniform across all states. The Act cannot be directly applied to every state in the country. Instead, its direct applicability is limited to specific states.

Case Law on Clinical Establishment Act

The question of whether one can operate a registered clinical establishment in residential premises is not a straightforward yes or no.

It depends on various factors, and unless there are objections, it may be permissible. However, if objections arise, a change of use may be required. This matter was addressed in the case of Sri Bhaskar Ghosh versus State of West Bengal, heard in the Calcutta High Court. In this case, it was alleged that a registered clinical establishment was being operated on the ground and first floors of a residential building in gross violation of various provisions of the law. Despite these violations, the establishment had been registered under the CEA. The central issue before the court was whether the license of the said clinical establishment should be quashed, and any further renewal of such a license should be denied. After considering the facts and legal arguments, the court arrived at a decision. The court ruled that in the event that the private respondent, identified as respondent No. 13, rectifies all the loopholes as pointed out in the present judgment, they may apply for a fresh license to run a clinical establishment from the building in question. However, this application must be made in compliance with all legal formalities and will be considered by the appropriate authorities in accordance with the law. This case underscores the significance of adhering to legal requirements and addressing any violations when operating clinical establishments in residential premises. It also highlights the potential for rectification and compliance with the law when objections arise.

The practice of medicine with an invalid degree or diploma is strictly prohibited.

This principle was reinforced in the Rani Seva Sadan case, where it was unequivocally established that such practices are not permissible. This prohibition serves a crucial purpose in curbing quackery and ensuring that healthcare providers meet the necessary educational and professional qualifications—practicing medicine on invalid degree/diploma. The Rani Seva Sadan case, which was heard in the state of Jharkhand, serves as a significant legal reference. In this case, the CEA of 2010 was invoked. Specifically, Section 40(1) of the Act, which deals with penalties for violations, came into play. In accordance with the principles of natural justice, a chance was given to address and rectify the situation. However, the overarching message from this case remains clear: Practicing medicine with an invalid degree or diploma is against the law and can result in legal consequences. This serves as a deterrent to maintain the integrity and quality of healthcare services.

The question of whether unqualified pathologists can be registered to operate clinical establishment laboratories is met with a resounding "No, not at all." This clear stance was reinforced through legal cases and judgments.

In the case of the Indian Association of Pathologists and Microbiologists versus State of Bihar, heard in the Patna High Court, the violation of the CEA of 2010 and Bihar Clinical Establishment Rules of 2013 was highlighted. It addressed the unlawful operation of unauthorized pathological centers, emphasizing the immediate need for the closure of such establishments.

Similarly, the case of the Association of Practicing Pathologists, Haryana (Regd.) versus State of Haryana, heard in the Punjab and Haryana High Court, emphasized the importance of having qualified pathologists for the operation of pathology laboratories. It referenced a Gujarat High Court judgment that affirmed by supreme court of India is of significance for qualified pathologists signing reports.

It is compulsory to give emergency aid and is no bar to CEA?

These legal precedents underscore the non-negotiable requirement for qualified pathologists to run pathology laboratories within clinical establishments. The law and judicial decisions emphasize the critical role of qualified professionals in maintaining the integrity and quality of healthcare services.

The provision of emergency aid is a compulsory requirement, and it does not pose a hindrance to compliance with the CEA. This clarity stems from the legal case of Ramneek Singh Bedi versus Union of India, which was heard in the Punjab and Haryana High Court.

In this case, specific sections of the CEA, namely Sections 12(2) and 2(c), were under scrutiny. Section 12(2) of the Act mandates clinical establishments to provide facilities to stabilize the emergency medical condition of any individual who is brought to the establishment. The court's interpretation emphasized that the provisions of the CEA do not create an impossible situation for the practice of the medical profession. It affirmed that the Act does not violate the constitution and is not considered ultra vires. This legal perspective underscores the importance of emergency aid as a fundamental requirement that aligns with the objectives of the Act without impeding the medical profession's practice.

The authority vested with the power to cancel registration under the CEA is a matter of legal clarity. In the case of Medaxis Hospital versus State of UP, which was heard in the Allahabad High Court, this issue was addressed comprehensively.

Designated CEA authority holds the authorization to cancel the registration of clinical establishments.

The court's decision unequivocally established that only the designated CEA authority holds the authorization to cancel the registration of clinical establishments. The role of an Additional Chief Medical Officer (CMO) in this regard was explicitly clarified. The court ruled that the cancellation order issued by an Additional CMO was without jurisdiction and, therefore, liable to be quashed. This legal stance reaffirms the specific authority designated by the CEA to handle registration cancellations and underscores the need for adherence to legal procedures in such matters. It will be open to the petitioner to apply for renewal or fresh registration, as the case may be, in accordance with law to CEA.

Appointment of a doctor to the West Bengal Clinical Establishment Regulatory Commission with a history of negligence.

In the case of Dr Kunal Saha versus Principal Secretary (Calcutta) (DB), a significant legal question arose regarding the appointment of a doctor with a history of negligence to the West Bengal Clinical Establishment Regulatory Commission. This case, which was decided in 2018 and can be found in the 2018 AIR (Calcutta) 148, 2018(2) Cal. L.T. 65, 2018(2) Cal. H.C.N. 33, and 2018(5) WBLR 485, sheds light on the intricacies of the West Bengal CEA, 2017.

The petitioner in this case challenged the appointment of a senior doctor to the regulatory body, citing concerns about his past negligence. The central issue was whether a doctor who had been found negligent in the past could be appointed to a position of authority within the Clinical Establishment Regulatory Commission. The court's decision in this matter was clear and definitive: There was no explicit legal bar preventing the appointment of a doctor with a history of negligence to the commission. In other words, the West Bengal CEA, 2017 did not contain any provisions that disqualified such individuals from serving on the commission.

Is nonregistration under CEA bailable?

The question of whether offences under nonregistration are bailable is an important one in the realm of legal proceedings. In the case of Padum Lal Sahu versus State of Chhattisgarh, which is documented in 2015(3) MPHT 38, 2015(14) R.C.R. (Criminal) 433, and 2015(3) C.G.L.J. 153, this very issue came to the forefront. The context of this case revolved around offences related to non-registration under the CEA. Specifically, the alleged offences were committed by a doctor, and the question of whether bail should be granted became a critical point of contention. In its decision, the court ruled that bail had to be granted in this case.

Can registered radiology clinic under clinical establishments be locked for stray deficiencies?

The question of whether a registered radiology clinic under the CEA can be locked due to stray deficiencies was addressed in the case of Vinod Kumar Khator versus State of Madhya Pradesh (Gwalior Bench). This case, which can be found in 2013(5) MPHT 417, 2013(3) M.P.W.N. 247, and 2013(45) R.C.R. (Civil) 138, provides valuable insights into the legal aspects surrounding CEA registered clinics. In this case, the petitioner was a radiologist who also served as a Medical Officer in District Hospital Morar. Additionally, he was running a medical consultancy chamber in his house, which was duly registered under the CEA. However, following an inspection, his clinic was locked by the authorities, raising questions about the legality of this action. The petitioner, dissatisfied with the locking of his clinic, decided to challenge this decision through a writ petition. The central issue was whether the locking of the clinic was illegal, given that it was a registered establishment under the CEA. The court, in its judgment, declared the locking of the clinic to be illegal. The respondents were directed to forthwith open the lock on the clinic.

What will happen if one wants to survive under CEA?

Navigating and surviving under the CEA can be a challenging endeavor, given the complexities and potential pitfalls associated with healthcare regulations. While the intention behind such regulations is often to ensure quality and safety in healthcare delivery, the practical implications can sometimes be burdensome. Here are some key considerations:

- *Impractical provisions:* The CEA, like many regulatory frameworks, may contain provisions that are perceived as impractical or difficult to adhere to. Some of these provisions might not align well with the realities of healthcare practice, leading to challenges in implementation.
- *Resorting to "jugaad":* In response to impractical provisions or stringent regulations, individuals within the healthcare system may resort to *"jugaad"* or finding creative workarounds. While this might help them continue their operations, it can also lead to a lack of transparency and accountability.
- *Corruption and inspector raj:* The presence of strict compliance requirements can sometimes foster an environment where individuals feel compelled to pay bribes or engage in corrupt practices to maintain their registration or compliance status. This "inspector raj" mentality can undermine the intended goals of regulation.
- *Increased prosecution:* Over-regulation can add another layer of potential prosecution against doctors and hospitals. This can create a sense of fear and uncertainty within the healthcare system, potentially affecting the quality of care provided.

SUMMARY

The NMC Act repeals the Indian Medical Council Act 1956. The NMC as an umbrella regulatory body. The NMC will subsume the MCI and will regulate medical education and practice in India. NMC Act to provide for a medical education system that improves access to quality and affordable medical education, ensures availability of adequate and high quality medical professionals in all parts of the country that promotes equitable and universal healthcare that encourages community health perspective. NMC adopts ethics 2002 of MCI act. Ethical code under NMC 2019 was rolled out on 02-08-23 and held in abeyance on 24-08-23 so situation is

CHAPTER 24: Understanding National Medical Commission Act 2019 and Professional Conduct...

as it was till next Central Government, Gazette notification.

The CEA 2010 is a landmark legislation in India that aims to regulate and standardize the quality of healthcare services provided by clinical establishments across the country. It applies to all types of clinical establishments, including hospitals, nursing homes, clinics, and diagnostic centers.

LEARNING KEY POINTS/ DOS AND DON'TS[9-11]

- RMP should obtain registration number before practice in the state.
- RMP should complete least 30 hours CME every 5 years required for renewal of license.
- RMP should display the registration number in clinic and in all prescriptions, certificates, and money receipts.
- RMP shall display as suffix only recognized medical degrees.
- RMP should obtain written "consent" before operation.
- RMP should be ever ready to respond to treat in emergency.
- Prime object is to render service to humanity and reward or financial gain is a subordinate consideration.
- RMP should display charges.
- It is unethical to enter into a contract of "no cure no payment".
- RMP should maintain the medical records of inpatient department (IPD) for a period of 3 years.
- RMP shall not indulge in cut practice for referring patients.
- RMP shall not receive valuable gifts, travel facilities, and monetary grants from Pharma Co.
- RMP shall not do advertising.
- RMP should not run shop for sale of medicine and surgical appliances.
- RMP shall not indulge in secret remedial agents.
- Clinical drug trials or other research involving patients or volunteers as per the guidelines of ICMR and schedule-Y of Drugs and Cosmetics rules 1945.
- On no account sex determination test shall be undertaken.

MUST AVOID THINGS

A RMP shall not do advertising.

ONLY ONE FACT TO REMEMBER

A RMP should obtain registration number before practice in the state.

DO NOT DO

It is unethical to enter into a contract of "no cure no payment".

WARNINGS

A RMP s shall display as suffix only recognized medical degrees.

MEDICAL NEGLIGENCE PEARL

A RMP should maintain the medical records of IPD for a period of 3 years.

MUST DO THING

A RMP shall not indulge in cut practice for referring patients.

MESSAGES WHICH THE READER MUST BE AWARE

A RMP should complete least 30 hours CME every 5 years required for renewal of license.

BALDWA'S DICTUM

Better qualified and skillful doctors take higher risks in medical field and get prosecuted.

REFERENCES

1. National Medical Commission Act, 2019.
2. The Indian Medical Council Act, 1956 (102 of 1956) repealed.
3. The Indian Medical Council (Professional conduct, Etiquette and Ethics) Regulations, 2002 with approval of Central Government, Gazetted on 6th April, 2002.
4. The National Medical Commission (Manner of Appointment and Nomination of Members, their Salary, Allowances and Terms and Conditions of Service, and Declaration of Assets, Professional and Commercial Engagements) Rules, 2019.
5. The National Medical Commission, Autonomous Boards (Manner of Appointment of Fourth Member and the Salary, Allowances and Terms and Conditions of Service, and Declaration of Assets, Professional and Commercial Engagements of President and Members) Rules, 2019.
6. The National Medical Commission (Submission of List of Medical Professionals) Rules, 2019.
7. The National Medical Commission, Medical Advisory Council (Qualification and Experience of Residuary Member) Rules, 2019.
8. The National Medical Commission (Annual Statement of Accounts, Submission of Annual Report and Other Reports and Statements) Rules, 2019.
9. Baldwa M, Baldwa S, Padvi N, Gupta V. Frequently Asked Questions Related to MCI "Code Of Ethics". [online] Available from: https://www.imlea-india.org/journal/Oct-Dec15.pdf. [Last accessed December, 2023].
10. Baldwa M, Baldwa V, Padvi N, Baldwa S. Legal Issues in Medical Practice, 2nd edition. New Delhi: CBS Publishers and Distributors Pvt. Ltd.; 2023.
11. Baldwa M, Baldwa V, Padvi N, Baldwa S. Legal Issues in Critical Care, 1st edition. New Delhi: CBS Publishers and Distributors Pvt. Ltd.; 2022.

Professional Indemnity and Out-of-Court Settlement

Satish Tiwari

Keywords: Indemnity, Medical establishment policy, Out-of-court settlement

Aim: Asset protection and financial erosion are prevented by professional indemnity (PI) and out-of-court settlement (OCS).

Objective: PI insurance and OCS are both important tools for professionals in India. PI insurance can help to protect professionals from the financial consequences of professional liability claims, while OCS can be a more cost-effective and time-efficient way to resolve disputes.

INTRODUCTION

The age-old doctor–patient relationship is no exception to the negative changes in the society. The enactment of Consumer Protection Act (CPA) initially in 1986 and again in 2019 and its subsequent application to medical practitioners have added fuel to the fire.[1] The process of liberalization and globalization has resulted in mushrooming of many insurance companies.

DEFINITIONS

Indemnity means "to make good the loss sustained by the insurer". The doctor's indemnity policy provides insurance protection to the doctors against their legal liability to pay damages arising out of their negligence in the performance of professional duties. The insured includes the policyholder and his qualified assistants or employees named in the proposal.

TYPES

The different types of professional indemnity (PI) or hospital insurance policies are:
- Doctor's indemnity policy
- *Doctor's composite package policy:* These policies also cover loss or damage to the property as the case may be.
- *Doctor's protection shield:* It includes protection from various hazards to which doctors are exposed such as buildings, computers, other appliances, and electronic equipment.
- *Doctors' and medical establishment policy:* These policies include nursing homes, hospitals, or medical establishments.

SCOPE

It applies to claims arising out of bodily injury, illness, and/or death of any patient caused by or alleged to have caused by an error, an act of omission or an act of commission during the professional service/duty. The other policies cover loss or damages to property, building, equipment, etc. One must inform the insurance company when you shift your nursing home or consulting room. Disclose your attachments with other hospitals or nursing homes otherwise company may refuse to take liability arising in that places.[2]

■ LEGAL ASSISTANCE SCHEME

- The member of this scheme is on yearly basis. The member can renew to remain continuous insured person of this scheme by paying renewal fees every year. The scheme shall assist the member *Only* as far as the medical negligence is concerned.
- This scheme shall be *assisting the members* by:
  - *Medicolegal guidance* in hours of crisis. A committee of subject experts shall be formed, which will guide the members in the hours of legal crisis.
  - *Expert opinion* shall be obtained if there are cases in court of law.
  - *Guidance of legal experts:* A team of legal and medicolegal experts shall be formed, which will help in guiding the involved members in the hours of legal crisis.
  - *Support of crisis management committee* at the city/district level.
- The money contribution toward the scheme shall be decided in consultation with the indemnity experts. The same will depend on the type and extent of practice, number of bed in case of indoor facilities, and depending upon the other liabilities.
- The hospital establishment can become the member of this scheme only if all the members associated with the hospital have their personal PI under the scheme.
- A trust/committee/company/society shall look after the management of the collected money.
- The financial assistance will be like as per Medical Indemnity Scheme, where indemnity part shall be covered by government/Insurance Regulatory and Development Authority (IRDA)-approved companies or any other private company.
- Any compensation/cost/damages awarded by judicial trial shall be looked after by government/IRDA-approved insurance companies.
- Experts will be involved so that we have better vision and outcome of the scheme.
- The payment to the experts, legal and medicolegal experts, shall be done as per the predecided remuneration.
- If legal notice/case are received by member he should forward the necessary documents.
- Reply to the notice/case should be made only after discussing with the expert.
- A discontinued member if he wants to join the scheme again will be treated as a new member.
- *Most of the negligence litigations related to medical practice shall be covered under this scheme. The scheme will not cover the damages arising out of fire, malicious intension, natural calamity, or similar incidences.*
- The scheme can cover untrained hospital staff by paying extra amount as per the decision of expert committee.
- A District/State/Regional level committee can be established for the scheme.
- It shall be established on what happens when a member approaches with a complaint made against him or her [Doctors in Distress (DnD) processes].
- *Telephone help line*: Setting up and manning will be done.
- A team of medical consultants/Medicolegal consultants and advocates shall be formed which will help the members in hours of legal crisis.
- Efforts will be made to spread preventive medicolegal aspects with respect to

record keeping, consent, and patient communication, and this shall be integral and continuous process undertaken for beneficiary of scheme by suitable medium.

ADVANTAGES

- With the prior permission of insurance company, the legal expenses incurred by the insured for defending the case are also payable.
- The insurer is bound to pay as per the coverage, if those parties were liable to pay at the end. The nonjoining of insurance company could not vitiate the trial, this was held in *S Panchori versus Dr K Pandey I (1999) CPJ 332.*
- The insurance company will always have the right to take over the conduct of the defense of any proceedings filed against the insured before the medical councils or any other criminal proceedings against the doctor connected with his professional capacity.

LIMITATIONS

- No liability for any claim prior to the retroactive date specified in the policy.
- It has been observed that if the patient or their advocate knew that the doctors are insured, there are more chances of negligence suits.
- After the CPA 2019, the jurisdiction at District, State, and National levels has been enormously increased as per the amount of bill services charged. So, most of the cases will be in District Commission. The companies may be hesitant in indemnifying such a big amount or give only part payments, especially if there are suits pending against the doctors.

What should be the amount of indemnity?

During the last few years the claims for compensation have increased phenomenally. The cases are filed in the court of law for exaggerated amount. So that even if the court does not sanction the exaggerated amount still the complainants get sufficient amount. The amount can be decided depending upon:

- Whether the clinic/hospital is in Metro/big cities/taluka places, etc.
- Whether you are specialist/superspecialist or general practitioner.
- Amount recommended by legal/medicolegal consultants
- Other criteria as per your scope of practice.

Which company's policy shall be taken?

The present era of consumerism almost all the companies promise for many benefits, but once it comes to provide services they start if and buts and fault findings. Hence, this is a very important decision and shall be taken based on:

- Our own previous experiences
- Experiences of our friends and colleagues
- Services received in the past
- Reliability of company.

OUT-OF-COURT SETTLEMENTS

Many times the relatives of patient, insurance companies, even some of our own colleagues are thinking for the out-of-court settlement (OCS). In CPA 2019 also there is a provision for mediation in case of consumer disputes. Such settlements can be planned if we want to avoid long drawn court cases. The following points shall be kept in mind before settling for any proposals:

- The terms and conditions for OCS shall be clearly and firmly decided.

- Though the name is OCS, the terms/conditions shall be decided in the Court itself.
- The decision maker relatives, the team of doctors, and some legal personalities where the case is filed (preferably the commission chairman/senior member) shall be involved in deciding the criteria for the settlements.
- Representatives from insurance companies shall be informed and involved in the settlement.
- An official document of OCS shall be prepared and registered by the court authorities.
- The payment shall be done by cheque or deposited in the Court and not directly handed over to the patient/relatives.
- An agreement shall be signed that this amount settles all the claims, and hence, the complainant will withdraw all other cases filed at other places like National Medical Commission (NMC) and civil/criminal courts.

Doctors are very soft target for any financial institutions. The role of insurance companies may not be controversial or questionable, but one must be alert and involve them whenever there is a medicolegal difficulty. The PI may not protect from legal problems, but it may turn out to be a protector for financial losses.[3] Thus it gives mental peace over and above financial relief. While signing a contract for PI, hospital insurance or risk management one must read in between the lines.

The insurance companies are coming with newer and newer policies for attracting the beneficiaries. It is desirable for a doctor or hospital to have a full insurance in present era.

Note: The minute details and legal intricacies related with most of the insurance policies are beyond the scope of this article. It is advisable that the doctor's colleagues should consult a reliable insurance agent or advocates before signing any policy.

SUMMARY

Professional indemnity insurance is a type of insurance that protects professionals from financial losses arising from claims of negligence or malpractice. In India, PI insurance is particularly important for healthcare professionals, such as doctors, lawyers, and engineers, as they are frequently exposed to the risk of professional liability claims. OCS offers several advantages over traditional court proceedings, including cost-effectiveness, time efficiency, and confidentiality. By avoiding the costly involvement of lawyers, expert witnesses, and court fees, OCS significantly reduces financial burdens. Additionally, OCS expedites dispute resolution by circumventing the lengthy and intricate procedures of the court system. Moreover, OCS maintains privacy by keeping settlement details confidential, shielding professionals' reputations from public scrutiny.

LEARNING KEY POINTS

- An adequate and sufficient amount of indemnity is essential in the present era of medical practice.
- Have a policy from reliable company and inform them whenever crisis occurs.
- Out-of-court settlement may seems to be an easier option; but should not be preferred frequently.
- Remember that medical practitioners can be soft targets for patients, relatives, policy makers, judiciary and so called social workers also.

TAKE-HOME MESSAGES
An adequate and sufficient amount of indemnity is essential in the present era of medical practice.

MUST AVOID THINGS
Break in indemnity policy.

ONLY ONE FACT TO REMEMBER
Check retroactive date in policy.

DO NOT DO
Never ever practice for single day without PI and errors and omissions insurance (E&O) for protection of financial assets.

WARNINGS
Intimate in writing insurance company moment medicolegal case comes up.

MEDICAL NEGLIGENCE PEARLS
Out-of-court settlement maintains privacy by keeping settlement details confidential, shielding professionals' reputations from public scrutiny.

MUST DO THING
An official document of OCS shall be prepared and registered by the court authorities.

MESSAGES WHICH THE READER MUST BE AWARE
Remember that medical practitioners can be soft targets for patients, relatives, policy makers, judiciary, and so called social workers also.

REFERENCES
1. Tiwari S, Baldwa M. What is medical negligence. In: Baldwa M, Tiwari S, Tiwari M, Shah N (Eds). Legal Problems in Day-to-day Pediatrics Practice, 2nd edition. Hyderabad: Paras Publishing; 2010. pp. 14-39.
2. Joshi MK (Ed). a-z Medical Law 2000, 1st edition. Ahmedabad; 2000. pp. 289-92.
3. Tiwari SK, Baldwa M. Medical negligence. In: Gupte S (Ed). Recent Advances in Pediatrics, volume 14. New Delhi: Jaypee Brothers Medical Publishers; 2004. pp. 311-29.

Index

A

Abdomen, pain in 265
ABO-Rh incompatibility 275
Abscess
　destabilizing vitals 183
　drainage 256
Accidental extubation 227
Accidental injury 269
Acetaminophen 234
Acharya Vinoba Bhave Rural
　　Hospital 268
Act of Medical Negligence 129
Acute crisis, lack of treatment
　　pushing child in 183
Acute ill patients, medicolegal
　　aspects of
　　transferring 225
Adenoidal hypertrophy 268
Administrative agencies 132
Admission
　advance deposit before 147
　consent 60
Adrenaline 217
Adverse event following
　　immunization 215
　types of 216
Advertisements 140
Affidavit 108
　complaint without 118
Agitation 227
Airway 61, 227
　assessment of 216
Algorithmic exercise 63
Allegations, classification
　　of 113
Alleged duty restriction, medical
　　certification for 81
Alleged harm 133
Alleged medical negligence 125
　case 108, 110
Alleged negligence 109
　money for 109
Allergies 32
Allopathic medicine 8
Alternative dispute
　　resolution 136
Ambulance 188
Ambulatory basis 140
Aminoglycosides 242
Amputation 161
Anal canal atresia 264

Anaphylactic reactions, emergency
　　management of 216
Anaphylaxis 189
　aggravating scenarios of 199
　catastrophic 212
　occurrence of 195
Anesthesia
　fitness 255, 256
　　certificate 83
　vegetative state after 262
Anesthetist's acceptance 76
Anesthetist's details 72
Animal anatomical waste 296
Anthropometry 278
　measurements 140
Antibiotics, use of wrong 275
Anticipatory bail 104
Anticonvulsant 234, 236
Antidepressant, off-label use of 236
Antihistamines 216
Antipsychotic medications 236
Antisnake venom 234
Anti-tetanus serum 234
Anxiety, reduction of 239
Apex court 156, 157, 162, 167, 175
　held 170, 174
　stated 155
　to medical professionals 175
Appeal 120
　and review 119
　cross 119
　filing complaint and 120
Appellant 172
Appendectomy 256
Appendicitis 269
　surgery 264
Appendix, removal of 205
Arena, treatment 183
Arguments 108
Arresting doctors, guideline for 166
Arrhythmia 227
Asepsis maintenance 277
Ashtang ayurveda 307
Aspiration 227
Assaults, threats of 194
Asthma 257
Attitude 12
　of relatives, circumstance
　　of 109
　sympathetic 182
Audio and videography, consent
　　taken by 57

Audio-video
　consent 41
　recorded 41
Audio-visual recording facility 41
Augmented informed consent 63,
　　137, 138
Authoritative clinical
　　guidelines 132
Awareness, lack of 20
Ayurveda 307
Ayushman Bharat 91

B

Bail 104
　provisions 104
Bailable offence 104
Baldwa's dictum 323
Barrier-free environment,
　　creation of 251
Bed head ticket 40
Bed rest 81
Bhartiya Nagarik Suraksha
　　(Second) Sanhita Bill 98
Bhartiya Nagarik Suraksha
　　Sanhita 98
Bhartiya Nyaya Sanhita 98
　(Second) Bill 98
Bhartiya Sakshya Sanhita 98
　Bill 98
Bills, recovery of 147
Biomedical waste 295
　management 295
Bio-waste management 289
Bird's eye view 3
Birth
　certificate 83
　injuries 275
　registration 84
Blanket consent 60
Bleeding 257, 271
　tendencies 257
Blood 256
　counts, lowering of 56
　pressure 185
　　monitoring 277
　sugar
　　levels 271
　　monitoring 277
　supply, blockage of 162
　transfusion 267
Bolam law 96

Bolam principle 9
Bolam test 28
Bombay Nursing Home Registration Act 296
Bombay Shops and Establishments Act 295
Bone, fracture of 267
Boyle's apparatus 256
Brainstem-evoked response audiometry 278
Breach of duty 5, 130
Breathing 61, 216, 227
Bronchopneumonia 266
Bronchospasm 227
Burn
 injuries 267
 significant 186

C

Capillary filling time 277
Cardiac arrest 227
Cardiopulmonary resuscitation 61, 209, 216, 266
Care
 amount of 7
 average standard of 163
 degree of 7
Case transfer, application for 120
Casual connection 140
Cataract surgery 263
Catheter ablation 174
Cautery tools 256
Central Protection Councils 94
Certificate
 issued, record of 39
 record keeping of 80
 types of 82
Challenge damages claimed 133
Charitable hospitals 93, 94
Chemical liquid waste 297
Chemical waste 297
Chief information commission 46
Child Labor (Prohibition and Regulation) Act 252
Child patient, identification of 257
Child's overall health 140
Children
 consent for 77
 with developmental disorders, laws related to 249
Chloramphenicol 161
Cholecystokinin 239
Circulation 227
Civil court 3

Civil laws 92
Civil pre-litigation and litigation process, dealing with 108
Civil Procedure Code 44
Civil wrong 129
Claims 71, 75
Cleft palate surgery 262
Clinical drug trials 316
Clinical Establishment Act 43, 319
Clinical Establishment Regulatory Commission 321
Clinical Establishments (Registration and Regulation) Act 295, 317
 application 318
Clinical Establishments Act 294
Closed circuit television 58
Clotting time 257, 271
Code of civil procedure 135
Code of criminal procedure 98
Code of ethical conduct-license to practice medicine 4
Cognizable offences 104
Coincidental event 216
Collaborative healthcare environment 29
Coma 262
Commission and cut practice 315
Common law, integral part of 152
Common vaccination errors 217
Communication 1, 11, 194, 258
 allegations 182
 audio recording of 18
 barriers 20
 basic process models of 11
 breakdowns 16
 clarification 33
 clear and compassionate 14
 cycle 11, 12
 documentation of 17
 electronic 21
 elements of 11
 facilitate effective 14
 failures 20
 foster open 274
 handoff 32
 in medical practice, core elements of 12
 interprofessional 14
 justified 18
 lack of
  poor 193
  proper 193
 medicolegal 13
 methods 15

 mode of 16
 nonverbal 11, 16
 official 16
 open 210
 patient 327
 practicing open 255
 privileged 55
 process, elements of 11
 record 19
 skill 20, 199
 strategies for effective 22
 supportive 22
 tool 27
 types of documentation of 17
 verbal 16
 written 16
Community health providers 310
Company's policy 327
Compensation 5
 calculation of 125, 130
 capping of 125
 granted consent 65
 highest ever 172
 policy for vaccine related injuries and death 220
 respondent claimed 172
Competence 111
Complaint
 allegations in 113
 classifying allegations of 114, 115
 copy 108, 112
 in court 120
 study of 112
 without affidavit, file objection for 118
Complex body of laws 202
Complex supravalvular defect 263
Compliance with standards 30
Complication
 consent for 61
 medical 109
Comprehensive care 253
Conciseness and clarity 31
Confidentiality 11
 and privacy 15
 concerns 13
 issues 21
Congenital birth defects 277
Congenital defects 275
Congenital esophageal atresia 266
Congenital heart disease 261, 266
Consciousness, level of 216

Index

Consent 1, 122, 169, 214, 258
  discussions 15
  formats 69
    component contents of 69
    logical basis of 68
  high-risk 71, 185
  printed form 60
  protects doctors 64
  standards for 188
  subject matter of 55
  types of 59
  validity of 56
  with disclaimers 61
Consolidated Omnibus Budget Reconciliation Act 229
Constitution of India 15
Constitutional Validity of Consumer Protection Act 91
Constitutionality of Clinical Establishments Act 318
Consult medicolegal adviser 175
Consultation 148
Consumer 87, 89
  cases, record maintenance for 45
  commission 91
  forum 167
  vendor includes medical services 157
Consumer Court 3, 158
  disposal of 120
Consumer Protection (e-commerce) Rules 90
Consumer Protection Act 10, 44, 45, 89, 91, 94, 95, 99, 108, 143, 150, 158, 181, 194, 212, 219
Contempt of Court 152, 155
Continuous monitoring system readings 185
Conviction by court of law 316
Copy-paste errors 30
Coronavirus disease-2019
  advent of 212
  vaccination 212
  vaccine 136, 219
Corruption 322
Counseling 19
  on medical communication skills 19
  professional providing 19
  various aspects of 19

Court fees 120
Court of law 141, 186
Court settlement 109
Court's observations 164
Crawford's principle 7
Criminal action, case of 166
Criminal cases to medical practitioner, defenses available in 103
Criminal court 167
  defenses 108
Criminal law 87, 92, 99
  applies 98
  on medical negligence 4
  to medical practice, application of 98
Criminal Procedure Code 44, 184
Criminal prosecution, expert witness mandatory for 163
Crisis Management Committee 199
  support of 326
Crisis, acute 182, 184
Critical analysis 158
Critical care 181, 182
  consent in 204
Critically ill
  care of 228
  children 226
  patients 189
  transport of 226
Critically sick children 184
Critique 168
Cultural sensitivity 13, 15
Custody, chain of 30
Customary practice 7
Cytomegalovirus infection 278

D

Daksha 110
Damage Payments Act 220
Day care
  clinics 256
  procedures 147, 148
  surgeries 148
Day-to-day practice 199
Dead body 150
Death
  case of unnatural 207
  causing 99, 106
  declaration certificate 84
  declare 187
  medical certification of 84

professional 152
summary 229
time of 84
transit 225, 232
Death certificate 83
  and postmortem, issuing of 232
  newborn 84
  perinatal 83
Decision makers 18
Defendant's breach 130
Defendant's assert 127
Defenses 6
Defensive medicine 173, 174
Defibrillator 188
Deficiency, allegations of 217
Degree qualification 174
Delhi Medical Council 79
  guidelines 79
Delhi Nursing Homes Registration Act 296
Delivery 282
Denture use 271
Deny consent 115
Deoxyribonucleic acid analysis process 285
Department for Works and Pensions 220
Depo-Medrol's chemical structure 172
Deserving compensation 129
Destroy records 47, 143
Deterioration, transfer risks of 226
Developmental disabilities 248
Developmental disorders 248
Developmental pediatrics, legalities in 248
Diabetic mother 277
Diagnostic opinion 75
Diaphragmatic hernia 275
  surgery 267
Diclofenac 234
Digoxin 234
Diligence, evidence for 110
Diphtheria 216
Disability
  certificate 83
    issuing government authorities 83
  professional 152
Disabled, unemployment allowance for 251

Discharge
    administrative procedures of 226
    against medical advice 143
    bill on 147
    card 40
        and discharge 40
        referral, and transfer notes record, importance of 39
    summary 140, 229
Disciplinary action and punishment, procedure for 316
Disorganization 30
Disputes Redressal Commission 219
Disseminated intravascular coagulation 187
District Commission 92, 119, 120
    decision 264
Diversity awareness 15
Doctor Protection Act 196
Doctor Violence Protection Act 193
Doctor/hospital, allegation against 117
Doctor's composite package policy 325
Doctor's conduct 96
Doctor's point of view 90
Doctor's protection shield 325
Doctor-based disease statistics 37
Doctor-patient
    and medicolegal contexts 11
    relationship 20, 21
        establishing 130
Doctors' and Medical Establishment Policy 325
Doctrine of precedents 152
Doctrine of respondent superior 93
Document changes, failure to 30
Documentation 1, 14, 194, 214, 226, 227, 274
    and record-keeping 14
    by qualified personnel 31
    during medical emergency 31
    in neonatal resuscitation record 39
    role of 28
Documenting continuous monitoring, legal proof of 185

Dressings 148
Drug 256
    administration, consent for 56
    after expiry date 233
    allergies 271
    controller general 292
    essential 133
    expiry date 232
    inspector arrives 292
    liquid forms 234
    medicolegal aspects of 241
    parenteral 55
    uses of 236
Drug's Indian manufacturer 172
Drugs and Cosmetics Act 243, 293, 316
Drugs and Cosmetics Rules 244, 302
Drugs and Magic Remedies (Objectionable Advertisement) Act 244
Duplicate certificates 78, 80
Duty of care 129, 131
    in emergency room 188, 228
Dying-dying dead situation 61

E

Education 251
Education Law 249, 251
    and children with disabilities 250
Effective communication 11, 20, 22
    skills, significance of 21
    strategies 14, 16
Electrocardiograph 185
Electronic health record 29
    standards 48
Electronic record 31
    keeping 41
Elements of consent 55
Emergency 61, 140, 142, 147, 149
    blood transfusion 189, 206
    department 61
        managements 14
    exit 196
    fees 148
    medical
        care 231
        condition 147, 230
        service 216, 231
        system 216
    medicolegal cases 203
    omission 189

patient
    care, refusal of 202
    transport of 206
pediatric surgical procedure 257
room 188, 196, 228
situations 6
surgery 259
treatment 181, 182, 202
Emergency Medical Treatment and Labor Act 229
Emotional distress 13
Employees Provident Fund Act 294, 295
Employment 251
Enactment of Consumer Protection Act 184, 325
Encoding 12
End-of-life care 202, 280
Environmental condition 227
Epilepsy 84
Epinephrine 216
    autoinjectors 234
Equal before law 251
Equip doctor 125
Equipment 256
    functionality of 256
Estimated treatment cost certificate 83
Estradiol 234
Ethical concerns 18
Ethical misconduct 317
Ethical standards 202
Ethics 195, 307, 311
    basics of 308
Euthanasia 209, 316
Evade legal restrictions 316
Evidence 108
    affidavit of 119
    courts, nature of 110
    file affidavit of 119
Execution petition 119
Ex-gratia compensation, challenging 135
Experience, evidence of 110
Expert doctors and scientific literature, affidavits of 116
Expert opinion 326
Expert testimony 31
Expert witness 92, 108
    discovery 122
Expertise 115
Expired drugs, health hazard of 234

Index

Expired medicine, safely dispose of 235
Expired vaccine 219
  dose of 218
Expiry drug
  inadvertently 235
  issues with 233
  medicolegal aspects of 232
  use of 235
Explicit consent 57, 59
Expression 199
Eye
  affidavits of 118
  camp 160
  drops 234
  of ethics, consent in 312
Eyewitness, affidavit of 115

F

Facility policies and procedures 132
Factual causation 130
Factual defense 115, 121
Fake certificates 78, 84
Fake medical leave certificates 78, 79
Family law 249
Family members 280
Fear
  and anxiety, levels of 13
  of litigation 20
Fecal fistula 270
Feedback 12
Fibroids, multiple 175
File application objecting additional pleas 119
Filing written statement 111
Fine-needle aspiration cytology 58
Fire prevention compliance 301
First information report 100, 184, 291
Fissure 256
Fistula treatment 256
Fit to work certificate 80
Fitness certificate 39, 83
  issuance of 81
Fitness-related medical certification 81
Floxacins, judicious use of 241
Food and drug administration 56
Food and public distribution 89
Free medical services 94

Friern Hospital Management Committee 28
Fundamental healthcare 36
Fundamental right 173

G

Gangrene 161
Gas 256
  gangrene 186
Gastrointestinal issues 276
General Medical Council 27
General practitioner 82
General waste 297
Geographic practice 7
Glucometer 141
Government and Regulatory Bodies 18
Government hospitals, retention period for 43
Grievance redressal 251
Growth assessment 213
Guardianship laws 249, 250

H

Hair transplant, consent for 70
Hammurabi's code 126
Handle free service 93
Handle OPD load 141
Head
  circumference 278
  injury 186, 269
Health
  care 37
  certification of 80
Health Insurance Portability and Accountability Act 27
Health law 249
  and children with disabilities 250
Healthcare
  administrators 18
  and legal professionals 14
  cost of 194
  facility 36
  lawyers 19
  practitioner 76
  professionals 18, 29
  providers 13, 16, 28, 32, 248
  service providers 49
  setups 19
  statistics, production of 35
  systems 26
Hearsay 31

Heart
  disorder 271
  rate 185
Hemogram 271
Hemophilia 276
Hemorrhagic disorders 276
Hepatitis
  B 218, 271
  C 271
Hernia repair 256
Herniotomy 267
High-risk newborn 278
  discharge card 278
  screening 213, 274, 276-279
Hindu Succession Act 250
Hiring of medical services
  contract for 66, 125, 131
  switching to contract for 63
Home care 279
Hospital
  insurance policies 325
  refuse emergency cases 203
  rendering services 158
Huge compensation, culprit for 137
Human affairs, conduct of 5
Human anatomical waste 296
Human culture 309
Human error 227
Human immunodeficiency virus 66, 313
  testing 257
Human life, preservation of 156
Human papillomavirus 218
Human Rights 316
Humanitarian judgments, kinds of 128
Hyaline membrane disease 284
Hydrocele repair 256
Hypersensitivity reaction 74
Hypertension 276
  severe 227
Hypoglycemia 275, 277, 278
Hypotension, severe 227
Hypothermia 227
Hypothetical ordinary doctor 7
Hypothyroidism 277
Hypoxia 227
Hypoxic encephalopathy 268
Hypoxic-ischemic encephalopathy 278
Hysterectomy 175
  operation 174

Index

I

Ideal medical record 37
Ideal OPD practice, elements of 140
Ignoring working environment 128
Illegible handwriting 30
Illness 12
Immunization 214, 216
　anxiety 216
　　related reaction 216
　error 216
　　related reaction 216
　need of 212
　process of 218
Impersonal document 48
Implied consent 59
Impractical provisions 322
In vitro fertilization 90, 312
Inadequate protection, responsibility for 218
Income Tax Act 44, 215, 249
Income Tax Laws and Children with Disabilities 251
Indemnity 325
　amount of 327
　policies 255
　　for surgeons and anesthetists 256
　professional 325
Indian Constitution 157
Indian Contract Act 4, 10, 63, 64
Indian Council of Medical Research 316
Indian Doctors Going Digital 58
Indian Evidence Act 47, 57, 98, 106
Indian Judiciary on Safe Transfer of Patients 230
Indian Medical Association 93, 104, 122, 136, 137, 193, 237
Indian Medical Council (Professional Conduct, Etiquette and Ethics) Regulations 17, 243
Indian Medical Council Act 309, 322
　Regulation 39
Indian Penal Code 98, 181, 202, 212
Individual communicates 54
Indoor case register 215
Indoor documents comprise 142
Indoor medical record, retention period of 45
Indoor pediatric prescriptions 142
Industrial Disputes Act 294
Infant milk substitute 274, 279
　Act 280
Infection 275, 278
　catching 275
　death caused by 284
Inform consent 131
Inform Insurance Company 120
Inform law enforcers, mandatory to 186
Information
　adequate 169
　administrative 57
　incorrect 30
　patient 32
　sensitive 14
　vital 37
　witness 32
Information Technology Act 21, 22
Informed consent 15, 26, 54, 57, 64, 68, 185, 202, 238
　augmentation of 131
　charge, lack of 96
　documentation of 27, 30
　protects 55
　purpose of 63
Informed decision making 33
In-hospital management 174
Injectables in pediatric, consent for 56
In-patient department 40, 60, 70
Inspector Raj 322
Institute of Child Health 284
Insurance cover 121
Insurance Regulatory and Development Authority 326
Intensive care
　management 62
　unit 225
Intercostal drainage 279
Interhospital transfer 225
Interprofessional collaboration 14
Intracranial hypertension 227
Intrauterine growth restriction 277
Intravenous fluids 217
Intussusception 261
　surgery 268
Irrefutable evidence and defense 259

J

Jaundice 257, 278
　physiological 283
Jeremy Bentham's utilitarian theory 137
Judgment, error of 102
Judicial impropriety 152, 155
Judicial precedents 152
　binding effect of 152
　of Supreme Court, binding effect of 153
Junior doctors, negligence of 206
Jurisdiction 75, 76
Juvenile Justice (Care and Protection) Act 252

K

Karnataka Private Medical Establishments Act 296
Kernicterus 283
Knowledge
　level of 7
　light of basis legal 190

L

Labor
　and drug inspectors 289
　progress of 276
Language
　barriers 11, 13, 20
　offensive 194
　unfamiliar 12
Laparoscopic surgeries, setup for 256
Laparotomy 256
Last menstrual period 39
Law and Children with Developmental Disabilities 249
Law for capping on compensation 136
Law of limitation 6, 108, 171
Law of tort 129
　and civil law 3
Law presumes 8
Lawful medical communication 18
Lawyers attitude 109
Leaking per vaginum 276
Leave against medical advice 51, 143, 204, 207, 229
Leave ambiguity 41

Index

Leaving hospital 40
Left kidney, reporting
    missing 262
Legal and compliance
    professionals 18
Legal and ethical
    considerations 32
    requirements 32
Legal aspects 19
    emergency 61
Legal Assistance Scheme 326
Legal binding, consent form 64
Legal contract 63
Legal experts, guidance of 326
Legal hurdles of police 289
Legal liability, admissions of 135
Legal notice 108, 109
Legal opportunity 117
Legal proceedings, evidence
    in 27
Legal provisions 103
Legal purposes 79
Legal reason 37
Legal remedies 101
Legal review 33
Legal safeguard 33
Legal technical defenses 115
Legal view regarding
    diagnosis 185
Legibility and accuracy 30
Legibility and completeness 29
Liability 125, 129, 140
Life support, withdrawal of 208
Lifesaving
    interventions, delivery of 32
    techniques 61
Life-threatening 61
Limit liability 87, 125
Linen, discarded 297
Litigation
    avoid 121
    phase 108
    process 87
Liver
    biopsy 187
    function tests 257
Lok Adalat and Mediation in
    Consumer Protect
    Act 136
Low blood sugar levels 275
Lower segment cesarean section
    81, 266, 276
Lumber puncture 187, 279
Lung disorder 271

M

Malpractice
    and negligence, allegations
    of 28
    claims 122
    liability, threat of 136
Manpower development 251
Marathon 122
Mathew guidelines, application
    of 166
Mattresses 297
Mature minor exception 206
Measles 217
    mumps, rubella, and
    varicella 217
MeCkel's diverticulum 261
Meconium aspiration 275, 285
Meconium plug confused 264
Mediation 92
Mediation in Consumer Protect
    Act 136
Medical and legal
    professionals 16
Medical and medicolegal
    communication 18
    implications 16
Medical Assessment and Rating
    Board 310
Medical Association 197
    Managing Police 196
Medical care
    demonstration of 6
    standards of 228
Medical certificate 82
    legal cases on 82
Medical consent 54
Medical consultants, team of 326
Medical Council 78, 93, 110
Medical Council Act
    Regulation 42
Medical Council of India 215
Medical documentation 17, 26,
    27, 30, 34, 81
    challenges in 29
    errors in 29
    essence of 26
    for legal defense 33
    legal importance of 27, 28
    medicolegal importance
    of 27, 28
    of telephonic consultation and
    tele-consultation 32
    section 22
Medical documents 28

Medical emergency 142, 202,
    203, 205
    law related to 156
Medical establishment policy 325
Medical facility 60, 72, 75, 285
Medical indemnity insurance
    policy 186
Medical information, consent for
    release of 57
Medical jargon 13
Medical jousting 145
Medical leave 82
    certificates 79
Medical literature 122
Medical malpractice
    allegations of 35
    lawsuits 122
    stress syndrome 122, 152
Medical management error 275
Medical negligence 3, 6, 9, 29, 98,
    143, 181, 202, 284
    basis of 1
    calls 96
    cases of 5, 19
    claim 129
    during vaccination 219
    essentials of 5
    guidelines for 170
    high liability in 126
    in critical care,
    complaint of 209
    judicial decisions on 4
    lay concept of 7
    litigation 127, 135, 136
    pearls 10, 52, 67, 77, 85, 97,
    106, 124, 138, 151, 176,
    190, 201, 211, 222, 245,
    253, 271, 287, 303,
    323, 329
    prosecutions for 182
    reasons of high liability in 127
    silent epidemic of 3
    under contract 4
    various scenarios in 179
Medical Negligence Law 3
Medical officers, guidelines to 230
Medical practice 289
    bio-waste in 289
    legal liabilities in 140
Medical practitioner 171, 283
    in monitoring, part of 228
Medical problems 58
Medical procedure 59
Medical profession and medical
    practice, nature of 307

Index

Medical professional 8, 18, 171, 182, 183, 185, 187, 188, 189
   wearing good 182
Medical publication 57
   consent for 57
Medical reason 37
Medical record 34-36, 292
   and RTI Act 46
   as per various acts, retention period of 43
   confidentiality of 48
   department 42
   documentation 202
   essential components of 38
   evidentiary value of 47
   issuing of 45
   officer 42
   preservation period for 42
   purpose of 37
   question credibility of 40
   retention of 43
   types of 37
Medical Registration Board 311
Medical research 316
   consent for 57
Medical service
   deficiency in 131
   hiring of 63, 66
   providing of 63
Medical Termination of Pregnancy Act 44, 163, 296
Medical work, delegation of 93
Medications 32
Medicine
   discarded 296
   expired 296
Mediclaim Insurance Companies 57
Medicolegal
   action group 89
   advice 110
   advisor 109
   aspect 225
   case 47, 202
      decided 282
   communication, challenges in 13
   considerations 255
   context 11, 16
   guidance 199, 326
   issues 208, 212
   litigation 35, 152, 277

   actual 20
   facing 35
   risks of 23
   pearl 145
   prospective 276
   situation 181
Memory 239
Meningitis 278
Menstrual problem 175
Mental handicap, irreversible 283
Mental Health Act 249, 252
Mental Retardation, and Multiple Disabilities Act 249
Message 12
Metabolism, inborn errors of 276
Minimum Wages Act 294
Minor's kidney, negligent removal of 262
Miscellaneous application 120
Miscellaneous Provisions Act 294
Miscommunication 13
Misunderstanding 13
Mob mentality 194
Mob violence 193
   recreated, actual scene of 198
Monetary issues 147
Monitoring and record keeping 189
Monitoring during transport 226
Monitoring equipment 184
   stethoscope 188
Morbidity 274
Mortality 274
Mothers consent stamp 280
Motivation 239
Motor vehicular 186
Mumps 217

N

Napier's record survives 35
Narrow therapeutic index drugs 234
Nasal septal deviation surgery 268
National Commission 92, 119, 120, 162, 170
National Consumer Disputes Redressal Commission 29, 126, 169
National exit test 310
National Exit Test Under National Medical Commission 310

National Medical Commission 4, 17, 57, 255, 307, 328
   Act 307, 309
   Registered Medical Practitioner 15
National Medical Council 110, 143
National Rare Disease Policy 274, 281
National Trust for Welfare of Persons with Autism, Cerebral Palsy, Mental Retardation and Multiple Disabilities Act 252
National Vaccine Injury Compensation 220
Nebulizer 141
Necrotizing enterocolitis 276
Negative consent 61
Negligence 89, 91, 92, 102, 129, 133, 158, 171, 283
   actual 136
   antonyms of 6
   benchmark of 102
   claims 11, 129
   concept of 5, 102
   contributory 6
   degree of 7
   doctor 163
   exclude 64
   jurisprudential concept of 5, 165
   nonintentional 93
   offence 6
   per se 8
   suits 129
   synonyms of 6
Neonatal and preterm care 286
Neonatal intensive care unit 62, 181, 182, 274, 275
Neonatal jaundice 275, 278
   picking late of 275
Neonatal klebsiella infection 284
Neonatal obstructive jaundice 277
Neonatal period 274
Neonatal resuscitation 276
Neonatal unit, discharge from 277
Neonate 277
Neonatology practice
   challenges in 274
   consent in 279
   criminal liability in 280
   ethical dilemma in 280
   medicolegal issues in 275

Neonatology
  legalities in 274
  negligence in 274
Neurobiological mechanisms 239
Neurodevelopmental delay 278
Neurodevelopmental
      sequelae 274
  risk of 278
Neurosonogram 278
Newborn
  burn injury 282
  care, facility based 277
  child 283
  discharge of 277
  with multiple congenital
      anomaly 281
Nidan Kendras 282
Night duties 81
No-fault liability 125
Noise 12
  physical 12
Nonaffordability 149
Nonbailable offence 104
Noncognizable 291
  offences 104
Non-emergency state consent 62
Nonformal education 251
Nonmaleficence 309
Nonsteroidal anti-inflammatory
      drug 56, 234
Nosocomial infection 277
Not paying hospital bills 208
Novus actus interveniens 6, 96, 97
Nursing homes 126

O

Obligation of civil society 171
Offences and penalties 317
Offered prenatal
      screening test 282
Off-label drug 237
  use of 225, 235-237
Old ethos and new changing
      values, conflicts
      between 308
Omission
  and commission under tort,
      negligence of 93
  insurance 329
Operation theater
  infrastructure of 116
  supporting 276
Opioid antagonist naloxone 239
Optimize resource allocation 274

Oral contraceptives 234
Otoacoustic emission 278
Outdoor and indoor practice 140
Out-of-court settlement 325,
      328, 329
Outpatient department 39, 56,
      70, 315
  emergency setup at 141
  prescription 213
  record keeping, issues in 41
Outside court settlement 108, 109
Oxygen
  saturation 185
  supply 141, 256

P

Pain protocol, observation of 277
Panchnama 292
Paraldehyde 234
Paralytic polio 216
Paralytic poliomyelitis, vaccine-
      associated 212, 220
Paroxysmal supraventricular
      tachycardia 174
Partial thromboplastin time 257
Patent and copyrights 316
Patient
  and healthcare providers,
      miscommunication
      between 13
  audio recordings of 58
  care continuity 26
  particulars 38
  party, contributory negligence
      of 108
  privacy 31
  refusal 61
  safety first 31
  transfer of 225
Patient Anti-dumping Act 229
Patient-ventilator
      dyssynchrony 227
Payment of Bonus Act 294
Payment of Gratuity Act 294
PCPNDT Act 44
Pediatric clinic 68
Pediatric consultations 140
Pediatric critical care, medicolegal
      issues in 202
Pediatric health services 141
Pediatric Intensive Care
      Society 226
Pediatric intensive care units 181,
      182, 202, 204

Pediatric orthopedic surgery 256
Pediatric outpatient
      department 140
Pediatric physician fitness 257
Pediatric surgeons, skills of 255
Pediatric surgery 255
  medicolegal aspects for 255
Pediatric surgical
  care 261
  procedure, planned 257
Perinatal asphyxia 275
Personal declaration proforma 38
Personal document 48
Personal medical records 48
Persons with Disabilities (Equal
      Opportunities,
      Protection of Rights
      and Full Participation)
      Act 251
Persons with Disabilities Act 249
Persons with disability,
      rehabilitation of 251
Pertussis vaccination 216
Physical assaults 194
Physical harm claimed,
      documentary
      proof of 133
Placebo
  controlled trials, ethics of 239
  drugs 225
      medicolegal aspects of 238
  effect, factors influencing
      power of 239
  in children, ethics of 240
  mechanism of action of 239
  use of 239, 241
Plaster of Paris 159
Platelet count 257, 271
Pneumonia 275
Pneumothorax 227
Policies and guidelines 132
Polio vaccine, inactivated 216
Pollution Control Committee 295
Poor laborer woman 162
Post-death diagnostic
      procedure 207
Post-expiration date 234
Postmortem 195
Potential litigant 6
Potential postsurgical
      improvements 256
Practice procedure 207
Pradhan Mantri Jan Arogya
      Yojana 282

Preanestheia 83
Preconceptions 12
Preconsent counseling and forewarning 59
Precounseling 158
Pregnancy, high-risk 276
Pre-litigation phase 108
Premature child 282
Prematurity 275
Preparing defense, proactive in 110
Prescription
  digitalization of 141
  paper 215
Preterm baby, screening of 287
Preterm birth 278
Pretransport coordination and communication 226
Primary Healthcare Center 203
Privacy to patient, automatic grant of 54
Privacy violations 30
Procainamide 234
Procedural defenses 118
Product liability 94
Professional indemnity
  prevention by 121
  types of 325
Prohibition of Child Marriage Act 252
Proposed treatment 55
Prosecution, increased 322
Protected health information 49
Protection of Children from Sexual Offences Act 252, 300-302
Prothrombin index 271
Prothrombin time 257
Provisional diagnosis 141
Proxy consent 60, 77
Prudence of doctor, evidence of 110
Psychiatric diseases
  certificates 78
  diagnosis of 81
Public interest litigation 319
Pulmonary function tests 257
Pulse oximeter 141, 256
Pyloric stenosis correction 256

Q

Quality assurance 33

R

Real consent 54, 60, 169
Real-time specific consent 60
Reasonable care, principle of 5
Reasonable medical care in emergency rooms, legal standards of 188
Receiving legal notice and replying 109
Record
  alleged manipulation of 50
  alleged tempering of 50
  benefits of 19
  incomplete 30
  maintenance, laws related to 49
  preservation of 31
  protection of 47
Record keeping 35, 36, 78, 215
  importance of 37
  training of 42
Redress grievances, different platforms to 3
Reflect self-advertising 141
Registered medical practitioner 21, 42, 57, 78
  performing medical procedures 100, 106
  teleconsultation by 43
  to paramedical profession, duties of 316
  to public, duties of 316
Registration counter 140
Registration of Births and Deaths Act 83
Regular team meetings 15
Rehabilitation Council 249
  Act 252
Renal function test 257
Res ipsa loquitur 91, 159, 160, 166
Research
  and manpower development 251
  project, consent for 70
Residual defenses 116
Respiratory distress 275
Respiratory rate 185
Retention of Record as per Income Tax Act 44
Retinopathy of prematurity 278, 287
  screening for 6
Reusing text 34
Review petition 119
Revised pecuniary jurisdiction 91
Right document 143
Right drug 143
Right of Doctor 142
Right of Patient 312
Right to Die with Dignity 173
Right to Education 250
Right to Information Act 46, 289, 302
Right wrist, dorsal aspect of 162
Risk bond 54
Road side accident 188
Rubella 217
Rules of drafting of reply, basics of 116

S

Safe transfer
  key elements of 226
  medicolegal aspect of 229
Schoolchildren 80
Secret drug formulations, use of 243
Secret remedies 316
Seizures 257, 278
Self-declaration proforma 131
Sepsis 278
Septicemia 183, 275
Serum
  creatinine test 257
  glutamic-pyruvic transaminase 257
Service, deficiency of 91
Sham treatment 187
Shelf Life Extension Program 225, 234
Shock, acute 184
Sick
  and leave certificates, record of 80
  attendant 232
  babies 274
  newborn
    transport of 275
    survived 274
Siddha 307
Skill
  and care, degree of 3
  plead prudence of 111
  prudence of 111
Slow-moving procedure 122
Social security 251
Soiled waste 296
Soliciting practices 141

Special professional tasks, legal
      presumption for 8
Speech, freedom of 199
Spoken conversation 16
Squint eye, corrective surgery
      for 266
Standard of care 7, 8, 27, 130,
      132, 236
   case laws 8
   short of 96
Standard operating
      procedure 101
Standard Treatment Guidelines
      Committee 278
State Commission 92, 119
   nor National Commission 175
State Medical Council 3, 110, 317
State Pollution Control Board
      295, 297
Stevens-Johnson syndrome 56
Still birth 281
Substantial injustice 129
Succession law 249
Succession law and children with
      disabilities 250
Sudden death 145, 147, 149, 150,
      193, 199
   occurrence of 195
Supreme Court
      judgments 152, 154
Supreme Court judicial
      precedents, violation
      of 155
Surgery 147, 149
   indication for 256
   moderate 256
Surgical problems 58, 277
Surgical site and side of operation,
      marking of 257
Surrogate
   consent 77
   decision-making 202
Symptom complexes and medical
      professional 185
Syrup nimesulide 242

T

Table deaths, occurrence of 196
Tacit consent 59
Teachers' training institutions 251
Technical defense 121, 133
Teleconsultation, consent in 57
Telemedicine 33, 279
   practice guidelines 207

Telephonic advice 207
Telephonic consultation 38
Temperature 275
   monitoring 277
Territorial jurisdiction 112, 123
Tetanus 186, 216, 278
Tetracyclines 234
Thalassemia 285
Therapeutic privilege 60,
      62, 102
Third party administrator 57
Thumb impression 80
Thyroid 276
   preparations 234
Tortuous liability, essential
      components of 131
Toxic epidermal necrolysis 173
Training 115
Transfer against medical
      advice 40
Transfer consent 57
Transfer notes 40
Transferring counseling 57
Transport equipment 226
Treatment certificate 83
Treatment facility 72, 75
Treatment not negligence, failure
      of 162
Tubectomy 162
Typhoid perforation 270

U

Ultrasonography scans 281
Unani Tibb 307
Understaffed emergency
      department 194
Unethical conduct 141, 181,
      182, 186
Unexpected death
   and insurance, difficult
      situation of 186
   difficult situation of 181, 183,
      184, 186-188
   in ML cases, difficult situation
      of 186
   in poisoning, difficult situation
      of 186
   situation of 184, 187-189
Unforgivable errors 260
Uniformity and consistency, lack
      of 128
Unqualified persons, association
      with 315

Unused medicine, safely dispose
      of 235
Unverified certificates 84
Urinalysis 257
Urinary infection 268
Urinary tract infection 78
Uterus, removal of 163

V

Vaccination 279
   card 215
   consent for 224
   duties during 213
   error 218, 219
      medicolegal issues in 219
      preventing and
         managing 217
   information statements 214
   medicolegal aspects of 212
   records 84
Vaccine
   after expiration date 218
   injury 220
   product 216
      related reaction 216
   quality defect-related
         reaction 216
   regulatory authority for 216
   type of 215
   wrong 217
Vaccine Injury Compensation
      Program 212
Valid consent, ideal components
      of 58
Varicella 217
Vasovagal syncope 216
Ventilation 278
Ventilator 188
Verapamil 234
Verbal communication,
      disadvantages of 16
Vicarious liability 93, 160
   legal concept of 93
Victim, income of 127
Violence 193
   against children, laws related
      to 252
   against doctors,
      prevention of 193
   against medical personnel 133
   and preparations, anticipation
      of 196
   causes of 193
   types of 194

Visheshgya 110
Vital monitoring 277
Vital signs 32, 216
   description of 39
Vitamin K deficiency
       bleeding 276
Voice recording on mobile 41

W

Warfarin 234
Water activities 84
Weight charting 277
White blood cell 257
Wilful judicial impropriety 155
Witness 185
   cross-examination of 118
   name 76
Workmen's compensation
       cases 48
Workplace modifications 81
Write legibly 17
Writing, prognosis in 70
Written arguments 119
Written consent 55, 59
   and dissents 184
   logic and reasoning for 58
Written proxy consent 70
Written refusal 62
Written statement 108, 110
   Under New Consumer
       Protection Act 113

Y

Your advice needs, refusal of 258

EU GSPR Authorised Reprsentative
Logos Europe, 9 rue Nicolas Poussin
1700, La Rochelle, France
Phone: +33 (0) 6 67 93 73 78
E-mail: contact@logoseurope.eu

www.ingramcontent.com/pod-product-compliance
Ingram Content Group UK Ltd.
Pitfield, Milton Keynes, MK11 3LW, UK
UKHW050456150426
5217IPUK00025B/1711